MW00843739

# Condensed Psychopharmacology 2020

## *Past, Present & Future*

# A Pocket Reference for Psychiatry, Neurology and Psychotropic Medications

*By:*
**Leonard Rappa, PharmD, BCPP**
Professor of Psychiatric Pharmacy Practice
Florida A&M University
College of Pharmacy and Pharmaceutical Sciences
Board Certified Psychiatric Pharmacist
**Fort Lauderdale, Florida**

*Published by RXPSYCH LLC, Ft. Lauderdale, FL*
*© January 2020*

# FOREWORD

Psychopharmacology, the study of psychiatric drugs, has evolved exponentially since the dawn of man. Early knowledge from experiments with various chemicals sourced from plants, animals, and the earth have accumulated over the millennium to what we know today. The pace accelerated greatly in the last 200 years, with the pinnacle at today, and every day after. Many monumental discovers in the treatment of psychiatric illnesses were serendipitous, and even today, we depend upon trial and error approaches to medication effectiveness. Having a comprehensive knowledgebase of these medications can help narrow down the choices to what we believe will be most efficacious for our patients and reducing undo harm. This book is a culmination of thousands of hours of scouring and researching the contemporary medical literature. I have culled the literature so that you don't have to, in order to give you a current synopsis of psychopharmacology, as it exists today.

Today's psychiatric medications are far from perfect. They are as good as we can get with our current knowledge and technology. Considering that most psychotropic medications were discovered by accident, it is a miracle that we even have these treatments for mental illness to be begin with. It is also very true that we have no real idea of how these medications actually work. We speculate our mechanisms of action based on theories and conjecture, and only time will truly disclose their real therapeutic pathways.

Every medication that exists today does so at some cost, be it financial or side effect on the body. The goal in treating any illness is to control the disease or symptoms with the least risk to the patient. For some, the costs are great, with addiction, exacerbation of other diseases, or long-term physical effects on the body. Each drug must be weighed in the context of such costs in consideration of treating an individual patient. It is also imperative that patients are included in the decision about their medications. This "informed consent" process must include the costs, benefits, and alternatives to the therapies being considered. Many prescribers today do not obtain true informed consent from their patients, because they fail to include all the elements needed for such. Many state laws include legal definitions of informed consent, which often include a provision about the patient's competence to provide a rational informed consent. Elements often include informing the patient the consequences of "doing nothing" or refusing medications altogether. An important component of informed consent that is often not discussed with patients is the long-term side effects of a psychotropic medication.

In decades past, most psychiatric patients were denied basic human rights and experimented upon or treated like criminals. Although we are much more conscientious about our patients' rights today, such contentious treatment still does occur, albeit to a far lesser degree. Our jails, however, are still utilized for the care of the mentally ill. In the United States, jails and prisons are the number one treatment providers for the mentally ill. A deficit in healthcare funding for mental illness combined with a privatized prison system has primed America for this endpoint. Historically, just like addiction, the treatment of chronic mental illness in punitive, rather than medical. That in and of itself decries the failing of our healthcare system today. But history also teaches us that we will continue to make improvements on that which exists today, so evolutionary steps may be small, but are inevitable.

Most of the psychotropics used today are far safer than the ones available 50 years ago, but still incur some potentially dangerous risks. For example, the risk of permanent body movements is less than with our older agents, but the increased risk for exacerbating diabetes, hyperlipidemia, and weight gain is the tradeoff. In such, the costs have simply shifted, but arc not eliminated altogether.

Twenty years ago I authored an article on the history of psychiatric medications and speculated that we may have a cure for mental illnesses in the next few decades. My optimism far exceeded reality, because now such hope for cure seems farther away than ever. The focus of today's research is more pharmaceutical treatment options, considering that there is more profit to be made in treating a chronic illness than curing it. Within the pages of this book, I have researched drug trials and potential future therapies, in part to give hope to those suffering from mental illness whose current medications have not helped them. Even with the dozens and dozens of medications available today, some people's mental illness resists all attempts to treat them, and we must continue to provide more options for their future. The good news is that no new medications (hopefully) will be FDA approved for mental illnesses that are toxic in overdose or with worse side effects than those that preceded it.

Psychotropics are not cures, and most take weeks to work, so their true efficacy has been difficult to measure. Today, our knowledgebase grows faster than ever. Combined with psychotherapy, an explosion of new medications, and new indications for existing medications, the potential to reduce suffering is limitless.

# TABLE OF CONTENTS

# NOTES:

# 1. QUICK REFERENCE CHARTS OF PSYCHOTROPIC MEDICATIONS

## I. ADHD MEDICATIONS / PSYCHOSTIMULANTS (*FOR FULL LIST SEE PAGE 32*)

| Generic Name | Brand Name | Usual Daily Dose (mg) | Other Uses |
|---|---|---|---|
| 4 mixed amphetamine salts: [N] (Dextroamphetamine sulfate & saccharate + Amphetamine sulfate & aspartate) | Adderall® / XR[1,2] | 2.5-40 | Weight loss |
| Amphetamine sulfate [N] | Evekeo™[3] | 2.5-40 | Obesity / narcolepsy |
| Atomoxetine [A] | Strattera™[4] | 0.5-1.4 mg/kg/day or up to 100 mg/d | |
| Clonidine | Catapres®[5] / Kapvay™[6] | 0.05 mg up to 25 mcg/kg/d | HTN / tics / Tourette's |
| Dexmethylphenidate [N] | Focalin® / XR[7] | 2.5-20 ÷ BID | |
| Dextroamphetamine[8] [N] | Dexedrine®/ Dextrostat®/ ProCentra® / Zenzedi®[9-13] | 5-60 | Weight loss, narcolepsy |
| Guanfacine | Intuniv™[14]/ Tenex® | 1-4 | HTN / tics / Tourette's |
| Lisdexamfetamine [N] | Vyvanse™[15] | 10-70 | Binge Eating Disorder |
| Methamphetamine [N] | Desoxyn®[16] | 5-25 | Exogenous obesity |
| Methylphenidate[17] [N] | Adhansia XR™/ Aptensio XR™ / Concerta®/ Cotempla XR®/ Daytrana™/ Focalin®/ Jornay PM™/ Metadate®/ Methylin® ER /Quillichew® / Quillivant XR®/ Relexxii™ / Ritalin® [18-30] | 5-60 | Weight loss / narcolepsy |
| Mixed levo- & dextro-amphetamines [N] | Adzenys®XR/ Dyanavel® XR / Evekeo ODT™/ Mydayis® [31-35] | 2.5-50 (varies by product) | |

## II. BENZODIAZEPINES [Y]

| Generic name | Brand name | Approved dosage range (mg/d)* | Other indications |
|---|---|---|---|
| Alprazolam [Y] | Xanax®[36]/XR®/Niravam® | 0.75-10 | Panic disorder / Anxiety-depression |
| Chlordiazepoxide [Y] | Librium®[37] | 25-200 | Anxiety / alcohol withdrawal |
| Clonazepam [Y] | Klonopin®[38] | 0.125-20 | Panic disorder / seizures |
| Clorazepate [Y] | Tranxene T-Tab®[39] | 7.5-90 | Anxiety / seizure disorders |
| Diazepam [Y] | Valium®[40]/Diastat®[41]/Valtoco®[42] | 2-40 | Anxiety / alcohol withdrawal |
| Estazolam [Y] | ProSom®[43] | 1-2 | Sedative-hypnotic |
| Flurazepam | Dalmane®[44] | 15-30 | Anxiety |
| Lorazepam [Y] | Ativan®[45] | 0.5-10 | Anxiety / pre-op sedation |
| Oxazepam [Y] | Serax®[46] | 30-120 | Anxiety / alcohol withdrawal |
| Quazepam [Y] | Doral®[47] | 7.5-15 | Sedative-hypnotic |
| Temazepam [Y] | Restoril®[48] | 15-30 | Sedative-hypnotic |
| Triazolam [Y] | Halcion®[49] | 0.125-0.25 | Sedative-hypnotic |
| * Elderly patients are usually treated with approximately one-half of the dose listed | | | |

## III. NON-BENZODIAZEPINE ANTI-ANXIETY AGENTS ("*ATARACTICS*")

| Generic name | Brand name | FDA-approved for Anxiety | Usual dosage range (mg/d) | Other Uses |
|---|---|---|---|---|
| Buspirone | BuSpar®[50] / Dividose® | Yes | 15-60 | |
| Hydroxyzine HCL | Atarax®[58] | No | 10-30 | Allergy / itching |
| Hydroxyzine pamoate | Vistaril®[60] | Yes | 50-100 (per PRAC recomm.) | Agitation |
| Meprobamate[61] | Equanil® / Miltown® | Yes | 400-1600 | (C-V) Anticonvulsant |
| Propranolol | Inderal®[51] | No | 10-160 (÷ up to QID) | Impulsivity / aggression |

[A] to [Z] - See Black Box Warnings on Page 9

1

## IV. NON-BENZODIAZEPINE SEDATIVE AND WAKE-PROMOTING AGENTS

| Generic name | Brand name | FDA-Approved for Insomnia | Usual dosage range (mg/d)* | Other Uses |
|---|---|---|---|---|
| Armodafinil | Nuvigil®[52] | No | 50-250 | Narcolepsy/Shift work |
| Diphenhydramine | Benadryl®[53] | Yes | 25-200 | Allergy |
| Doxepin[54] [A] | Sinequan® / Silenor®[55] | Yes | 3-6 | |
| Doxylamine | Nyquil® | Yes | 25-50 | |
| Eszopiclone [T] | Lunesta™[56] | Yes | 1-3 | |
| Hydroxyzine HCL[57] | Atarax®[58] / Ucerax®[59] | No | 10-30 | Allergy / itch |
| Hydroxyzine pamoate | Vistaril®[60] | No | 50-100 | Acute agitation |
| Meprobamate | Equanil® / Miltown®[61] | No | 400-1600 | Anticonvulsant (Note: C-IV C. S.) |
| Modafinil | Provigil® / Sparlon®[62] | No | 85-225 | Narcolepsy |
| Pitolisant | Wakix®[63] | No | 8.9-35.6 | Narcolepsy |
| Ramelteon | Rozerem®[64] | Yes | 8 | |
| Solriamfetol | Sunosi®[65] | No | 37.5-150 | Narcolepsy |
| Suvorexant | Belsomra®[66] | Yes | 5-20 | (Note: C-IV Controlled Substance) |
| Sodium oxybate [N,R] | Xyrem®[67] | No | 3-9 gm/d | Cataplexy |
| Tasimelteon | Hetlioz®[68] | Yes | 20 | |
| Trazodone [A] | Desyrel®[69] | No | 5-150 | Depression |
| Zaleplon [T] | Sonata®[70] | Yes | 5-20 | |
| Zolpidem [T] | Ambien®/CR®/ Zolpimist®/ Intermezzo®/ Edluar® [71-74] | Yes | 2.5-10 | |

* Elderly patients are usually treated with approximately one-half of the dose listed

## V. GERIATRIC PSYCHIATRY MEDICATIONS

| Generic name | Brand name | Usual daily dose (mg/d) |
|---|---|---|
| Amantadine | Symmetrel /Osmolex ER™[75] / Gocovri™[76] | 100-400 |
| Apomorphine | Apokyn®[77] | 2-6 |
| Bromocriptine | Cycloset®[78] / Parlodel®[79] | 2.5-100 (÷ BID) / Avg. 40 a day |
| Cabergoline | Dostinex®[80] | 0.25-1 twice a week |
| Carbidopa | Lodosyn®[81] | 25-100 |
| Carbidopa + Levodopa | Sinemet® / CR®[82] / Parcopa®[83] / Rytary®[84] / Duopa®[85] | 25-2450 (levodopa) |
| Carbidopa + Levodopa + Entacapone | Stalevo®[86] | 50-1200 (levodopa) |
| Donepezil | Aricept®[87] | 5-23 QAM |
| Entacapone | Comtan®[88] | 200-1600 (÷ 8x/d) |
| Galantamine / Galantamine ER | Razadyne® / Razadyne ER®[89] | 8-32 (÷ BID for IR forms) |
| Istradefylline | Nourianz™[90] | 20-40 |
| Levodopa | Inbrija™ inhalation powder[91] | 84-420 (÷ up to 5x/d) |
| Memantine / Memantine XR | Namenda® / Namenda XR®[92] | 5-20 (÷ BID for IR forms) XR: 7-28 |
| Memantine XR + Donepezil | Namzaric™[93] | 14/10 to 28/10 |
| Pergolide | Permax®[94] | 3-5 (÷ TID) |
| Pramipexole | Mirapex®[95] | 0.375-4.5 (÷ TID) |
| Rasagiline | Azilect®[96] | 0.5-1 |
| Rivastigmine | Exelon®[97] | 1.5-6 po BID / 4.6-9.5/24h patch |
| Ropinirole | Requip®[98] | 0.75-24 (÷ TID) |
| Rotigotine | Neupro®[99] | 2-8/24 hour |
| Safinamide | Xadago[100] | 50-100 |
| Selegiline | Eldepryl®[101] / Zelapar®[102] ODT / Emsam[103] | 2.5-10 |
| Tolcapone | Tasmar®[104] | 300-600 (÷ TID) |

[A] to [Z] - See Black Box Warnings on Page 9

## VI. EPS TREATMENT MEDICATIONS AND ANTICHOLINERGICS

| Generic Name | Brand Name | Equivalent dose (mg) | Dosage range (mg/d) |
|---|---|---|---|
| **Antimuscarinics** | | | |
| Benztropine ▪ | Cogentin®[105,106] | 1 | 1- 8 ⅄ (÷ up to BID) |
| Orphenadrine ▪ | Norflex® | 50 | 50 - 200 (÷ up to BID) |
| Trihexyphenidyl | Artane®[107] | 2 | 2 - 15 (÷ up to TID) |
| **Antihistamine** | | | |
| Diphenhydramine ▪ | Benadryl® | 50 | 50 - 400 (÷ up to QID) |
| **Dopamine Agonist** | | | |
| Amantadine[108] | Symmetrel®[109] | N/A | 100-400 (÷ up to QID) |
| **Benzodiazepines** | | | |
| Lorazepam ▪ᵞ | Ativan® | N/A | 1- 8 (÷ up to TID) |
| Diazepam ᵞ | Valium® | N/A | 2 - 20 (÷ up to QID) |
| Clonazepam ᵞ | Klonopin® | N/A | 2 - 8 (÷ up to TID) |
| **Beta-Blocker** | | | |
| Propranolol | Inderal® | N/A | 20 - 160 (÷ up to TID) |
| **VMAT2 Inhibitors** | | | |
| Deutetrabenazine ᶜ | Austedo®[110] | N/A | 12 - 36 (÷ BID) |
| Valbenazine ᴮ | Ingrezza®[111] | N/A | 40 - 80 |
| Tetrabenazine ᶜ | Xenazine®[112] | N/A | 12.5 - 50 (÷ BID) |

▪ Injectable dosage form can be given intramuscularly for relief of acute dystonia
⅄ Dosage may be titrated to 12 mg with care; non-linear pharmacokinetics have been demonstrated

## VII. BIPOLAR MEDICATIONS / MOOD STABILIZERS

| Generic Name | Brand Name | Usual Daily Dose (mg) | Other Indications / Uses |
|---|---|---|---|
| Carbamazepine ᴱ,ᶠ | Tegretol®/XR / Epitol®/ Equetro™ / Carbatrol® / Carnexiv (injection)[113-116] | 200-1200 | Aggression / Epilepsy / peripheral neuropathy |
| Lamotrigine ᴶ | Lamictal®[117] / XR[118] / ODT | 50-500 | Epilepsy / Bipolar maintenance |
| Lithium ᴰ | Eskalith®[119]/ Lithobid®[120]/ Cibalith-S® | 300-2700 | Cluster headache / Bipolar |
| Olanzapine + fluoxetine ᴬ,ᴷ | Symbyax®[121] | 3/25 to 12/50 | Bipolar depression / Treatment-resistant depression |
| Valproic Acid ᴳ,ᴴ,ᴵ | Depakote®/ ER / Stavzor® /[122] Depakene® / Depacon® | 500-3000 | Epilepsy / migraine headaches / hiccups |

## VIII. OLDER COMBINATION PRODUCTS

| Generic Name | Brand Name | Usual Daily Dose (mg) | Other Indications/Uses |
|---|---|---|---|
| Chlordiazepoxide + amitriptyline ᴬ,ᴷ | Limbitrol® / Limbitrol DS® | 5/12.5, 10/25 up to QID | Depression / schizophrenia anxiety / psychotic depression |
| Perphenazine + amitriptyline ᴬ,ᴷ | Etrafon® / Etrafon-A® | 2/10, 2/25, 4/10 up to QID | |
| Perphenazine + amitriptyline ᴬ,ᴷ | Triavil® | 2/10, 2/25, 4/10, 4/25, 4/50 up to QID | |

ᴬ to ᶻ - See Black Box Warnings on Page 9

## IX. ANTICONVULSANTS

| Generic Name | Brand Name | Usual Daily Dose (mg) | Other Uses / Important Notes |
|---|---|---|---|
| Brivaracetam | Briviact®[123] | 1 mg/kg/d up to 100 mg BID | |
| Cannabidiol | Epidiolex®[124] | 2.5 to 20 mg/kg p.o. BID | |
| Clobazam [Y] | Onfi®[125] | 5-40 | (Note: C-IV Controlled Substance) |
| Eslicarbazepine | Aptiom®[126] | 400-1200 | |
| Ethotoin | Peganone®[127] | 500-3000 divided Q 4-6 h | |
| Ethosuximide | Zarontin®[128] | 500-1500 divided TID | |
| Felbamate [C,F] | Felbatol®[129] | 1200-3600 | |
| Fosphenytoin sodium [M] | Cerebyx®[130] | 75-600 I.V. | |
| Gabapentin | Neurontin®[131] /Gralise™[132] / Horizant®[133] | 900-1800 | ALS / neuralgias (post-herpetic) |
| Lacosamide | Vimpat®[134] | 100-400 mg ÷ BID | (Note: C-V Controlled Substance) |
| Levetiracetam | Keppra®/XR®/[135] Elepsia XR™[136] / Roweepra[137] / Spritam[138] | 1000-3000 ÷ BID | (Note: Spritam® is the 1st drug ever to be 3D printed)[139] |
| Methsuximide | Celontin®[140] | 300-1200 | |
| Midazolam [Y] | Versed / Nayzilam®[141] | 5-10 | |
| Oxcarbazepine | Trileptal®[142] / Oxtellar XR®[143] | 300-2400 ÷ BID (4-16 y.o.: 8-10 mg/kg/d ÷ BID/TID up to 1800) | Genetic testing of at risk patients required before initiation |
| Perampanel [X] | Fycompa®[144] | 2-12 HS | (Note: C-III Controlled Substance) |
| Phenobarbital[145] | Luminal® | 30-240 | (Note: C-IV Controlled Substance) |
| Phenytoin | Dilantin®[146]/ Phenytek®[147] | 50-400 | |
| Pregabalin | Lyrica®[148] /CR[149] | 150-600 ÷ BID/TID | (Note: C-V Controlled Substance) |
| Primidone | Mysoline®[150] / Sertan® | 100-2000 | (Note: C-IV Controlled Substance) |
| Rufinamide | Banzel®[151] | 400-3200 ÷ BID | |
| Stiripentol | Diacomit®[152] | 50 mg/kg up to 3000 mg/d | |
| Tiagabine | Gabitril®[153] | 4-56 (peds: 2-32) ÷ BID-QID | |
| Topiramate | Topamax®[154] / Trokendi XR™[155] / Qudexy™ XR[156] / Topiragen® | 50-1600 ÷ BID (avg=200 BID) | Migraine prophylaxis |
| Trimethadione | Tridione[157] | 900-2400 ÷ TID-QID | |
| Vigabatrin [Z] | Sabril®[158] / Vigadrone®[159] | 25-75 mg/kg/day po BID 500-1500 ÷ BID | High risk of vision loss |
| Zonisamide | Zonegran®[160] | 100-600 ÷ BID | |

Between Phenobarbital and Phenytoin/Primidone: *metabolized to* (arrow)

→ Anticonvulsant metabolized to the other (following the arrow)

[A] to [Z] - See Black Box Warnings on Page 9

# X. ANTIDEPRESSANTS [A]

| Class | Generic Name | Brand Name | Dose range (mg/d) | Other Indications / Uses |
|---|---|---|---|---|
| Tertiary (3°) amine TCAs<br><br>*Inhibit*<br>*5HT > NE* | Amitriptyline [161] [A] | Elavil®* | 25-300 | Nocturnal enuresis / anxiety / OCD / insomnia / Panic Disorder / neuropathic pain / headaches |
| | Imipramine [162] [A] | Tofranil®** | 25-300 | |
| | Doxepin [54] [A] | Sinequan®/Adapin®/Silenor® | 3-300 | |
| | Trimipramine [A] | Surmontil® [163] | 25-300 | |
| | Clomipramine [A] | Anafranil® | 25-250 | |
| Secondary (2°) amine TCAs<br><br>*Inhibit*<br>*NE > 5HT* | Nortriptyline [164] [A] | Pamelor®* [165] | 25-<u>150</u> | |
| | Desipramine [A] | Norpramin®** [166] | 25-300 | |
| | Protriptyline [A] | Vivactil® [167] | 15-60 | |
| | Amoxapine [A] | Asendin® [168] | 50-600 | |
| | Maprotiline [A] | Ludiomil® [169] | 50-225 | |
| Monoamine Oxidase Inhibitors (MAOIs) | Phenelzine [A] | Nardil® [170] | 15-90 | Atypical depression / psychotic depression / anxiety |
| | Tranylcypromine [A,L] | Parnate® [171] | 10-60 | |
| | Selegiline [A] | Emsam® | 6-12 (patch) | |
| | Isocarboxazid [A] | Marplan® [172] | 20-60 | |
| Selective Serotonin Reuptake Inhibitors (SSRIs) | Fluoxetine [A] | Prozac® / Sarafem® [173] | 10-80 | OCD / Bulimia / PTSD / PMDD / hot flashes / Panic Disorder / headaches / premature ejaculation / various anxiety disorders |
| | Sertraline [A] | Zoloft® [174] | 25-200 | |
| | Paroxetine [A] | Paxil® [175] / Pexeva® [176] / Brisdelle™ [177] | 10-50 | |
| | Fluvoxamine [A] | Luvox®/CR® [178] | 50-300 | |
| | Citalopram [A] | Celexa® [179] | 10-40 | |
| | Escitalopram [A] | Lexapro® [180] | 5-20 | |
| SSRI + serotonin receptors antagonists (SARIs) | Nefazodone [A,G] | Serzone® [181] | 100-600 | Anxious depression |
| | Trazodone [A] | Desyrel®/Oleptro™ [182] | 50-450 | Insomnia |
| | Vortioxetine [A] | Trintellix® [183] | 5-20 | |
| Serotonin Norepinephrine Reuptake Inhibitors (SNRIs) | Venlafaxine [A] | Effexor [184] / XR®*** | 37.5-375 | Neuropathic pain / Diabetic neuropathy Fibromyalgia / GAD |
| | Desvenlafaxine [A] | Pristiq™ [185]*** | 50-100 | |
| | Duloxetine [A] | Cymbalta® [186]/Irenka™ [187]/ Drizalma Sprinkle™ [188] | 20-120 | |
| | Milnacipran [A] | Savella® | 12.5-200 (÷BID) | |
| | Levomilnacipran [A] | Fetzima® [189] | 20-120 | |
| Alpha$_2$ & 5HT$_{2/3}$ antagonist | Mirtazapine [A] | Remeron® [190] / Sol-tab® | 15-45 (at HS) | Insomnia / ↑ appetite |
| NE/DA reuptake inhibitor (NDRI) | Bupropion [A] | Wellbutrin® [191] /SR/XL/ Aplenzin® / Forfivo™/ Zyban®/ Budeprion® | 75-450 (÷ up to TID) | ADHD / seasonal affective disorder / smoking cessation |
| 5HT$_{1A}$ autoreceptor partial agonist + SSRI (SPARI) | Vilazodone [A] | Viibryd™ [192] | 10-40 (with FOOD) | |
| NMDA receptor antagonist | Esketamine [A,N,U] | Spravato™ [193] | 56-84 from 2 x a week to Q 2 weeks | Treatment-resistant depression (TRD) |
| GABA$_A$ receptor positive modulator | Brexanolone [U] | Zulresso™ [194] | 60-hr IV infusion of 30-90 mcg/kg/hour | Postpartum depression (PPD) |
| Medical food | L-methylfolate | Deplin® [195] / Cerefolin NAC (combo) | 7.5-15 mg/d | |

\* and \*\* and \*\*\* → antidepressants that are metabolized to the other (following the arrows)

[A] to [Z] - *See Black Box Warnings on Page 9*

## XI. TYPICAL ANTIPSYCHOTICS (FGAs) (aka: NEUROLEPTICS / ANALEPTICS)

| Generic Name | Brand Name | Usual Daily Dose (mg) | Other Indications / Uses |
|---|---|---|---|
| Chlorpromazine [K] | Thorazine® [196] | 25-1600 | Hiccups / bipolar / dementia / anxiety / N&V / agitation |
| Fluphenazine [K] | Prolixin® [197] / Decanoate [198] | 1-40 | Acute psychosis / psychotic depression / agitation |
| Haloperidol [K] | Haldol® [199] / Decanoate [200] | 0.5-40 | Acute psychosis / ADHD / Tourette's / agitation / autism / delirium / migraine / N&V / hiccups |
| Loxapine [K] | Loxitane® [201] / Adasuve® [202] [O] | 10-100 | Agitation |
| Molindone [K] | Moban® [203] | 10-100 | |
| Perphenazine [K] | Trilafon® [204] | 2-64 | N&V / acute psychosis / psychotic depression / hiccups |
| Thioridazine [B,K] | Mellaril® [205] | 10-800 | Anxiety / agitation |
| Thiothixene [K] | Navane® [206] | 2-30 | Acute psychosis / agitation / psychotic depression |
| Trifluoperazine [K] | Stelazine® [207] | 1-30 | Anxiety |

## XII. ATYPICAL ANTIPSYCHOTICS (SGAs) (aka: NEUROLEPTICS / ANALEPTICS)

| Generic Name | Brand Name | Usual Daily Dose (mg) | Other Indications/Uses |
|---|---|---|---|
| Aripiprazole ⊚♦+ | Abilify® [208] [A,K] | 10-30 | Adjunct for MDD / agitation / bipolar / autism |
| Aripiprazole ⊚♦+ | Abilify Maintena ™ [209] [A,K] | 300-400 | Acute psychosis |
| Aripiprazole lauroxil ⊚♦+ | Aristada ™ [210] / Initio ™ [211] [A,K] | 441-882 (studied) | |
| Asenapine ⊚♦ | Saphris® [K] SL [212] / Secuado® [213] [K] | 10-20 (÷ BID) | Bipolar disorder |
| Brexpiprazole + | Rexulti® [214] [A,K] | 2-4 | Adjunct for MDD |
| Cariprazine ⊚ | Vraylar® [215] [A,K] | 1.5-6 | Bipolar mania |
| Clozapine [F,K,P,Q,R] | Clozaril® / Fazaclo® / Versacloz ™ [216-218] | 25-900 | Treatment-resistant schizophrenia / tremor / schizoaffective disorder / bipolar / agitation |
| Iloperidone | Fanapt® [219] [K] | 12-24 (÷ BID) | |
| Lurasidone ⊚♦ | Latuda® [220] [A,K] | 40-160 (with FOOD) | Bipolar depression |
| Olanzapine ⊚♦+ | Zyprexa® [221] / Zydis® [K] | 2.5-20 | Agitation / acute psychosis |
| Olanzapine ⊚♦ | Zyprexa Relprevv ™ [222] [K,S] | 300-405 Q 4 weeks | |
| Paliperidone ⊚♦ | Invega® [223] [K] | 6-12 | Schizoaffective disorder |
| Paliperidone ⊚♦ | Invega Sustenna® [224] [K] | 78-234 Q 4 weeks | Schizoaffective disorder |
| Paliperidone ⊚♦ | Invega Trinza ™ [225] [K] | 273-819 Q 3 months | |
| Pimavanserin | Nuplazid ™ [226] [K] | | |
| Quetiapine ⊚♦+ *metabolized to* | Seroquel® / XR® [227] [A,K] | 25-800 | Bipolar depression / adjunct for MDD / acute psychosis / agitation |
| Risperidone ⊚♦ | Risperdal® / M-Tabs® [228] [K] | 1-16 | Autism / ADHD / psychotic depression / acute psychosis / Tourette's Syndrome / agitation |
| Risperidone ⊚♦ | Risperdal Consta® [229] [K] | 12.5-50 Q 2 weeks | Bipolar Disorder |
| Risperidone | Perseris ™ [230] [K] | 90 or 120 | |
| Ziprasidone ⊚ | Geodon® [231] [K] | 20-160 (÷ BID with FOOD) | Agitation / acute psychosis / Tourette's |

⊚ Approved for Bipolar Disorder / ♦ Approved in children &/or adolescents / + Approved as add-on therapy in depression
→ Antipsychotic metabolized to the other (following the arrow)

[A] to [Z] - See Black Box Warnings on Page 9

# 2. COMMONLY USED PSYCHIATRIC ACRONYMS, TERMS, & ABBREVIATIONS
## (unless otherwise defined herein)

If you see an abbreviation used in this book that you're not familiar with, it's likely here:

- ≈ or ~ = approximately
- ↑ = Increase
- ↓ = Decrease
- 5HT = Serotonin (5-hydroxytriptamine)
- Ψ = Psi = Unapproved abbreviation for PSYCH
- ABW = Actual body weight
- AchEls = Acetylcholinesterase Inhibitors
- ADD / ADHD = Attention Deficit Disorder / Hyperactivity Disorder
- ADR = Adverse Drug Reaction
- AKA = Also Known As
- ALF = Assisted Living Facility
- ALP = Alkaline Phosphatase
- ALT or SGPT = Alanine Transaminase
- AMA = Against Medical Advice
- ANC = Absolute Neutrophil Count
- APA = American Psychiatric Association
- ASD = Autism Spectrum Disorder
- AST or SGOT = Aspartate Transaminase
- BA = "Baker Act" (law in Florida)
- BBB = Blood Brain Barrier
- BBW = Black Box Warning
- BDNF = Brain-Derived Neurotrophic Factor
- BP = Blood Pressure
- BPAD = Bipolar Affective Disorder
- BPD = Borderline Personality Disorder (some clinicians use it for Bipolar D/O, so caution)
- BUN = Blood Urea Nitrogen
- BZD = Benzodiazepine
- C/O = Complains of
- CAD = Coronary Artery Disease
- CAT / CT = Computerized Axial Tomography
- CBC = Complete Blood Count
- CBZ = Carbamazepine
- CGI = Clinical Global Impressions scale
- CNS = Central Nervous System
- CR = Controlled-release
- CrCl = Creatinine Clearance
- CV = Cardiovascular
- CVA = Cerebrovascular Accident
- CXR = Chest X-Ray
- CYP = Cytochrome P450 Enzyme System
- D or DA = Dopamine
- D/O = Disorder
- D/T = Due to
- DBPCT = Double-blind placebo-controlled trial
- DCF = Department of Children and Families
- Def. = Deferred
- Diff = Differential
- DJJ = Department of Juvenile Justice
- DRESS = Drug Reaction with Eosinophilia & Systemic Symptoms
- DT = Delirium Tremens
- EBM = Evidence-Based Medicine
- ECT = Electroconvulsive Therapy
- EEG = Electroencephalogram
- EKG = Electrocardiogram
- EP = Elopement precautions
- EPS = Extrapyramidal Side Effects
- ER or XR = Extended-Release
- ESRD = End Stage Renal Disease
- ETO = Emergency Treatment Order
- EtOH = Ethyl Alcohol
- FDA = Food and Drug Administration
- Fx or Fxn = Function
- GABA = Gamma Aminobutyric Acid
- GAD = Generalized Anxiety Disorder
- GFR = Glomerular Filtration Rate
- GGT = Gamma Glutamyl Transpeptidase
- GI = Gastrointestinal
- H&P = History and Physical
- H/I = Homicidal Ideation
- H1 = Histamine-1 receptor
- HIV = Human Immunodeficiency Virus
- HTN = Hypertension
- IBW = Ideal Body Weight
- IM = Intramuscular
- INR = International Normalized Ratio
- IR = Immediate-release
- LAIA = Long-acting Injectable Antipsychotic
- LFTs = Liver Function Tests (e.g., ALT/AST)
- MA = Marchman Act
- MAO / MAOI = Monoamine Oxidase / Inhibitor
- MDD = Major Depressive Disorder
- MI = Myocardial Infarction
- MMSE = Mini Mental State Examination
- MOA = Mechanism of Action
- MR = Mental Retardation
- MRI = Magnetic Resonance Imaging
- MSE = Mental Status Exam
- NDA = New Drug Application (to the FDA)
- NE = Norepinephrine
- NMDA = N-Methyl-D-aspartate
- NNH = Number Needed to Harm
- NNT = Number Needed to Treat
- NOS = Not Otherwise Specified
- NPO = Nothing By Mouth
- NTE = Not To Exceed
- N/V or N&V = Nausea & Vomiting (+ D for diarrhea)
- OCD = Obsessive-Compulsive Disorder
- OCPD = Obsessive-Compulsive Personality Disorder
- OOB = Out of Bed
- OROS = Osmotic Controlled-Release Oral Delivery System (e.g., Invega®/Concerta®)
- CYP450 = Cytochrome P450 Enzyme System
- PCOS = Polycystic Ovarian Syndrome
- PD = Panic, Parkinson's or Personality Disorder
- PDD = Pervasive Developmental Disorder
- PEG = Percutaneous endoscopic gastrostomy
- PET = Positron Emission Tomography Scan
- Pgp or P-gp = P-glycoprotein
- PMS / PMDD = Premenstrual Syndrome / Dysphoric Disorder
- prn = As needed = "*pro re nata*" in Latin
- PSA = Polysubstance Abuse
- PT = Prothrombin Time
- pt. = Patient
- PTH = Parathyroid Hormone
- QD / BID / TID / QID / HS = Daily / 2X a day / 3X a day / 4X a day / Bedtime
- RCT = Randomized Clinical Trial
- REMS = Risk Evaluation and Mitigation Strategy
- RR = Regular-Release
- rTMS = Repetitive Transcranial Magnetic Stimulation
- Rxn = Reaction

7

- S/I = Suicidal Ideation
- SAD or SCAD = Schizoaffective Disorder (Schizophrenia + Bipolar/mood component)
- SAD = Seasonal Affective Disorder (depends on geographic location)
- SCPT = Schizophrenia Paranoid Type
- SCr = Serum Creatinine Level
- SCUT = Schizophrenia Undifferentiated Type
- SEs = Side Effects
- SIADH = Syndrome of Inappropriate Antidiuretic Hormone
- SJS = Steven Johnson's Syndrome
- SL = Sublingual
- SNDRI = 5HT, NE, DA reuptake inhibitor
- SNF = Skilled Nursing Facility
- SNRI = Serotonin Norepinephrine Reuptake Inhibitor
- SP = Suicide precautions
- SR = Sustained-release
- SubQ = Subcutaneous
- SSRI = Selective Serotonin Reuptake Inhibitor

- Sx = Symptom
- SZ = Seizure
- T½ = Half-life
- TB = Tuberculosis
- TBI = Traumatic Brain Injury
- TCA = Tricyclic Antidepressant
- tDCS = Transcranial Direct Current Stimulation
- TEN = Toxic Epidermal Necrolysis
- TRD =Treatment-Resistant Depression
- TSH = Thyroid Stimulating Hormone
- Tx. = Treatment
- UDP = Uridine diphospho
- UGT = Uridine diphospho-glucuronyl transferase
- UNSPEC = Unspecified
- VPA = Valproic acid
- W/D = Withdrawal
- WBC = White Blood Cells
- XR or ER = Extended-release
- Y.O. = Year(s) Old
- Yr or Yrs = Year(s)

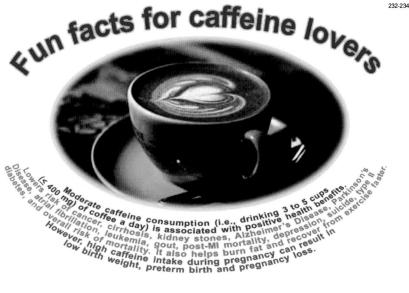

232-234

**Fun facts for caffeine lovers**

Moderate caffeine consumption (i.e., drinking 3 to 5 cups (≤ 400 mg) of coffee a day) is associated with positive health benefits. Lowers risk of cancer, cirrhosis, kidney stones, Alzheimer's Disease, Parkinson's Disease, atrial fibrillation, leukemia, gout, post-MI mortality, depression, suicide, type II diabetes, and overall risk of mortality. It also helps burn fat and recover from exercise faster. However, high caffeine intake during pregnancy can result in low birth weight, preterm birth and pregnancy loss.

---

### *DID YOU KNOW*???    **INTERESTING FUN FACTS:**

**The color of the medication (tablet/capsule) can influence its perceived efficacy[235]**
  1. Blue pills = sedatives
  2. Red or orange pills = stimulants
  3. Yellow = antidepressants
  4. Green = anxiolytic and pain medications
  5. Embossed brand names = more effective

The power of the "placebo effect"[236]
  ► The placebo effect is a real thing
  ► Placebos can objectively improve symptoms
  ► The placebo effect is highest in the United States
  ► Confidence in the prescriber boosts the placebo effect[237]
  ► A negative placebo ("nocebo") can worsen symptoms if that's what the person is told
  ► Telling patients that they're taking a placebo still gives the placebo efficacy
  ► "Placebo" in Latin means "I will please"

# 3. BLACK BOX WARNINGS

A - Suicidality and Antidepressant Drugs - Antidepressants ↑ the risk compared to placebo of suicidal thinking and behavior (suicidality) in children, adolescents, and young adults in short-term studies of Major Depressive Disorder (MDD) and other psychiatric disorders. Anyone considering the use of an antidepressant in a child, adolescent, or young adult must balance this risk with the clinical need. Short-term studies did not show an ↑ in the risk of suicidality with antidepressants compared to placebo in adults beyond age 24; there was a reduction in risk with antidepressants compared to placebo in adults aged 65 and older. Depression and certain other psychiatric disorders are themselves associated with increases in the risk of suicide.

B - Proarrhythmic Effects - QT-Prolongation and *Torsades de Pointes (TdP)*

C - Increased risk of depression and suicidal thoughts and behavior (suicidality) in patients with Huntington's disease

D - Lithium toxicity is closely related to its serum levels and can occur at dose close to therapeutic levels

E - Serious dermatologic reactions and HLA-B*1502 Allele - including toxic epidermal necrolysis (**TEN**) and Stevens-Johnson syndrome (**SJS**); the risk is 10x greater in Asian countries; the allele is almost exclusively in Asian patients

F - Aplastic Anemia/Agranulocytosis

G - Hepatoxicity and hepatic failure

H - Teratogenic Fetal Risk, particularly neural tube defects, other major malformations, and decreased IQ

I - Pancreatitis - cases of life threatening pancreatitis has been reported in both children and adults

J – Life-threatening Serious Rashes - Serious rashes including Stevens-Johnson syndrome may occur requiring hospitalization and discontinuation of treatment

K - Dementia-Related Psychosis - elderly patients with dementia-related psychosis treated with antipsychotic drugs are at an increased risk of death; not approved for the treatment of patients with dementia-related psychosis

L - Excessive consumption of foods or beverages with significant tyramine content or certain drugs can precipitate hypertensive crisis. Monitor blood pressure, allow for medication free intervals, and advise patients to avoid foods and beverages with high tyramine content.

M - Cardiovascular Risk with Rapid Infusion - infusion not to exceed 150 mg/min (adults) or 2 mg/kg/min whichever is slower (in pediatric patients); increased risk of severe hypotension and cardiac arrhythmias above recommended infusion rate; Careful cardiac monitoring is needed during and after administration

N - High Abuse Potential, Dependency - high abuse potential; avoid prolonged tx, may lead to drug dependence; potential for non-therapeutic use or distribution to others; prescribe/dispense sparingly; serious cardiovascular adverse events and sudden death reported w/ misuse

O - Bronchospasm that has the potential to lead to respiratory distress and respiratory arrest

P - Seizures

Q - Myocarditis

R - Other cardiovascular and respiratory effects (orthostatic hypotension, respiratory/cardiac arrest, collapse, CNS depression)

S - Post-injection Delirium/Sedation Syndrome. Patients are at risk for severe sedation (including coma) and/or delirium after each injection & must be observed for at least 3 hours in a registered facility with ready access to emergency response services.

T - Complex sleep behaviors including sleep-walking, sleep-driving, and engaging in other activities while not fully awake may occur

U - Risk for severe sedation and dissociation

V - Retinal abnormalities and/or permanent vision loss. Baseline and periodic eye exams required

W - Thrombocytopenia or reduced platelet counts

X - Serious or life-threatening psychiatric and behavioral adverse reactions including aggression, hostility, irritability, anger, and homicidal ideation and threats have been reported

Y - Concomitant use of benzodiazepines and opioids may result in profound sedation, respiratory depression, coma, and death

Z - Permanent Vision Loss

# 4. DOSING FREQUENCY OF PSYCHOTROPIC MEDICATIONS

| Brand Name | Generic Name | Dosing Frequency | Brand Name | Generic Name | Dosing Frequency |
|---|---|---|---|---|---|
| **ANTIDEPRESSANTS** | | | | | |
| Anafranil® | clomipramine | 1-2 | Parnate® | tranylcypromine | 1-2 |
| Asendin® | amoxapine | 2-3 | Paxil®/Pexeva®/ Brisdelle™ | paroxetine | 1 |
| Trintellix® | vortioxetine | 1 | Pristiq™ | desvenlafaxine | 1 |
| Celexa® | citalopram | 1 | Prozac®/ Sarafem® | fluoxetine | 1 |
| Cymbalta®/Irenka™ | duloxetine | 1-2 | Remeron® / Sol-tab® | mirtazapine | HS |
| Desyrel®/ Oleptro™ | trazodone | QHS-2 | Savella® | milnacipran | 2 |
| Effexor | venlafaxine | 2-3 | Serzone® | nefazodone | 2 |
| Effexor XR® | | 1 | Sinequan®/ Silenor® | doxepin | 1-2 |
| Elavil® | amitriptyline | 1-3 | Spravato | esketamine | Q 1-2 w |
| Emsam® | selegiline | 1 (patch) | Surmontil® | trimipramine | 1-3 |
| Fetzima® | levomilnacipran | 1 | Tofranil® | imipramine | 1-3 |
| Lexapro® | escitalopram | 1 | Viibryd™ | vilazodone | 1 (w/ food) |
| Ludiomil® | maprotiline | 2-3 | Vivactil® | protriptyline | 3-4 |
| Luvox®/CR® | fluvoxamine | 1-2 | Wellbutrin® / Aplenzin® | bupropion | 3 |
| Marplan® | isocarboxazid | 2-4 | Wellbutrin® SR/ Zyban® | | 2 |
| Nardil® | phenelzine | 3-4 | Wellbutrin® XL/ Forfivo™ | | 1 |
| Norpramin® | desipramine | 1-2 | Zoloft® | sertraline | 1 |
| Pamelor® | nortriptyline | 3-4 | Zulresso® | brexanolone | one time |
| **TYPICAL (FGAs) AND ATYPICAL (SGAs – IN ITALICS) ANTIPSYCHOTICS (AKA: NEUROLEPTICS)** | | | | | |
| *Abilify Maintena™* | *aripiprazole* | Q 4 w | Nuplazid® | pimavanserin | 1 |
| *Abilify®* | | 1 | *Perseris™* | *risperidone* | Q 4 w |
| *Aristada™* | *aripiprazole lauroxil* | Q 4-8 w | Prolixin® | fluphenazine | 2-3 |
| *Clozaril® / Fazaclo®* | *clozapine* | 2 | Prolixin® Decanoate | | Q 2-3 w |
| *Fanapt®* | *iloperidone* | 2 | *Rexulti®* | *brexpiprazole* | 1 |
| *Geodon®* | *ziprasidone* | 2 (w/ food) | *Risperdal® Consta®* | *risperidone* | Q 2 w |
| Haldol® | haloperidol | 2-3 | *Risperdal®/ M-Tabs®* | | 1-2 |
| Haldol®Decanoate | | Q 4 w | *Saphris® SL* | *asenapine* | 2 |
| *Invega Sustenna®* | paliperidone | Q 4 w | *Seroquel XR®* | *quetiapine* | 1 |
| *Invega Trinza™* | | Q 3 mo. | *Seroquel®* | | 2 |
| *Invega®* | | 1 | Stelazine® | trifluoperazine | 2-3 |
| *Latuda®* | *lurasidone* | 1 (w/ food) | Thorazine® | chlorpromazine | 2-3 |
| Loxitane®/Adasuve® | loxapine | 2-3 | Trilafon® | perphenazine | 2-3 |
| Mellaril® | thioridazine | 2-3 | *Vraylar®* | *cariprazine* | 1 |
| Moban® | molindone | 2-3 | *Zyprexa®/ Zydis®* | *olanzapine* | 12 |
| Navane® | thiothixene | 2-3 | *Zyprexa Relprevv™* | | Q 2-4 w |
| **BIPOLAR MEDICATIONS / MOOD STABILIZERS** | | | | | |
| Depakene®/ Stavzor®/Depacon® / Depakote® | valproic acid | 2-3 | Symbyax® | olanzapine + fluoxetine | 1 |
| Depakote® ER | | 1 | Tegretol® / Epitol® | carbamazepine | 3-4 |
| Eskalith® / Lithobid® | lithium | 2-3 | Tegretol® XR / Equetro™ / Carbatrol® | | 2 |
| Lamictal® | lamotrigine | 1-2 | | | |
| **NON-BENZODIAZEPINE SEDATIVE-HYPNOTIC AGENTS** | | | | | |
| Ambien® & CR®/ Edluar®/Zolpimist®/ Intermezzo® | zolpidem | QHS | Lunesta™ | eszopiclone | QHS |
| Belsomra® | suvorexant | QHS | Rozerem® | ramelteon | QHS |
| Hetlioz® | tasimelteon | QHS | Sonata® | zaleplon | QHS |
| **DEMENTIA MEDICATIONS** | | | | | |
| Aricept® | donepezil | QAM | Namenda XR® | memantine XR | 1 |
| Exelon® | rivastigmine | 2 | Namzaric™ | memantine XR + donepezil | 1 |
| Exelon® Patch | | 1 | Razadyne® | galantamine | 2 |
| Namenda® | memantine | 2 | Razadyne ER® | galantamine ER | 1 |

## KEY: 1 = QD  2 = BID  3 = TID  4 = QID

# DOSING FREQUENCY OF PSYCHOTROPIC MEDICATIONS (cont.)

| Brand Name | Generic Name | Dosing Frequency | Brand Name | Generic Name | Dosing Frequency |
|---|---|---|---|---|---|
| **ANTICHOLINERGICS AND OTHERS** | | | | | |
| Akineton® | biperiden | 4 | Inderal® | propranolol | 1-4 |
| Artane® | trihexyphenidyl | 3 | Kemadrin® | procyclidine | 3 |
| Atarax® | hydroxyzine HCl | QHS-4 | Norflex® | orphenadrine | 2 |
| Benadryl® | diphenhydramine | 4 | Symmetrel® | amantadine | 4 |
| BuSpar®/ Dividose® | buspirone | 3 | Vistaril® | hydroxyzine pamoate | QHS-4 |
| Cogentin® | benztropine | 2 | | | |
| **BENZODIAZEPINES** | | | | | |
| Ativan® | lorazepam | 1-4 | Restoril® | temazepam | QHS |
| Halcion | triazolam | QHS | Serax® | oxazepam | 1-4 |
| Klonopin® | clonazepam | 1-3 | Tranxene® | clorazepate | 1-4 |
| Librium® | chlordiazepoxide | 1-4 | Valium® / Valtoco® | diazepam | 2-4 |
| Paxipam® | halazepam | 1-4 | Xanax® / Niravam® | alprazolam | 3-4 |
| ProSom® | estazolam | QHS | Xanax® XR® | | QAM |
| **ANTICONVULSANTS** | | | | | |
| Aptiom® | eslicarbazepine | 1 | Gralise™ | gabapentin | 1 |
| Banzel | rufinamide | 2 | Horizant® | gabapentin enacarbil | 1-2 |
| Dilantin® | phenytoin | 3 | Onfi® | clobazam | 1-2 |
| Felbatol® | felbamate | 3-4 | Sabril | vigabatrin | 2 |
| Fycompa® | perampanel | QHS | Topamax® | topiramate | 2 |
| Gabitril® | tiagabine | 2-4 | Trokendi XR™ / Qudexy™ XR | | 1 |
| Keppra® XR®/ Elepsia™ XR | levetiracetam | 1 | Trileptal® | ox-carbazepine | 2 |
| Keppra® | | 2 | Oxtellar XR® | | 1 |
| Luminal® | phenobarbital | 1-3 | Vimpat | lacosamide | 2 |
| Lyrica® | pregabalin | 2 or 3 | Zarontin® | ethosuximide | 2 |
| Mysoline®/ Sertan® | primidone | 1 | Zonegran® | zonisamide | 2 |
| Neurontin® | gabapentin | 3 | | | |
| **ADHD MEDICATIONS / PSYCHOSTIMULANTS** | | | | | |
| Adderall® Adderall® XR / Mydayis™/ Dyanavel® XR / Adzenys ER & XR-ODT / Evekeo™ ODT | mixed amphetamine salts | 1-2 | Kapvay™ / Catapres® | clonidine | 1-3 |
| Dexedrine® / ProCentra® / Zenzedi® | dextro-amphetamine | 1-3 | Adhansia XR™ / Aptensio XR™ / Concerta® & XL / Cotempla XR-ODT / Daytrana™ / Jornay PM® / Methylin® ER / Quillivant XR™ / Ritalin® LA / Quillichew ER™ / Relexxii™ | methyl-phenidate | 1 |
| Desoxyn® | meth-amphetamine | 2 | Ritalin® / Methylin® | | 2-3 |
| Evekeo™ | amphetamine sulfate | 1 | Ritalin® SR / Metadate® CD/ER | | 1-2 |
| Focalin® | dexmethyl-phenidate | 2 | Strattera™ | atomoxetine | 1-2 |
| Focalin® XR | | 1 | Tenex® / Intuniv™ | guanfacine | 1-3 |
| Provigil®/ Sparlon® | modafinil | 1 | Vyvanse™ | lisdex-amfetamine | 1 |

## KEY: 1 = QD  2 = BID  3 = TID  4 = QID

## I. DIAGNOSTIC AND STATISTICAL MANUAL OF MENTAL DISORDERS (DSM)
A. Published by the American Psychiatric Association and provides diagnostic criteria for mental disorders within specified time frames
  1. DSM-I (1952)
  2. DSM-II (1968), revised in 1974
  3. DSM-III (1980), revised DSM-III-R (1987)
  4. DSM-IV (1994), revised DSM-IV-TR (2000)[244] is still frequently used today
   i. **Multi-axial diagnosis from the DSM-IV-TR**
    a. Axis I: Main psychiatric diagnosis
    b. Axis II: Personality Disorders or Mental Retardation
    c. Axis III: Co-morbid medical disorders (supposedly related to psychiatric diagnosis)
    d. Axis IV: Psychosocial stressors (listed)
     1. i.e. Divorce, school issues, job-related stress
    e. Axis V: Global Assessment of Functioning (GAF)
     1. Scale of function from 0 to 100 (0=lowest / 100=highest)
  5. DSM-5 (2013) 5th edition[245]
   i. The 5 Axes from DSM-IV-TR have been removed
   ii. Most diagnostic criteria is unchanged from DSM-IV-TR, but some categories refined or added
    a. Removed *NOS* (not otherwise specified) and *NED* (not elsewhere defined)
     1. Replaced with *other* or *unspecified disorder*
    b. Removed sub-types of Schizophrenia
    c. Mental retardation now called *intellectual disability / developmental disorder*
    d. Removed *PTSD* and *OCD* from anxiety chapter and placed into their own sections
    e. All types of *autism* are now diagnosed as *Autism Spectrum Disorder*
    f. New diagnosis: *DMDD* (Disruptive Mood Dysregulation Disorder)
     1. People with frequent temper tantrums and irritability
   iii. Corresponds to ICD-10 (International Statistical Classification of Diseases and Related Health Problems)
   iv. The severity of the current mental illness should be addressed
    a. Qualifier: Mild, Moderate, Severe
    b. Descriptive features: e.g., with good insight; in a controlled environment
    c. Course of illness: e.g., in partial remission, in full remission, recurrent

## II. "BAKER ACT" (Florida Mental Health Act of 1971) - SPECIFIC TO FLORIDA!
A. Most states have very analogous laws about mental health patients, so many of these terms and definitions may be similar in other states (e.g., "51/50")
B. Definition: A law that protects the patient's rights while in a psychiatric hospital
  1. Florida Statutes – Chapter 394 (summary can be found at: http://www.floridasupremecourt.org/pub_info/documents/BakerSummary.pdf)
C. Terminology:
  1. Informed Consent
   i. Informed consent must satisfy the following elements[246]
    a. Patient must be provided information (i.e., given full disclosure about treatment options, medication side effects, alternative therapies, etc.)
    b. Patient has to have the decisional capacity (i.e., ability to make a decision)
    c. Patient must be free from coercion in making their decision
   ii. Consent to treatment – Patient agrees to be in the hospital
    a. The capacity of a patient to understand and agree is up to psychiatrist
    b. If psychiatrist deems patient not able to give expressed and informed consent, a Proxy or Guardian Advocate must be found
   iii. Consent for medication
    a. Patient should be informed of purposes of prescribed medication, common side effects, risks, and alternatives to medication, and benefits of therapy
    b. Even if patients are admitted involuntarily, he/she can consent or not consent to medications
    c. If psychiatrist deems patient not able to give expressed and informed consent, a Proxy or Guardian Advocate must be found
     1. A patient is never force-medicated if no consent is given, unless in the event of an emergency or a guardian or judge gives permission
  2. *Ex Parte* – Court-issued order for involuntary examination in a psychiatric hospital (up to 72 hrs)
  3. Typical "Baker Act" – Involuntary hospitalization for up to 72 hours by law enforcement or the judicial system (Time can be extended by a court hearing)
  4. Voluntary Admission
   i. Patient consents to treatment or admitting self to hospital setting
  5. Application for Discharge (FL Statute Section 394.4625(2))
   i. If a patient is hospitalized and voluntarily consents to treatment, then he/she may revoke consent at any time. The attending psychiatrist has up to 24 hours to discharge the patient AMA (Against Medical Advice) or make the patient involuntary (becomes "Baker-Acted" and goes to court)

6. Florida Marchman Act - An involuntary admission due to substance abuse impairment
   i. See Chapter 397 of the Florida Statutes
7. Emergency Treatment Orders (ETOs) - (order valid for only 24 hours)
   i. If a patient needs emergency psychiatric medication because they are at risk of hurting themselves or another person, and that patient is deemed by their psychiatrist to be unable to consent to treatment or medications (and a guardian or proxy cannot be obtained in a timely manner), the physician can order emergency medication to be given
   ii. Order is a response to violent patient behaviors (not a prn)
   iii. Order should be discontinued by prescriber after patient's behavior improves
   iv. Usually consists of IM antipsychotic + anticholinergic + benzodiazepine
      a. Called a "cocktail" or "B-52" (for the ingredients: Benadryl/benztropine + 5 mg haloperidol + 2 mg lorazepam)
8. Guardian Advocate or Proxy
   i. Assigned when a patient is deemed unable to consent to treatment to protect the patient's rights and consent for medications under principles of beneficence
9. Court-ordered Detainment
   i. After the 72 hour period of the "Baker Act" is up, a psychiatrist must either discharge the patient or petition the court for more time to treat the patient (involuntarily)
      a. Petition must be filed before the "Baker Act" expires (within initial 72 hours)
   ii. The court can decide to discharge the patient or retain them for an indeterminate amount of time for treatment
   iii. The patient can still refuse medication if capable of consenting unless court-ordered to be force-medicated
      a. A Guardian Advocate may consent for the patient's medications at this point, even if against the patient's will

## III. PSYCHOPHARMACOLOGY MEDICATION ALGORITHMS (JUST A FEW...)
A. The National Guideline Clearinghouse™ - U.S. Department of Health & Human Services - Agency for Healthcare Research and Quality - http://www.guideline.gov (searchable)
B. International Psychopharmacology Algorithm Project (IPAP) (www.ipap.org)
C. American Association of Child and Adolescent Psychiatry (AACAP)
   1. www.aacap.org/publications/pubcat/guideline.htm
D. American Psychiatric Association (APA)
   1. https://www.psychiatry.org/psychiatrists/practice/clinical-practice-guidelines
E. National Institute for Health and Clinical Excellence (NICE) (www.nice.org.uk/guidance/)
F. Veteran's Administration / Department of Defense (VA/DoD)
   1. https://www.healthquality.va.gov/guidelines/
G. World Federation of Societies of Biological Psychiatry (WFSBP) (http://wfsbp.org)

## IV. PSYCHOPHARMACOLOGY TERMINOLOGY
A. Nov. 2014 - A new psychotropic drug classification system is proposed[247]
   1. Collaborative effort between the European College of Neuropsychopharmacology (ECNP), American College of Neuropsychopharmacology (ACNP), the International College of Neuropsychopharmacology, the International Union of Basic and Clinical Pharmacology, and the Asian College of Neuropsychopharmacology
   2. Based on 4 Axes
      i. Pharmacologic target and mechanism of action
      ii. Indication and uses
      iii. Description of efficacy and major side effects
      iv. Neurobiological description of the drug
B. This resource book uses the current classification system for simplicity

## V. PSYCHOTROPIC DANGERS
A. Emergency room (ER) visits due to a mental illness or psychotropic medication has ↑ over 50%[248] in last 10 years[249]
   1. 9.6% of all drug-related ER visits by adults involve a psychotropic[250]
      i. Approx. 50% involve patients from 19-44 years old
      ii. Approx. 17% involve patients over 65-years-old
      iii. 62% women (mostly antidepressant-related) / 38% men (mostly antipsychotic-related)
      iv. Approx. 20% of the time, patient was admitted to the hospital (lithium >50% of time)
      v. 10 most common drugs responsible (in decreasing order of occurrences):
         a. Zolpidem > quetiapine > alprazolam > lorazepam > haloperidol > clonazepam > trazodone > citalopram > lithium > risperidone
         b. Account for almost 60% of psychotropic-related visits
         c. Benzodiazepines & other sedatives responsible for 75% of head injury & fall-related ER visits
         d. Ratio of drug to number of prescription visits shows haloperidol, lithium, and risperidone have the highest incidence of ER visits
   2. Women who are depressed AND/OR on psychotropics fall down more frequently[251]
      i. Overall = 5.3%
      ii. Depression ↑'s risk by 2.4 times
      iii. Psychotropics and benzodiazepines ↑'s risk by 2.8 and 3.4 times, respectively

**VI.** *SURPRISING FACTS AND STATISTICS*[252-262]
A. 60% of counties in America do not have a single practicing psychiatrist
  1. Shortage will continue to grow rapidly as demand outpaces supply (mostly in rural areas (80%))
B. **Mental illnesses and treatment**
  1. In **2018/2019**, 44 million (18.07%) of the US adult population had a mental illness
    i. Over 24 million (56.5%) adults with a mental illness received no treatment
      a. Approximately 43.3% received some treatment
      b. The average delay between onset of mental illness symptoms and treatment is 11 years
    ii. 4.2 million adults live with an Anxiety Disorder
    iii. 17 million adults live with Major Depression
    iv. Over 10 million (4.13%) of the population were classified as having a <u>serious</u> mental illness
      a. 64.1% of U.S. adults with <u>serious</u> mental illness did receive treatment in 2018
  2. 9.8 million (4.04%) adults reporting <u>serious</u> thoughts of suicide (increased 200,000 in a year)
  3. 40 million (16.7%) of adults have taken a prescribed psychotropic medication in the *last year*
    i. Based on the <u>latest</u> 2013 adult data (Data for children is over 10-years-old – from 2008)
  4. 50% of youth ages 11-17 and 20% of adults think about suicide or self-harm almost *<u>daily</u>*
    i. 9.4% of youth ages 12-17 in 2017 experienced at > 1 major depressive episode (MDE)
      a. Adolescent suicide attempts and rates are *increasing* each year[263]
    ii. Sexual minority youth (LGBTQ) are 3.5 times more likely to attempt suicide
      a. Highest in transgender population (5.9 times more likely to attempt suicide)
C. **Substance statistics from SAMHSA's 2018 National Survey on Drug Use and Health (NSDUH)**[256]
  1. 139.8 million (60%) of those > 12 y.o. <u>admitted</u> to drinking alcohol in the *past month*
  2. 53.2 million (19.4%) of those > 12 y.o. have <u>admitted</u> to using an illicit drug in the *past year*
    i. 43.5 million (15.9%) used marijuana
    ii. 9.9 million (3.6%) used prescription pain medicine illicitly
  3. >19.3 million (7.93%) of adults <u>admitted</u> to having any substance use disorder in the *last year*
    i. 7.5 million (2.76%) has an Illicit Drug Use Disorder (55% of which is marijuana)
    ii. 16.7 million (6.09%) has an Alcohol Use Disorder (use is increasing)
    iii. 1.7 million (0.6%) has a Pain Reliever Use Disorder
  4. 4.61-5.13% of *youth* reported a substance use disorder or alcohol problem in the *past year*
    i. 3.3 million youth reported the use of Marijuana, Cocaine, and/or Heroin
    ii. Approx. 1 in 200 (0.5%) 12-17 y.o.'s engage in binge drinking on > 5 days in the *past month*
D. **State of Healthcare in America** (at the end of **2018**)
  1. 45% (87 million) of U.S. adults ages 19 to 64 are inadequately insured
    i. i.e., their out of pocket expenses are between 5-10% of their annual income
    ii. Nearly the same as in 2010
  2. 12.4% of the population remains uninsured, despite the Affordable Care Act (ACA) availability
  3. 35% of adults are not able to receive the treatment they need because of limited insurance,
    insufficient number of healthcare providers, unavailable inpatient/outpatient/individual therapy
    services, and insufficient money to cover treatments or medication
  4. Adults with sufficient insurance are more likely to have cancer screenings & preventative care
  5. Over 5.3 million (11.3-12.2%) American adults with a mental illness are uninsured
    i. 13.4% of U.S. adults with *serious* mental illness had no insurance coverage in 2018
  6. 50.6% of U.S. youth (aged 6-17) with any mental health disorder received treatment in 2016
    i. 1.8 million (60.1%) of youth with major depression receive absolutely no treatment
    ii. Only 505,000 (25.1%) of youth with severe depression receive consistent treatment
    iii. Over 2 million (8.7%) youth experienced severe major depression (↑ of 100,000 in 1 year)
  7. Despite the enactment of the *Mental Health Parity and Addiction Equity* law (MHPAE), private
    insurances have found subtle ways to limit coverage for mental health services, declaring
    some as not "medically necessary"
    i. National Alliance for the Mentally Ill (NAMI) survey showed that 29% reported that they were
    denied treatment because it was not "medically necessary"[254]
E. Racial disparities
  1. Recognition and treatment of minorities with mental illness
    i. African Americans and Hispanics seek out treatment for depression less than Caucasians[264]
    ii. African Americans are diagnosed with Schizophrenia 9 times more than Caucasians[265]
      a. The actual rate of Schizophrenia may truly be a little higher in African Americans
      b. The diagnosis of Schizophrenia in African Americans is over-utilized
    iii. Dosing of antipsychotics <u>is much higher</u> in black male schizophrenia patients, compared to
    whites[266]
      a. Pharmacogenetic differences in drug disposition may or may not explain this
      phenomenon[267,268]
      b. Cultural mistrust, based on the historical abuse of African Americans, may be mis-perceived
      as paranoia
    iv. The incidence of anxiety and depression is comparable among all ethnic and racial groups
    v. African Americans are less likely to exhibit or convey affective symptoms[269]
  2. Side effects
    i. Risk of diabetes is 66-77% higher in African Americans and Hispanics than Caucasians[270]
      a. Consideration must be given to metabolic risks with antipsychotic options

## VII. PSYCHOTROPIC CLINICAL TRIALS, STUDIES, AND EXPERIMENTAL TREATMENTS

A. Clinical trial information (from https://clinicaltrials.gov)
  1. FDA categories
    i. Early Phase I (formerly listed as Phase 0), Phase I, Phase II, Phase III, and Phase IV
      a. Not Applicable is used to describe trials without FDA-defined phases, including trials of devices or behavioral interventions
  2. Phase I - Focuses on the safety of a drug, usually with healthy volunteers, to determine adverse events and drug pharmacokinetics in humans
  3. Phase II - Gathers preliminary data on whether a drug is effective (vs. placebo) for a certain condition/disease
  4. Phase III - Gathers more information about a drug's safety and effectiveness in different populations and at different dosages or combinations with other drugs
    i. Usually DBPCTs (double-blind placebo-controlled trials) are Phase III
    ii. Can also be RCTs (randomized controlled trials)
  5. Phase IV - After FDA approval (i.e., post-market evaluation) to gather data on a drug's safety, efficacy, or optimal use

## VIII. RENAL AND HEPATIC IMPAIRMENT

A. Renal dysfunction is determined by calculating the CrCl using the Cockcroft and Gault equation[271]
  1. CrCl is also called "glomerular filtration rate" (GFR) or "estimated GFR" (eGFR)
  2. Must have patient's SCr, sex, height and weight

$$CrCl = [(140 - age) \times IBW] \div (SCr \times 72) \ (\times 0.85 \text{ if female})$$
Note: Use ABW if less than the IBW

  3. To estimate Ideal Body Weight in (kg)
     IBW = (50 kg for males or 45.5 kg for females) + 2.3 kg for each inch > 5 feet (60" or 152 cm)

  4. Abbreviations: ABW (actual body weight)   SCr (serum creatinine level)
                    IBW (Ideal body weight)   CrCl (creatinine clearance)
B. Hepatic dysfunction is measured from liver enzymes, bilirubin, albumin, ascites, INR and PT
  1. Used to calculate a Child-Pugh score classification (also called Child-Turcotte-Pugh score)
    i. Developed in 1973 to predict surgical outcomes in patients with bleeding esophageal varices
    ii. Pneumonic: "PIA-BEA" for PT, INR, Ascites, Bilirubin, Encephalopathy, Albumin
    iii. Package inserts for drugs use this classification for adjustments to drug dosing

| Child-Pugh Class | Points | Expected 1 year survival rate | Expected 2 year survival rate |
|---|---|---|---|
| A | 5–6 | 100% | 85% |
| B | 7–9 | 80% | 60% |
| C | 10–15 | 45% | 35% |

  iv. Add up the points for each correct assessment and then total them up

| Measured Assessment | 1 point | 2 points | 3 points |
|---|---|---|---|
| Albumin (serum) in g/dL | > 3.5 | 2.8–3.5 | < 2.8 |
| Ascites | None | Mild to moderate (diuretic responsive) | Severe (diuretic refractory) |
| Bilirubin (total) in μmol/L or mg/dL | < 34 (< 2) | 34–50 (2–3) | > 50 (> 3) |
| Hepatic encephalopathy | None | Mild to moderate (grade 1 or 2) | Severe (grade 3 or 4) |
| INR | < 1.7 | 1.7–2.3 | > 2.3 |
| TOTAL SCORE | | | |

C. Recently, scores using the MELD and MELD-Na score are used for better prognostic value[272]
  1. Model For End-Stage Liver Disease (MELD) predicts survival for advanced liver disease
  2. United Network for Organ Sharing (UNOS) changed the policy on scoring for transplants
  3. New scores are calculated by determining the traditional MELD initial score (MELD$_{(i)}$)
    i. If MELD$_{(i)}$ ≥ 12, the score is adjusted by including the serum sodium (Na) value (MELD-Na)
  4. Formulas used
    i. MELD$_{(i)}$ = round[1][0.378 X log$_e$(bilirubin)) + (1.120 X log$_e$(INR)) + (0.957 X log$_e$(creatinine)) + 0.643] X 10 (where round[1] means to round everything in the brackets to 2 decimal places)
    ii. MELD-Na = MELD$_{(i)}$ + 1.32 X (137-Na$^+$) - [0.033 X MELD$_{(i)}$ X (137-Na$^+$)]
    iii. MELD utilizes logarithmic scale calculations. Any value < 1 is automatically given a lower limit value of 1 to prevent generating a negative score.
    iv. Serum sodium (Na$^+$) must be between 125 and 137 in the calculation
    v. The max upper limit of serum creatinine is 4
      a. If the patient is on dialysis at least twice a week, the value for SCr will be adjusted to 4.0
    vi. The maximum MELD score is 40
  5. Abbreviations
     AST or SGOT (aspartate transaminase)   ALP (alkaline phosphatase)
     ALT or SGPT (alanine transaminase)   GGT (gamma glutamyl transpeptidase)
     INR (international normalized ratio)   PT (prothrombin time)

## IX. USEFUL TIPS
A. If a patient's ALT is $\geq$ 2 times greater than AST, then check patient for hepatitis
B. If a patient's AST is $\geq$ 2 times greater than ALT, then it may be alcoholic liver disease

## X. NEURONAL DEFINITIONS
A. Neuroplasticity – *positive changes* in gene regulation, intracellular signaling, neurotransmitter release, synaptic number and strength, dendritic and axonal architecture
  1. Generation of new neurons in some parts of the CNS
B. Neurotoxicity – the opposite of neuroplasticity

## XI. MEDICATION COUNSELING FOR PSYCHOTROPIC MEDICATIONS
A. Practically every psychotropic medication should be taken with FOOD
B. Food reduces GI upset and can enhance some drugs' absorption
  1. Some sedative hypnotics are recommended to be taken on an empty stomach
C. Avoid operating heavy machinery (e.g., driving) until you know how the medication affects you
D. Most psychotropic medications cause drowsiness (i.e., take at bedtime)
  1. If stimulation occurs (or insomnia results), switch to morning dosing
E. Medication adherence is very important
  1. Since most psychotropics take weeks to be effective, consistent dosing is important
  2. Once medications become effective, they must be continued for a fairly long time
  3. Sudden discontinuation of meds can result in untoward withdrawal and/or rebound effects
F. Communicate with the prescriber about side effects
  1. More than half of psychotropics are stopped within the first month because of side effects
  2. Many options exist today for switching medications or correcting side effects
  3. Counsel patients on the importance of full communication with all healthcare providers
G. Medication + psychotherapy achieves maximal benefits and are always recommended adjunctly[273]

---

# 6. TIME FRAME FOR MEDICATIONS TO SHOW EFFICACY

## I. ANTIDEPRESSANTS (*See page 46 for more information*)
A. Generally 2-6 weeks for maximum antidepressant efficacy, but may be up to 12 weeks[274-276]
  1. Early switching to another agent may not benefit patient more than waiting[277]
B. No drug is proven to take full effect faster than another, with the exception of mirtazapine[278]
  1. Exactly how much faster mirtazapine works is unknown, but it ↑ risks of weight gain
C. Some symptoms may improve in first few days to 1 week, but depression signs are still there

## II. ANTIPSYCHOTICS[279-281] (*See page 81 for more information*)
A. **Typical**
  1. 1-2 days: hyperactivity, combativeness, hostility
  2. 1-2 weeks: hallucinations, sleep, appetite, hygiene, delusions, social skills
  3. 1-2 months: judgment, insight
B. **Atypical**
  1. Effects on negative symptoms and cognition may take months

## III. ANXIOLYTICS[282,283] (*See page 20 for more information*)
A. **Benzodiazepines:** Usual onset from 10 minutes up to 1-2 hours
  1. Onset depends upon absorptive, distributive, and lipophilic properties of individual drug
  2. Rapid: diazepam, clorazepate, alprazolam
  3. Intermediate: chlordiazepoxide, lorazepam
  4. Slow: oxazepam, temazepam, clonazepam
B. **Buspirone:** $5HT_{1A}$ pre-synaptic agonist & post-synaptic partial agonist[50]
  1. Anxiolytic onset in 5 -14 days
  2. Not a prn drug

## IV. MOOD STABILIZERS / ANTIMANIC AGENTS[284-286] (*See page 38 for more information*)
A. **Lithium:** 7 to 14 days for onset of efficacy / maximal efficacy in 1 month
B. **Carbamazepine and Valproic Acid**
  1. Onset in first "several days" to weeks
  2. Maximal efficacy when steady state blood levels reach higher spectrum of therapeutic range
C. **Antipsychotics for Acute Mania**
  1. Onset in first "several days" to weeks

---

# 7. CLINICALLY SIGNIFICANT DRUG INTERACTIONS

## I. **Linezolid (Zyvox®)**[287] - This antibiotic is a monoamine oxidase inhibitor (MAOI)
A. Combined with an SSRI, TCA, or other MAOI can increase the risk of serotonin syndrome or hypertensive crisis

## II. **Ziprasidone (Geodon®)**[231] or **Iloperidone (Fanapt®)**[219]
A. Contraindicated if combined with other QT-prolonging drugs such as quinidine, thioridazine, moxifloxacin, and many others
B. Discontinue if QTc > 500 ms

## 8. DISEASES OF SIGNIFICANCE IN PSYCHIATRIC PATIENTS

I. **Parkinson's Disease (PD)** - high depression risk (may be an early indicator for PD)[288]
 A. Approx. 40% comorbidity
 B. Parkinson's medications can ↑ risk of psychosis
II. **Alzheimer's Disease** - high depression risk
 A. Atypical antipsychotics ↑ risk of death up to 1.7X
 B. Avoid benzodiazepines and anticholinergic drugs
III. **Crohn's Disease** - high comorbid anxiety
IV. **Infectious Diseases** (TB, Hep. C, HIV, Syphilis, Encephalitis) - high depression/psychosis risk
V. **UTIs and Upper Respiratory Infections** – may cause psychosis (especially in the elderly)
VI. **Dialysis** – psychosis and mood lability
 A. See www.renalpharmacyconsultants.com for dialysis help

## 9. EVIDENCE-BASED MEDICINE (EBM)

I. Using the strongest medical evidence based on scientific studies to make appropriate
 pharmacotherapy decisions
II. **Levels of Evidence** (i.e., quality of data) – in decreasing order of quality
 A. **Level I** (e.g., Cochrane Database of Systematic Reviews)
  1. At least 1 high-quality, randomized, double-blind placebo-controlled trial (DBPCT) with narrow
   Confidence Interval
  2. *Systematic review* of homogenous randomized controlled trials (RCTs) with or without meta-
   analysis
  3. Evidence-based *clinical practice guidelines* based on systematic reviews of RCTs
  4. Three or more RCTs of good quality that have similar results
 B. **Level II**
  1. At least 1 well-designed quasi-experimental study (e.g., non-randomized, case-control, cohort
   design, non-equivalent dependent variables designs, repeated treatment designs, outcomes
   research)
  2. Systematic review (with or without meta-analysis) that includes quasi-experimental studies
 C. **Level III**
  1. Non-experimental study
  2. Systematic review (with or without meta-analysis) of homogenous, well-designed comparative
   studies, correlation studies, case-controlled studies, case reports, descriptive and qualitative
   studies (meta-synthesis)
  3. Combination of poor quality RCTs, quasi-experimental, or non-experimental studies
 D. **Level IV**
  1. Opinion of respected authorities and/or nationally recognized expert committees/ consensus
   panels based on scientific evidence (e.g., clinical practice guidelines)
  2. Case series of poor quality cohort / case-controlled studies
 E. **Level V**
  1. Based on experiential and non-research evidence (e.g. literature reviews, quality improvement
   study, single descriptive case report)
  2. Bench research (test-tube, animal, or chemical)
III. **Grades of Recommendations** (i.e., quality of recommendation)
 A. **Grade A** – based on consistent Level I data
 B. **Grade B** – based on consistent Level II/III studies or extrapolated from Level I studies
 C. **Grade C** – Level IV studies or extrapolations from Level II/III studies
 D. **Grade D** – Level V evidence or inconsistent / inconclusive studies of any level

## 10. ACTIVE METABOLITES AND ENANTIOMERS[289-291]

In the R/S system, based on the specific atoms in the molecule, one configuration is called "rectus"
(*R*- for short) and the other is called "sinister" (*S*- for short), from the Latin words for right and left. In
the D/L system, which is related to how the molecule compares to the chiral molecule
glyceraldehyde, one version is called "dextro-" (D- for short) and its mirror image is called "levo-" (L-
for short) (from another pair of Latin words for right and left).
***Des*** -Often indicates a demethylated active metabolite of a compound. (Ex: Desvenlafaxine
(Pristiq™); Desipramine (Norpramin®); Desloratadine (Clarinex®)
***Es or Levo*** - (Ex: Escitalopram (Lexapro®), Eszopiclone (Lunesta™), Esomeprazole (Nexium®),
Levocetirizine (Xyzal®); Levofloxacin (Levaquin®)
***Ar or Dextro*** - (Ex: Arformoterol (Brovana®); Armodafinil (Nuvigil®); Dextroamphetamine
(Dexedrine®; Dextrostat®); Dextromethorphan (Robitussin DM®); Dexmethylphenidate (Focalin®)

## 11. METABOLITES WHICH ARE MARKETED AS OTHER DRUGS

| EFFEXOR® | → PRISTIQ™ | ELAVIL® | → PAMELOR® |
|---|---|---|---|
| Venlafaxine | → desvenlafaxine | Amitriptyline | → nortriptyline |

| TOFRANIL® | → NORPRAMIN® | VALIUM® | → SERAX® |
|---|---|---|---|
| Imipramine | → desipramine | Diazepam | → oxazepam |

| LOXITANE® | → ASENDIN® | VISTARIL / ATARAX® → ZYRTEC® |
|---|---|---|
| Loxapine | → amoxapine | Hydroxyzine → cetirizine |

RISPERDAL® → INVEGA®
Risperidone → paliperidone (9-hydroxyrisperidone)

## 12. KEY DRUG LEVELS[145,146,116,119,122164,166]

Must wait 3-7 days after a dosage change or it may not be accurate
Draw level first thing in the AM before giving a dose

| **Lithium – acute** | 0.8 – 1.2 mEq/L | draw level in 5 days (depending on CrCl) |
|---|---|---|
| **Lithium – maintenance** | 0.6 – 1.2 mEq/L | draw level in 5 days (depending on CrCl) |
| **Valproic Acid** | 50 – 125 mcg/mL | draw level in 3 days |
| **Carbamazepine** | 4 – 12 mcg/mL | draw level in 5 days |
| | *recheck carbamazepine level in 5 weeks due to auto-induction* | |
| **Phenytoin** | 10 – 20 mcg/mL | draw level in 5 days |
| **Phenobarbital** | 15 – 40 mcg/mL | draw level in 5 days |
| **Nortriptyline** | 50 – 150 ng/mL | draw level in 5 days |
| **Desipramine** | 125 – 300 ng/mL | draw level in 5 days |
| **Clozapine** | > 350 ng/mL preferred | draw level in 5 days |

Clozapine : norclozapine ratio > 2 : 1

## 13. PSYCHOTROPIC GHOST TABLETS[292,293]

Medications that use a tablet delivery system, which leaves leftover shells
in the GI tract, expelled in the stool.

- ✦ Aplenzin (bupropion HBr)
- ✦ Concerta (methylphenidate)
- ✦ Pristiq (desvenlafaxine)
- ✦ Tegretol XR (carbamazepine)
- ✦ Wellbutrin XL (bupropion)
- ✦ Invega (paliperidone)
- ✦ Some generic venlafaxine ER tablets

## 14. PSYCHOTROPIC MEDICATIONS THAT SHOULD NOT BE CRUSHED

- ⊕ Bupropion (any sustained-release form, such as Wellbutrin SR/XL, Zyban, Aplenzin, Forfivo XL)
- ⊕ Desvenlafaxine (Pristiq)
- ⊕ Duloxetine (Cymbalta delayed-release capsule)
- ⊕ Prozac Weekly®
- ⊕ Fluvoxamine CR (Luvox CR)
- ⊕ Levomilnacipran (Fetzima ER capsules)
- ⊕ Paroxetine (Paxil CR, Pexeva)
- ⊕ Selegiline (EMSAM patch, Zelapar ODT)
- ⊕ Venlafaxine (Effexor XR, venlafaxine ER, and generics)

# 15. PSYCHOTROPIC MEDICATIONS
## IMPORTANT SIDE EFFECTS AND MONITORING PARAMETERS

| Medication/ Class | Important Side Effects | Medical Monitoring Parameters | Important Notes |
|---|---|---|---|
| **ANTIDEPRESSANTS** | | | |
| **TCAs/MAOIs** | Sedation, anticholinergic, cardiac, sexual dysfunction | EKG | Useful for neuropathic pain |
| **SSRIs** | Stimulation, weight loss, sedation, nausea, vomiting, diarrhea, headache, sweating, sexual dysfunction, Celexa - QT prolongation at higher doses | None EKG with Celexa | Can also treat anxiety, panic attacks, OCD, PTSD, PMDD and eating disorders |
| **SNRIs** | Same as SSRI's May increase blood pressure | Blood Pressure Cymbalta - LFTs | Useful for neuropathic pain |
| **Mirtazapine** | Sedation, Weight Gain | Weight, Lipids, etc. | |
| **Bupropion** | Anxiety, stimulation, dry mouth, seizures, insomnia, ↑ BP | Watch for seizures | Doses > 200 mg at once ↑ risk for seizures (check on high doses) May ↑ psychosis due to ↑ DA |
| **ANTIPSYCHOTICS** | | | |
| **TYPICAL ANTIPSYCHOTICS** | EPS, anticholinergic, cardiac, weight gain | EKG, EPS | Some movement disorders can be permanent |
| **ATYPICALS:** | Metabolic Side Effects | *Baseline and periodic weight, glucose, lipids (refer to Schizophrenia chapter for details)* | Most atypicals are approved for bipolar disorder |
| **Clozapine** | Drowsiness, dizziness, diabetes, weight gain, dry mouth, seizures, akathisia | WBC, Seizure, Weight, Lipids, Glucose | Higher doses = ↑ seizure risk / Must monitor ANC weekly for 1st 6 months |
| **Olanzapine** | Drowsiness, dizziness, weight gain, diabetes, akathisia | Weight, Lipids, Glucose | Once daily dosing |
| **Risperidone** | Dose-related EPS, drowsiness, dizziness, akathisia | Weight, Lipids, EPS, Glucose, ↑ Prolactin | |
| **Quetiapine, Lurasidone, Asenapine, Aripiprazole, Brexpiprazole, Cariprazine** | Drowsiness, stimulation, GI, headache, dizziness, akathisia | Weight, Lipids, Glucose | Quetiapine XR=evening dose / (bipolar depression = QD dosing) / Watch for allergies with asenapine / DA agonist/antagonists may worsen psychosis if given with another antipsychotic (due to DA agonist properties) |
| **Ziprasidone or Iloperidone** | Drowsiness, dizziness, QT prolongation, akathisia | Weight, Lipids, Glucose, EKG | BID dosing |
| **MOOD STABILIZERS** | | | |
| **Lithium** | GI, ↑ thirst, ↑ urination, mild tremors, hypothyroidism | TSH, WBC, renal function | Pregnancy Category D |
| **Valproic Acid** | GI, decreased platelets, ↑ LFTs | Platelets, LFTs, pancreatic enzymes (amylase / lipase) | Teenage girls → polycystic ovarian syndrome Pregnancy Category D |
| **Carbamazepine** | GI, dizziness, ↓ Na⁺, diplopia | Na⁺ | Pregnancy Category D Enzyme induction / autoinduction |
| **Lamictal** | Rash, GI, headache | Rash | Must titrate *VERY* slowly to reduce risk of rash Pregnancy Category C |
| **BENZODIAZEPINES** | | | |
| **ALL BENZODIAZEPINES** | Drowsiness, dizziness, amnesia, depression, disinhibition | Watch for abuse | Counsel on withdrawal seizures |

## I. DSM-5 ANXIETY DISORDERS[245]
A. Most common mental illness in the U.S.
1. 18.1% of the adult population
2. 25.1% of children between 13 and 18-years-old
3. Only 36.9% of those receive treatment
4. People with an anxiety disorder are 3 to 5 times more likely to visit a physician and 6 times more likely to be psychiatrically hospitalized
5. Anxiety and depression are highly comorbid
B. Generalized Anxiety Disorder (GAD)
1. Affects 2.2 to 3.1% of the U.S. population
2. Most common anxiety disorder among older adults
3. Only 43.2% are receiving treatment
4. Women are 2-3 x more likely to be affected than men
5. DSM-5 diagnosis
   i. Lasting at least and typically 6 months or more in adults
   ii. Must have > 3 of the following 6 symptoms for most of the time over 6 months*:
      a. Restlessness or feeling keyed up or on edge
      b. Being easily fatigued
      c. Difficulty concentrating or mind going blank
      d. Irritability
      e. Muscle tension
      f. Sleep disturbance (difficulty falling or staying asleep, or restless, unsatisfying sleep)
      *Only 1 symptom is required for > 4 weeks in children and adolescents
C. Specific Phobia
1. Affects 8.7 to 10.3% of the U.S. population
2. Disproportionate fear or anxiety about a specific object or situation (e.g., flying, heights, dogs, injections, blood)
D. Panic Disorder (with or without agoraphobia)
1. Affects 2.7 to 6% of the U.S. population
   i. Approx. 11% of adults experience at least one panic attack each year
2. May be from overactivity of neural transmission from the raphe nuclei to the mesolimbic cortex and hippocampus[302]
3. A sudden surge of intense fear or intense discomfort that reaches a peak within a few minutes
4. DSM-5 diagnosis
   i. Must have 4 or more of the following symptoms plus > 1 month of worry about having an attack
      a. Palpitations, pounding heart, or accelerated heart rate
      b. Sweating
      c. Trembling or shaking
      d. Sensations of shortness of breath or smothering
      e. Feelings of choking
      f. Chest pain or discomfort
      g. Nausea or abdominal distress
      h. Feeling dizzy, unsteady, light-headed, or faint
      i. Chills or heat sensations
      j. Paresthesias (numbness or tingling sensations)
      k. Derealization (feelings of unreality) or depersonalization (being detached from one-self)
      l. Fear of losing control or "going crazy"
      m. Fear of dying
5. Agoraphobia
   i. Affects approx. 1.7% of adolescents and adults (and 0.4% of those > 65 y.o.) each year
   ii. Females are twice as likely as males
   iii. Incidence peaks in late adolescence (avg. 17 y.o.)
   iv. Heritability for agoraphobia is 61%
   v. Fear or anxiety about two (or more) of the following five situations with active avoidance
      a. Using public transportation (e.g., automobiles, buses, trains, ships, planes)
      b. Being in open spaces (e.g., parking lots, marketplaces, bridges)
      c. Being in enclosed places (e.g., shops, theaters, cinemas)
      d. Standing in line or being in a crowd
      e. Being outside of the home alone
E. Social Anxiety Disorder (SAD) / Social Phobia
1. Affects 2.7 to 6.8% of the U.S. population
2. Fear or anxiety about being exposed to possible scrutiny by others in social situations
   i. Recent study found association with overactive presynaptic serotonin system, with increased serotonin synthesis and transporter availability in SAD[303]
F. Separation Anxiety Disorder[245]
1. Distress when anticipating or experiencing separation from home or from major attachment figures
2. Occurs in 4% of children, 1.6% of adolescents and 0.9-1.9% of adults

3. Genetics: Concordance in 73% of identical twins
4. Girls > boys
5. Must last at least 4 weeks in children and adolescents and typically 6 months or more in adults

## II. ANXIETY OR TENSION ASSOCIATED WITH THE STRESS OF EVERYDAY LIFE USUALLY DOES NOT NECESSITATE TREATMENT WITH AN ANXIOLYTIC

*SURPRISING FACT*: Eating more fermented foods can help reduce social anxiety, due to their probiotic properties[297]

## III. Other related disorders (previously under Anxiety Disorders in the DSM-IV-TR)
A. Obsessive-Compulsive Disorder (OCD) -- *Refer to page 74*
B. Post-Traumatic Stress Disorder (PTSD) -- *Refer to page 78*

## IV. TRIGGERS OF ANXIETY[298-301]

| COMMON MEDICAL DISORDERS ASSOCIATED WITH ANXIETY & INSOMNIA SYMPTOMS | DRUGS ASSOCIATED WITH ANXIETY & INSOMNIA SYMPTOMS |
|---|---|
| *Cardiovascular/respiratory system* | *Withdrawal from CNS depressants* |
| Arrhythmias | Alcohol |
| Chronic obstructive lung disease | Anxiolytics/sedatives |
| Hyperdynamic β-adrenergic state | Marijuana |
| Hypertension | Narcotics |
| Hyperventilation | Nicotine |
| Mitral valve prolapse (high correlation to panic) | *Prescription products* |
| Myocardial infarction | Albuterol (Proventil®, Ventolin®) |
| Angina | Amphetamines (Dexedrine®) |
| Pulmonary embolus | Antidepressants/antipsychotics |
| *Endocrine system* | Corticosteroids |
| Cushing's disease | Diethylpropion (Tenuate®) |
| Hyper- or hypothyroidism | Fenfluramine (Pondimin®) |
| Hypoglycemia | Isoproterenol (Isuprel®, Medihaler Iso®) |
| Pheochromocytoma | Baclofen (Lioresal®) |
| *Gastrointestinal system* | Digitalis toxicity |
| Colitis | Dapsone |
| Irritable bowel syndrome | Cycloserine (Seromycin®) |
| Peptic ulcer | Quinacrine (Atabrine®) |
| Ulcerative colitis | Levodopa/methyldopa |
| *Psychiatric* | Levothyroxine |
| Alzheimer's | Modafinil/armodafinil |
| Delirium/dementia | Methylphenidate (Ritalin®) |
| Depression or Mania | *Non-prescription products* |
| Psychosis/Schizophrenia | OTC stimulants |
| *Miscellaneous* | OTC decongestants |
| Epilepsy | OTC weight loss drugs |
| Migraine | Caffeine |
| Pain | Illicit amphetamines/stimulants |
| Pernicious anemia | Cocaine |
| Porphyria | *Miscellaneous* |
| Cancer | Anticholinergic toxicity |
| Allergic conditions | |
| Vestibular disorders | |

## V. PHARMACOTHERAPY[304]
A. CBT (cognitive behavioral therapy) should always be used first with or without medication
B. SSRIs are considered first-line pharmacotherapy in children & adults along with psychotherapy
1. Fluoxetine (Prozac) is approved for acute treatment of Panic Disorder with/without agoraphobia
2. SNRIs are second-line, followed by TCAs, MAOIs, & buspirone
   i. Venlafaxine (Effexor) is FDA-approved for Panic Disorder, SAD, and GAD
   ii. **Drizalma Sprinkle™ & Irenka™** (duloxetine) approved for GAD in patients ≥ 7 y.o.
3. ALWAYS start at the lowest possible dose and titrate weekly (to reduce emergent anxiety)
4. Caution: Suicidal ideation in children & young adults (more so with SNRIs like venlafaxine)[305]
5. GAD treatment duration is not clearly defined, but guidelines suggest 6-24 months
   i. Antidepressant discontinuation after tx. shows 36.4% relapse rate (vs. 16.4% if continued)
   ii. Must weigh long-term benefits against specific medication side effects
   6. Risk of relapse in Panic Disorder after successful antidepressant treatment, then discontinuation
   is ≈ 2.9 x greater than if remained on medication

C. Buspirone (BuSpar®)[50,306]
 1. MOA- $5HT_{1A}$ pre-synaptic full agonist (which inhibits the synthesis and firing of 5HT) & post-synaptic partial agonist (hippocampus & cortex)
  i. ALSO: $5HT_{2B}$ agonist
   a. Presynaptic dopamine antagonist ($D_2$)
   b. Partial *alpha*$_{1,2}$ receptor antagonist
   c. Releases oxytocin
   d. Enhances activity in the locus coeruleus
 2. Approved for Generalized Anxiety Disorder and Acute anxiety
  i. Off-label uses: Major Depressive Disorder, sexual dysfunction, cerebellar ataxia, ADHD
  ii. Not shown to be effective in other anxiety disorders (e.g., panic, OCD, PTSD)
 3. Onset of action may be delayed for up to 2-4 weeks → Not for prn therapy
 4. Metabolized by CYP3A4 (inducers or inhibitors will significantly affect levels)
 5. Start at 7.5 mg po BID (or 5 mg TID) and ↑ by 5 mg/d every 2-3 days as tolerated (Max 60 mg/d)
  i. Avg. dose: 10-30 mg/d divided; anxiolytic effects: 10-60 mg/d
  ii. Give with FOOD to increase bioavailability
 6. Brand name BuSpar® is no longer available – only generic versions
 7. Half-life is 2-3 hours with non-linear kinetics
 8. Adverse reactions: nausea, dysphoria, headache, weakness, dizziness, nervousness, akathisia
 9. Drug interactions: triptans (for migraines), inhibitors or inducers of CYP3A4, grapefruit juice
  i. Contraindicated with MAOIs, linezolid, or methylene blue
 10. Not recommended in severe renal or hepatic impairment
 11. Pregnancy category B
 12. Studies of 559 children ages 6 and over showed no difference from placebo
 13. Compared to diazepam, buspirone is equally effective at the same doses[307,308]
 14. Buspirone may NOT be effective in previous users of benzodiazepines[309]
D. Hydroxyzine (Atarax®/Vistaril®)[58,60,306]
 1. FDA-approved for treating "anxiety and tension associated with psychoneurosis"
 2. Potent H1 receptor *inverse agonist* (i.e., antagonist effects)
 3. Acts as a $5HT_{2A}$, $D_2$, and $\alpha_1$-adrenergic receptor antagonist
 4. Minimal anticholinergic effects compared to diphenhydramine[310]
 5. Also used for allergic pruritis, muscle relaxation, and nausea
 6. Research suggests that 60-90% of individuals with GAD obtain significant therapeutic benefits[306,311]
 7. Dosage: 10 to 100 mg dosed up to QID prn (Max. U.S. daily dose: 400mg)
  i. Maximum total adult daily dose in Canada: 100mg[57]
  ii. Maximum geriatric daily dose: 50mg
  iii. Reduce doses 50% in renal impairment and 33% in hepatic impairment
  iv. Clinical effects are usually noted within 15 to 30 minutes after oral administration
 8. Dose-related sedation and tardive dyskinesia have been reported with its use
 9. Metabolized by alcohol dehydrogenase and CYP3A4/5[59]
  i. Primary metabolite: cetirizine (Zyrtec®)
  ii. High doses inhibit CYP2D6
  iii. Half-life: 20 hours (7 hours in children)
 10. Antagonizes effects of cholinesterase drugs
 11. Can potentiate the effect of opiates and barbiturates (and other CNS depressants)
 12. QTc prolongation warning
  i. European Medicines Agency (EMA) Pharmacovigilance Risk Assessment Committee (PRAC)[312,313]
  ii. Recommendations to minimize known heart risks of hydroxyzine-containing medicines
   a. Using at the lowest effective dose for as short a time as possible
   b. Use not recommended in the elderly (max dose: 50 mg in the elderly if use cannot be avoided)
   c. Maximum daily dose should not exceed 100 mg in adults, and 2 mg/kg in children (<40 kg)
   d. Avoid use in cardiac arrhythmia patients or with other QT-prolonging drugs
   e. Contraindicated with concomitant CYP3A4/5 inhibitors
   f. Caution with medications that ↓ potassium or cause bradycardia
 13. Long-term efficacy is superior to placebo and equal to benzodiazepines on anxiety scales[314]
E. Other effective agents for anxiety
 1. Propranolol (Inderal®) and other *beta*-blockers[315-317]
  i. May act as a central $5HT_{1A}$ and $5HT_{1B}$ (an autoreceptor) agonist / antagonist[318]
  ii. Propranolol is highly lipophilic and easily penetrates the BBB
  iii. There is a relative lack of well-designed clinical studies for anxiety
  iv. No statistical difference found for effects of benzo's vs. propranolol for generalized anxiety and panic attacks[319]
  v. 20-40 mg pre-surgery was statistically superior to placebo on levels of anxiety and stress[320]
  vi. Propranolol was ineffective for Simple and Social Phobias[319]
 2. Clonidine[321] (Catapres®/Kapvay™) and Guanfacine (Tenex/Intuniv™)
  i. Centrally acting *alpha*$_{2a}$ agonists
  ii. Stimulates presynaptic receptors that act as "autoreceptors" of noradrenergic release
   a. Attenuates sympathetic responses to stress and anxiety
  iii. Average daily doses of clonidine 0.2-0.4 mg were superior to placebo for GAD & panic[322]

iv. Extended-release guanfacine did not reduce or increase pediatric anxiety disorders (e.g., GAD, separation anxiety disorder (SAD), or social phobia/social anxiety disorder)[323]
  a. Clinicians rated guanfacine as superior to placebo on CGI score
3. Pregabalin (Lyrica®)[324] - See chapter on *Seizure Disorders* for more details
  i. Approved by the *European Medicines Agency* for GAD
  ii. A 2017 meta-analysis of 8 RCTs (n=2299) found it superior to placebo for GAD symptoms[325]
    a. Clinical response comparable to benzodiazepines, but with lower dropout rates
  iii. In patients with schizophrenia, 75-600 mg/d (divided) ↓ the severity of anxiety symptoms[326]
  iv. Sedation and other side effects may limit first-line use[327]

## F. Benzodiazepines (BZDs)
1. Leo Sternbach accidentally discovered chlordiazepoxide (Librium®) in 1955
  i. By the end of the 1970's, they were the #1 class of drug prescribed in the world
2. BZDs are drugs of choice for <u>short-term</u> **prn** treatment of Generalized Anxiety Disorder (GAD)
  i. Onset of effect is generally 15 to 60 minutes
  ii. The American Psychiatric Association (APA) and the National Institute for Health and Clinical Excellence (NICE) guidelines recommend SSRIs as best choices for Panic and GAD[328]
    a. BZDs should not be prescribed for more than 2 to 4 weeks
    b. Due to abuse potential, dependence, tolerance, and withdrawal use N.T.E. 4 months
      1. NOTE: physical dependence can occur in as little as 2 weeks
      2. Most BZD package inserts list 4 months as longest treatment duration
      3. 50% of patients treated daily with BZDs for 4 months become dependent[328]
      4. Overall risk of patients needing dose escalations over 2-years' time is ≈ 1.6%
    c. The recommendations to give preference to newer antidepressants are not based on direct comparison studies but rather on the known risks of benzodiazepines
3. HELPFUL ADVICE: Tell patients to think of BZDs like a 'fire extinguisher in a glass case'
  i. Only 'break the glass' in cases of emergency (i.e., only use a BZD as a last resort for episodic or breakthrough symptoms)
    a. Avoid BZDs in patients with comorbid Bipolar Disorder, PTSD, or Substance Use Disorders[329]
  ii. Each time a person uses a BZD, it becomes a little less effective
  iii. Patients should **NEVER** be prescribed *2 or more* BZDs, even if for different indications
    a. All BZDs work in exactly the same way
      1. If taken throughout the day, sedation wears off, so not an effective hypnotic
      2. All are similar in sedative, hypnotic, anxiolytic, muscle relaxant, and anticonvulsant activity
      3. They differ in their *pharmacokinetic* profiles
  iv. Abuse potential is greater with higher lipophilicity and a shorter half-life[330]
    a. Clorazepate and diazepam have highest lipid solubility
    b. Diazepam has the most abuse liability based on drug abuser reports

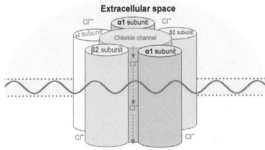

**Extracellular space**

**Intracellular space**

*The most common GABA$_A$ receptors subunit arrangement*

4. BZDs act on the Ionotropic GABA$_A$ Receptor Protein Complex ("GABA$_A$ receptor")[331-333]
  i. Binding causes a conformational change of the channel allows chloride ions in to nerve cells, thereby decreasing nerve conductivity and transmission
  ii. GABA$_A$ receptors have several subunits (e.g., $\alpha_{1-6}$ (alpha), $\beta_{1-3}$ (beta), $\gamma_{1-3}$ (gamma), $\delta$ (delta), $\varepsilon$ (epsilon), $\pi$ (pi), $\theta$ (theta), and $\rho_{1-3}$ (rho))
    a. Subunits are arranged in a cylindrical pentagonal shape around a chloride central channel
  iii. BZDs bind between $\alpha_1$ and $\gamma_2$ subunits
  iv. Natural GABA binds between the $\alpha_1$ and $\beta_2$ subunits
    a. Barbiturates, anesthetics, ethanol, neurosteroids (e.g., pregnenolone), and endocannabinoids also bind to the GABA$_A$ receptor
    b. Ethanol's effect on the cerebellum may be explained by the GABA$_A$ receptor having $\alpha_6$, $\beta_3$, and/or $\delta$ subunits[334]
  v. BZDs are highly specific in their site of action, and do not agonize other receptor sites - *even at high doses*
  vi. Death from a pure BZD overdose is rare unless mixed with other toxic drugs[335]

5. *Absorption* determines onset of action
   i. **Rapid:** diazepam, clorazepate, alprazolam
   ii. **Intermediate:** chlordiazepoxide, lorazepam
   iii. **Slow:** oxazepam, temazepam, clonazepam
6. Most BZDs are metabolized to active metabolites
   i. Except lorazepam, oxazepam, temazepam (LOT)
      a. LOT is ideal for elderly patients as no extensive metabolism occurs
      b. Minimal metabolism to Phase II conjugated metabolites via glucuronidation
         1. Lorazepam – UGT2B15 (Uridine diphospho-glucuronosyltransferase)
         2. Oxazepam – UGT2B15, UGB1A9, and UGT2B7
         3. Temazepam – UGT2B15, UGT2B7, CYP2C19 & CYP3A4 (to oxazepam)
      c. UGT inhibitors can ↑ LOT blood levels (e.g., NSAIDS, valproate, immunosuppressants)
   ii. Diazepam is converted to temazepam, then converted to oxazepam
   iii. Most BZDs utilize the CYP3A4 pathway; diazepam and quazepam also use CYP2C19
7. Adverse reactions: sedation, fatigue, disorientation, dizziness, ataxia, confusion, disinhibition, anterograde amnesia, respiratory depression, depressed mood
   i. Rare and unpredictable Paradoxical Reactions (more common in children & elderly)
      a. E.g., extreme disinhibition, stimulation, mania, irritability, restlessness, aggression, psychosis, hostility, rage, or hallucinations
   ii. Tolerance to sedation develops within weeks[336]
   iii. ↑ risk of developing dementia[337-340] / risk of Alzheimer's or vascular dementia is greater for short-term users (< 1 year) than long-term users (> 1 year)[341] [Adjusted odds ratio of 2.2-3.3]
      a. Dizziness & falls → can lead to broken bones
      b. Impaired driving ability
8. Pregnancy Category: D and X
9. Drug interactions: CNS depressants, alcohol, cimetidine (except LOT)
   i. Nefazodone and fluvoxamine drastically ↑ alprazolam/triazolam levels
10. Seizures are possible with acute withdrawal (**must taper!!**)
11. Long-term users of BZDs can successfully taper off[342, 343344]
    i. 2018 Cochrane Review[345] found that *withdrawal symptoms* may be reduced by pregabalin, captodiame (an antihistamine like diphenhydramine), paroxetine, TCAs and flumazenil[346]
       a. Quality of the evidence was very low
       b. Symptoms of anxiety *after withdrawal* may be reduced by carbamazepine, pregabalin, captodiame, paroxetine, and flumazenil
       c. Only valproate and cyamemazine (a phenothiazine antipsychotic with atypical features) seemed to reduce the proportion of participants that *relapsed* to benzodiazepine use, but quality of evidence was very low
    ii. If inpatient, a rapid taper (e.g., 5-7 days) can be used with PRNs per withdrawal symptoms
    iii. If outpatient, then a long-term taper schedule can be designed[347]
       a. Patients prefer a gradual reduction of their dose to a rapid, abrupt cessation
       b. **RULE OF THUMB:** For every year a patient has taken a BZD, extend taper by 1 month
       c. See https://www.benzo.org.uk/manual/index.htm for patient withdrawal information
G. Other therapies studied, but not approved, for various anxiety disorders with recommendations from WFSBP (World Federation Societies of Biological Psychiatry) for treatment-resistant or treatment-intolerant patients[327,348-356]
   1. Switch to a TCA, mirtazapine, quetiapine, phenelzine, risperidone, olanzapine, ziprasidone, levetiracetam, topiramate, tranylcypromine, gabapentin or pregabalin (only in GAD)
   2. Combined valproate and clonazepam
   3. Addition of buspirone to an f
   4. Addition of lithium to clomipramine
   5. Pindolol (Visken®) augmentation of an SSRI
   6. Can also consider a trial of:
      i. PRN trazodone (Desyrel®) or diphenhydramine
      ii. Vilazodone (Viibryd®), vortioxetine (Trintellix®), or tiagabine (Gabitril®)
      iii. d-cycloserine (Seromycin®) may hasten the onset of effect or ↑ overall effectiveness of CBT[357]
H. **Trifluoperazine (Stelazine)**[207] – a typical phenothiazine antipsychotic
   1. FDA-approved for the short-term treatment of generalized non-psychotic anxiety
      i. Doses should not exceed 6 mg a day, or be used for longer than 12 weeks
      ii. Risks of using an antipsychotic in anxiety do not outweigh the benefits

---

### A CAUTION ON COMPLEMENTARY AND ALTERNATIVE MEDICINES (CAM)

▶ Within this book are listed many of the CAM therapies tried for psychiatric disorders. A majority of them have low quality evidence to support their routine or first-line use in serious mental illness. They are provided for your information.

▶ In the United States, herbal supplements and other CAM therapies are not required to undergo the standard rigorous quality testing that prescription medicines are held to. In such, the quantities of active ingredients in the bottle can vary from zero to multiple times the doses listed. In addition, a multitude of contaminants have been found in locally sourced and imported products, mostly from products originating in India and the People's Republic of China. Among these are dust, heavy metals, bacteria, fungi, mold, pesticides, insects, rodents and actual prescription medication.[358] Please consider this before advising a person of CAM's utility.

## VI. COMPLEMENTARY AND ALTERNATIVE THERAPIES (CAM):[359-362]

A. Borage / Weevil head (Echium amoenum)
  1. Contains rosmarinic acid and thesinine
  2. Dose studied: 375 mg daily for 6 weeks
B. Brahmi / Bacopa monnieri (Water hysop)
  1. Contains bacoside A and bacoside P
  2. Acts as a cholinesterase inhibitor, antioxidant, and protects β-amyloid
C. California poppy (eschscholzia californica)
  1. Binds to GABA receptors and has shown effects in animal studies
D. Chamomile (Matricaria recutita/chamaemelum nobile)
  1. Doses studied: 220-1100 mg (standardized to 1.2% apigenine) divided up to 3 times a day
  2. Binds to GABA receptors and modulates neuroendocrine system & monoamine transmission
  3. May intensify BZDs' effects and may interact with warfarin, statins, and oral contraceptives
E. Eschium amoenum[363] ("ox-tongue") – an herb from Iran
  1. Flowers are brewed into a tea and used for mood enhancing & anxiolytic effects
F. Ginkgo (ginkgo biloba)
  1. Ginkolides and bilobalides modulate cholinergic & monoamine pathways and nitric oxide activity
  2. Also has antioxidant, anti-inflammatory, and GABAergic effects
  3. A 4-week RCT showed 240 and 480 mg/d to be superior to placebo
G. Gotu cola (centella asiatica)
  1. Active compound: asiaticoside - that inhibits GABA transaminase
  2. Human RCTs showed that it decreased the startle response to loud noises
H. Hops (humulus lupulus)
  1. Contain humulone, lupulone, and xanthohumol
  2. Bind to Melatonin-1 and -2 ($MT_1$ & $MT_2$) receptors
I. Kava-Kava (Piper methysticum) – NOT RECOMMENDED!
  1. Possibly hepatotoxic, based on over 25 reported cases of liver toxicity in Germany, Switzerland, France, Canada, and the UK
  2. Side effects: drowsiness, headache, GI upset, dizziness, sensitivity to ultraviolet light sources
J. Lavender (Lavandula augustifolia)
  1. Contains linalool and linalyl acetate
  2. Lavender was proven to be better as an additive to standard antidepressants than the standard antidepressants alone
  3. Silexan® is an oral capsule of lavender abstracts (80 mg each)[364]
    i. Found to bind to $5HT_{1A}$ receptors and potently inhibit voltage gated calcium channels
  4. Meta-analysis review of over 5000 patients showed overall significant reductions in anxiety[365]
K. Lemonbalm (melissa officinalis)
  1. Contains citranellal and geraniol
  2. Inhibits MAO-A and GABA transaminase
  3. Shown to reduce human stress levels acutely after dosing
L. Leonurus cardiaca (motherwort)
M. Mimosa (albizia julibrissin - contains julibrosides)
  1. Has receptor affinities for $5HT_{1A}$ and $5HT_{2C}$
N. Passionflower (passiflora incarnata, maypop, purple passionflower)
  1. Contains harman and chrysin
  2. BZD receptor partial agonist shown in animals to reduce anxiety without sedation
  3. In a 4-week RCT, 500 mg was shown as effective as oxazepam 30 mg
O. Rhodiola rosea (roseroot, rosewort, golden root, or arctic root, Hongjingtian, King's Crown)
  1. Side effects: headache, GI upset, drowsiness, dizziness, vivid dreams and insomnia
  2. Doses studied: 100-700 mg QD
  3. Active compounds: salidroside glycosides, rosarin, rosavin, rosin, flavonoids, phenolic acid: gallic acid and chlorogenic acid (an antioxidant), organic acids (succinic, citric, malic, oxalic), tannins, anthraquinones
  4. Inhibits Monoamine Oxidase A and affects the neuroendocrine system
P. Saffron (Crocus sativus)
  1. Active compounds: Safranal, crocin, and crocetin
  2. Found to activate BDNF and acts as a $GABA_A$ agonist & post-synaptic NMDA antagonist
  3. Saffron overdose can be fatal - vomiting, diarrhea, urogenital & GI bleeding
Q. Skullcap (scutellaria lateriflora)
  1. Active compounds: scutelaterin A and baicalin
  2. Believed to have $GABA_A$ binding affinity
  3. Superior to placebo in a small crossover RCT
R. Sour date (zizyphus jujuba)
  1. Contains jujuboside A & B which inhibit glutamate pathways in the hippocampus
S. Valerian (valeriana officinalis)
  1. Contains valepotriate and valerenic acid
  2. Various proposed mechanisms of action include GABA modulation, interaction with adenosine-1 (A1) receptors, $GABA_A$ (β3 subunit) receptor agonism, and $5HT_{5A}$ partial agonism
T. Withania (withania somnifera)
  1. Active compounds: withanolide and withaferin
  2. Has GABA binding activity similar to lorazepam in animal models

## VII. POTENTIAL FUTURE TREATMENTS FOR ANXIETY DISORDERS IN STUDY[366,367]

A. Aloradine nasal spray (**PH94B**) by Pherin Pharmaceuticals, Inc. / Vistagen Pharmaceuticals
  1. 4,16-androstadien-3β-ol - a positional isomer of androstadienol
  2. New class of drugs called pherines or vomeropherines
  3. Odorless synthetic neuroactive steroids that act on nasal chemosensory receptors & $GABA_A$
  4. Ultra-low doses (ng to low mcg quantities) showed rapid onset of anxiolytic effects (10-15 min)
  5. Pherines are minimally invasive (not systemically absorbed)
  6. Excellent safety and tolerability profile, and can be used on demand
  7. For Social Anxiety Disorder (as needed)
    i. Significant results seen in a Phase III trial of PH94B nasal spray used PRN up to QID
    ii. Self-administered 15-minutes before entering a "feared situation"
    iii. https://clinicaltrials.gov/ct2/show/NCT02622958?term=PH94B&rank=1
  8. Currently in Phase II studies for GAD and PTSD
B. Agomelatine (AGO-178; **Valdoxan**®)[302,368] by Novartis and Servier
  1. Refer to "*Potential Future Antidepressants*" for more info
  2. Melatonin $MT_1$ and $MT_2$ receptor agonist, & $5HT_{2C}$ receptor antagonist
  3. Development is currently suspended in the U.S. as of 2018 for GAD and OCD
C. Antioxidant drugs that have effects on cellular mitochondria (e.g., **Coenzyme Q10**)[369]
D. AVN-101 by Avineuro Pharmaceuticals (Phase II for GAD)
  1. $5HT_6$ receptor antagonist
E. BNC-210 (IW-2143) by Bionomics and Ironwood Pharmaceuticals
  1. "GABA modulator" – a negative allosteric modulator (antagonist) of the α7 nicotinic Ach receptor
  2. Doses of 150 mg, 300 mg and 600 mg BID for 12 weeks studied
  3. Also in Phase II trials for agitation in dementia and PTSD
F. Cannabidiol (CBD) Oil in Phase III trials
  1. 200 mg capsules up to a maximum of 800 mg total a day
G. D-cycloserine (**Seromycin**) for Social Anxiety Disorder, OCD and Panic Disorder[357]
  1. Glycine-gated NMDA partial agonist/antagonist
  2. In Phase III trials
H. FKW00GA by Fabre-Kramer Pharmaceuticals, Inc. (Phase II for GAD & social phobia)
  1. $5HT_{1A}$ agonist and $5HT_2$ antagonist
  2. May be beneficial for both anxiety and sexual dysfunction (Phase II trials on-going)
I. Gepirone ER (Travivo™) - Fabre-Kramer Pharmaceuticals[370]
  1. A $5HT_{1A}$ partial agonist (like buspirone, but stronger)
  2. Phase II trials completed for GAD
  3. Mission Pharmacal will pursue its future commercial manufacture
  4. Common adverse effects: transient lightheadedness, nausea, and headache (no weight gain)
    i. Found to improve symptoms of sexual dysfunction in men and women
  5. Status: currently unknown, but may be in pre-registration status with the FDA
J. JNJ-42165279/ JNJ-5279[371] by Janssen-Cilag
  1. Fatty acid amide hydrolase (FAAH) inhibitor
  2. Interacts with the human endocannabinoid system (cannabinoid receptor-based effects)
  3. Anti-inflammatory action in mice colitis models
  4. Also, antidiarrheal and antinociceptive effects (analgesic) in animal models
  5. Phase II completed for social anxiety (NCT02432703) & Pervasive child development disorders
K. Lorazepam extended-release capsules (**EDG004**) by Edgemont Pharmaceuticals
  1. Phase III trial for GAD was completed in 2017 (ClinicalTrials.gov Identifier: NCT02305797)
L. Melatonin in Phase III trials
M. Probiotics in Phase III trials
N. Riluzole sublingual (**BHV-0223**) by Biohaven Pharmaceutical Holdings Co.
  1. Post-synaptically potentiates $GABA_A$ receptors via an allosteric binding site
  2. Used for amyotrophic lateral sclerosis
  3. Phase III for Social anxiety and Performance anxiety
O. TGFK08AA by Fabre-Kramer Pharmaceuticals (Phase II for GAD)
  1. $5HT_{1A}$ receptor modulator
P. Tianeptine oxalate (**TNX-601**) by Servier and Vela Pharmaceuticals
  1. Atypical μ-opioid receptor agonist and AMPA receptor modulator
  2. Already marketed in Europe for Alcoholism, Anxiety disorders, and Major Depressive Disorder
     Europe under the brand names "Coaxil", "Stablon" and "Tatinol"
  3. Not currently in study in the U.S. – Phase I for PTSD planned for 2020
Q. Troriluzole (**BHV4157**) by Biohaven Pharmaceutical and Yale University
  1. Glutamate modulator
  2. 100 mg PO QD
  3. In Phase III trials for GAD and Phase II/III for Alzheimer's and OCD
R. Yohimbine for Phobias in Phase III trials

---

☆ Most anxiety disorders respond best to psychotherapy and/or antidepressants! ☆
BENZODIAZEPINES ARE **NOT** RECOMMENDED FOR LONG-TERM USE!!!

| Drug | Relative Potency | Peak Blood Level - oral (hours) | Metabolic pathway | Half-life (hours) | Equivalent Dose (mg) | Dosage range (mg/d) |
|---|---|---|---|---|---|---|
| Alprazolam (Xanax®) | High | 1 - 2 | CYP3A4 | 9 - 20 | 0.5 | 0.25 - 10 |
| Chlor-diazepoxide (Librium®) | Low | 1 - 4 | CYP3A4 | 100 | 10 - 25 | 5 - 400 |
| Clonazepam (Klonopin®) | High | 1 - 4 | CYP3A4 | 19 - 80 | 0.25 | 0.25 - 20 |
| Clorazepate (Tranxene T-TAB®) | Medium | 0.5 - 2 | CYP3A4 pro-drug (nordiazepam) | 100 | 7.5 - 10 | 3.75 - 90 |
| Diazepam (Valium®) | Medium | 1 - 2 I.V. = 1-5 min I.M. = erratic | CYP3A4 / CYP2C19 | 100 | 5 | 2 - 40 |
| Estazolam (ProSom®) | High | 0.5 - 1.5 | CYP3A4 | 10 - 24 | 0.5 - 2 | 0.5 - 2 |
| Flurazepam (Dalmane®) | Medium | 0.5 - 1 | CYP3A4 | 2 - 100 | 15 - 30 | 15 - 60 |
| Lorazepam (Ativan®) | High | 1 - 4 I.V. = 5-10 min I.M. = 15-30 min | Conjugated by UGT2B15 | 8 - 24 | 1 | 0.5 - 10 |
| Midazolam (Versed®) | High | 3 – 10 min | CYP3A4 | 1.8 - 6.4 | 2 - 5 | 2.5 – 10 IV/IM |
| Oxazepam (Serax®) | Low | 1 - 4 | Conjugated by UGT1A9, UGT2B7 & UGT2B15 | 6 - 25 | 15 | 10 - 120 |
| Quazepam (Doral®) | Medium | 2 | CYP3A4 / CYP2C9 / CYP2C19 | 39 – 73 (Avg. 40 - 50) | 10-20 | 7.5 – 15 |
| Temazepam (Restoril®) | Low | 1.5 - 3 | Conjugated by UGT2B7 & UGT2B15 | 6 - 16 | 10 - 30 | 15 - 60 |
| Triazolam (Halcion®) | High | 1 - 2 | CYP3A4 | 1.5 - 5 | 0.25 | 0.125 - 0.5 |

### I. BACKGROUND
  A. Approx. 20% of children in the US have some form of mental illness
  B. 80% receive no treatment
    1. Approx. 7.5% of children are prescribed psychotropic medications
    2. 85% prescribed by a pediatrician and not a trained Psychiatrist

### II. OFF-LABEL USE OF MEDICATIONS IN CHILDREN
  A. American Academy of Pediatrics has a policy statement[382]
    1. If a medication is not FDA-approved for use in children, prescribing information must specify "the safety and efficacy in pediatric patients have not been established"
    2. FDA does not monitor individual prescribers
    3. To be FDA-approved, a drug must show "substantial evidence," from "adequate and well-controlled investigations"
    4. Prescribers using off-label medications should document informed-consent about off-label use (i.e., prescribing done in "good faith", without fraudulent intent, and in best interest of the patient)
  B. In 2012, Congress passed the Food and Drug Administration Safety and Innovation Act
    1. Reauthorized and strengthened the Best Pharmaceuticals for Children Act (BPCA) and the Pediatric Research Equity Act (PREA), which mandates that almost all new drugs must be studied in children for approved uses (if there is potential for use of that drug in children)

### III. ATTENTION DEFICIT HYPERACTIVITY DISORDER (ADHD)[383-386]
  A. Onset is typically by age 3 and must be by age 7
    1. Approx. 9.2% of boys and 2.9% of girls (general prevalence is 6%)
    2. Girls generally display *inattentive* type; boys exhibit more *hyperactive* & *impulsive* type of ADHD
    3. Heritability of ADHD is substantial[245]
  B. Study found using acetaminophen while pregnant ↑ risk of "hyperkinetic disorders" and ADHD-like behaviors in children[387]
  C. Symptoms may persist into adulthood (30-70%)
  D. Adult prevalence is 4% by National Comorbidity Survey
  E. Clinical Presentation – Inappropriate inattention, impulsivity, hyperactivity
    1. Hyperthyroidism must be ruled out, because ~40-80% of these kids will meet criteria for ADHD[388]
  F. National survey results show that behavioral therapy greatly underutilized in lieu of medications[389]
    1. Half of preschoolers received the recommended first-line treatment of behavioral therapy
  G. 12 times more likely to have binge-eating behaviors[390]
  H. Increased risk of death from accidents (e.g., motor vehicle accidents, risk-taking behaviors)
    1. Treatment with ADHD medications can reduce the risk of injuries and ER visits by up to 45%[391]
      i. First-line therapy ALWAYS includes psychosocial interventions (Parent Management Training [PMT], Parent-Child Interaction Therapy [PCIT], Multisystemic Therapy [MST], and others)[392]
  J. MEDICATIONS USED IN ADHD
    1. **Psychostimulants (*SEE CHART ON PAGE* 32)**
      i. In 1887, *ma-huang* was discovered to contain ephedrine by Japanese scientist Nagai[393]
      ii. First amphetamine was synthesized in 1887 by Lazăr Edeleanu, a Romanian chemist while attempting to manufacture synthetic aliphatic amines[394]
        a. A congener of ephedrine
        b. Found to have bronchodilating, as well as sympathomimetic properties[395]
      iii. In the 1930's, reports were surfacing about its actions in the central nervous system[394,396]
        a. Found to "produce feelings of euphoria and relief from fatigue"
        b. Also noted to "improve performance on some simple tasks, increase activity levels, and produce anorexia"
        c. *Benzedrine* (amphetamine sulfate) marketed in 1930s for nasal congestion, asthma, ADHD, narcolepsy, depression, and other medical uses[397-399]
      iv. Amphetamines widely used in soldiers in WWII
      v. Not believed to be addictive or habit-forming[400]
      vi. February 2006 - An FDA Advisory Panel suggested a Black Box Warning (BBW) be placed on all stimulant medications, warning of increased risk of CV death and injury
      vii. Currently *required* BBW warning is about Abuse Potential (*See page 9 for* BBWs)
        a. Estimated 1 in 4 youth may be using their stimulant medication non-medically[401]
      viii. Other common warnings for stimulants
        a. Cardiovascular reactions (including sudden death), hypertension, tachycardia, psychosis or mania, priapism, peripheral vasculopathy (including Raynaud's Phenomenon), serotonin syndrome, and long-term suppression of growth
        b. Recent studies find no increased risk of cardiovascular events in children and young to middle-aged adults[402,403]
        c. Stimulants associated with ↑ risk of psychosis (62.5% vs. 27.4% no meds) (odds ratio 4.41)[404]
        d. A 10-year study found that stimulants ↑ HR by 4-5 beats per minute, but not BP in children/adolescents[405]
          1. Baseline cardiac safety screening is warranted before giving stimulants
          2. Other studies find no ↑ risk of CV events in children & young to middle-aged adults
      ix. Benefits of stimulant medication use in treating ADHD[406]
        a. Significantly reduced risk of developing depression, bipolar disorder, and conduct disorder

    b. Reduced suicide attempts and suicide-related events
    c. Reduced risk of smoking, substance use disorders, and criminality
    d. Lower rates of motor vehicle accidents and academic failure
  x. Stimulants inhibit reuptake of DA & NE from presynaptic neurons in the CNS[407]
    a. Amphetamines (*but not methylphenidate*) is taken up in the presynaptic intracellular neuron
      1. Amphetamines also increase the intracellular pool of neurotransmitters by displacing DA, NE
        and 5HT from storage vesicles and thus more is available for presynaptic release
  xi. Approximately 60-75% effective on ADHD symptoms
  xii. Off-label use includes: defiance, aggression, depression, and narcolepsy[408]
  xiii. Effects rapidly evident (Response seen in 15-30 minutes and lasts 2-12 hours orally)
  xiv. Side effects:
    a. May cause (or worsen) motor or vocal *tics* and ↑ BP
    b. May slow or permanently suppress growth
    c. Abdominal pain, weight loss, insomnia, agitation, tachycardia, irritability, blurred vision
      1. Oral doses should be given 30-45 min before meals to reduce anorexia
    d. Numbness and feeling of bugs crawling on the skin
2. **Amphetamines (psychostimulants)**[409]
  i. Most are approved for > 3 yrs old
  ii. Typical onset in 30-45 minutes / effects last 4-6 hours for IR and 8-12 hours for ER formulations
  iii. Metabolism (minor) by CYP2D6 (inhibitors will ↑ blood levels)
  iv. Interactions: amphetamine & metabolites are minor inhibitors of CYP2D6, 1A2, and 3A4
    a. Alkaline foods & urine PH – decreases excretion and ↑ amphetamine blood levels
    b. Acidic foods & urine PH – increases excretion and ↓ amphetamine blood levels
      1. In cases of overdose, acidify urine with ascorbic acid (Vitamin C) or potassium phosphate
  v. Evekeo[®3] (amphetamine sulfate / Benzedrine[®])
    a. Also indicated for Narcolepsy (5-60 mg/d divided) & Exogenous Obesity for those > 12-years-
      old (5-30 mg/d divided before meals)
    b. Currently in Phase III trials for adult ADHD
  vi. **Racemic mixture of dextro- & levo-amphetamine**
    a. Adzenys ER[®31]
      1. Racemic mixture of dextro- and levo-amphetamine, ratio of 3:1 respectively
      2. Approved in children > 6-years-old (as is Adzenys[®] XR-ODT)
      3. Orange-flavored suspension (shake well before administration)
      4. Do not mix with other liquids or foods
      5. Max dose is lower with adolescents (as is Adzenys[®] XR-ODT)

| 6. **Half-life** | Dextro-amphetamine | Levo-amphetamine |
| --- | --- | --- |
| Children | 12.7 hours | 15.3 hours |
| Adults | 11.4 hours | 14.1 hours |

    b. Adzenys[®] XR-ODT[32]
      1. Racemic mixture of dextro- and levo-amphetamine, ratio of 3:1 respectively
      2. Orange-flavored orally dissolving tablets
      3. Tablets should be dissolved in saliva, then swallowed

| 4. **Half-life** | Dextro-amphetamine | Levo-amphetamine |
| --- | --- | --- |
| Children | 9-10 hours | 10-11 hours |
| Adults | 11.4 hours | 14.1 hours |

    c. Dyanavel[®] XR[33]
      1. Racemic mixture of dextro- and levo-amphetamine, ratio of 3.2:1 respectively
      2. Suspension should be stored at room temperature and shaken vigorously before use
      3. Half-life is 12 hours for dextro- and 15 hours for levo-amphetamine
      4. Onset of action in about 1 hour / duration of approx. 13 hours
    d. Evekeo ODT™[34]
      1. A 1:1 ratio of dextro- and levo-amphetamine sulfate (not the same as regular Evekeo)
      2. Tablets should be dissolved in saliva, then swallowed
    e. Mydayis[®31] (amphetamine sulfate) - only approved for children > 13 y.o.
      1. Racemic mixture of dextro- and levo-amphetamine, ratio of 3:1 respectively
      i. 3 types of microbeads release drug at various intervals
        a. Immediately, in small intestine (pH 5.5), and in distal small colon (pH 7.0)
      2. Max dose in those with renal disease is 12.5 mg/d
      3. Longer duration of action than Adderall (up to 16 hours)
  vii. **Mixed amphetamine salts**
    a. Adderall[1] / Adderall XR[®1]
      1. 4 salts: dextroamphetamine saccharate & sulfate, amphetamine aspartate & sulfate
      2. Dextro- to levo- ratio of 3:1
      3. Based on bioequivalence data, patients taking divided doses of immediate-release Adderall
        may be switched to Adderall XR at the same total daily dose taken QD
      4. Adults with severe renal impairment: 15 mg QAM
      5. Not recommended for patients with ESRD

3. **Dextroamphetamines**
   i. Dexedrine[®9] / Dextrostat[®11]
     a. After initial morning dose, additional doses can be given at 4-6 hour intervals
   ii. Dexedrine Spansules[®9]
     a. Bi-phasic release of immediate- and controlled-release medication
     b. Initial peak plasma concentrations in about 3 hours, followed by another at 8 hours
   iii. ProCentra[®12] (dextroamphetamine oral solution)
     a. Also approved for Narcolepsy (dosed up to 60 mg/d divided)
   iv. Zenzedi[®9] (immediate-release dextroamphetamine)
     a. Also approved for Narcolepsy (dosed up to 60 mg/d divided)
   v. Vyvanse™ (lisdexamfetamine)[15]
     a. A prodrug of dextroamphetamine, so it has to be metabolized to be active
       1. Less risk of abuse, because it won't be active if snorted or injected
     b. FDA-approved for Moderate to Severe Binge Eating Disorder (BED) in adults in 2015
     c. With severe renal impairment: Maximum dose is 50 mg/day
     d. With End Stage Renal Disease (ESRD): Maximum dose is 30 mg/day
     e. Completed Phase II studies for treating ADHD in 4 to 5 year-olds
4. **Methamphetamine** (Desoxyn[®16])
   i. Also approved for Exogenous Obesity for those $\geq$ 12-years-old (5 mg before meals)
5. **Methylphenidate products**
   i. Most are approved for $\geq$ 6 yrs old
   ii. Recommended as 1st-line therapy in most guidelines[392]
   iii. Metabolism is by de-esterification to alpha-phenyl-piperidine acetic acid (PPAA) – not active
     a. Also known as "ritalinic acid" (60-80% excreted in urine)
   iv. Focalin[®] / Focalin XR[®7] (dexmethylphenidate)
     a. After AM dose, can repeat Immediate-release (IR) dose in 4 hours
     b. XR produces a bi-modal pharmacokinetic profile similar to IR given 4 hours apart, but with a lower 2nd peak concentration
       1. 1st peak in 1.5 hours (range 1 to 4 hours) and 2nd peak in 6.5 hours (range 4.5 to 7 hours)
   v. Adhansia XR™[18] (methylphenidate)
     a. Dosing is equivalent to immediate-release methylphenidate given TID (4 hours apart) producing two distinct peak concentrations
       1. 1st peak in 1.5 hours (range 1 to 2.5 hours) and 2nd peak in 12 hours (range 8.5 to 16 hours)
   vi. Aptensio XR™[19] (methylphenidate)
     a. Bi-phasic release of immediate (37%) and controlled-release (63%) microparticle beads
     b. Initial peak plasma concentrations in about 2 hours, followed by 4-6 hours of gradual descending levels
     c. Second peak plasma concentrations at approximately 8 hours and lasts ~ 16 hours
   vii. Concerta[®20] (methylphenidate)
     a. Recommended dose conversion from methylphenidate regimens to Concerta[®]
       • 5 mg Methylphenidate twice daily or three times daily $\approx$ 18 mg every morning
       • 10 mg Methylphenidate twice daily or three times daily $\approx$ 36 mg every morning
       • 15 mg Methylphenidate twice daily or three times daily $\approx$ 54 mg every morning
       • 20 mg Methylphenidate twice daily or three times daily $\approx$ 72 mg every morning
       • Other methylphenidate regimens: Use clinical judgment in selecting the starting dose
   viii. Cotempla XR-ODT[®21] (methylphenidate)
     a. Peak levels occur in 5 hours
     b. Pharmacokinetics of 51.8 mg (2 x 25.9 mg tabs) QD mirror methylphenidate ER 60 mg caps
   ix. Daytrana™[22] (methylphenidate in adhesive) patch
     a. Contraindicated in those with marked anxiety or agitation, glaucoma, tics or Tourette's, and concomitant MAOI therapy
     b. Starts working 2 hours after applied and lasts 3 hrs after removed
       1. After removed, patch still contains > 60% of active drug – handle with caution
     c. Avoid heat on external patch (can increase rate of absorption)
     d. May cause visual disturbances (blurry vision, difficulty in accommodation)
     e. Do not cut patches or adhere with tape/bandages
     f. Hematologic monitoring is suggested (e.g., CBC with differential, platelets)
     g. May cause skin irritation and permanent skin lightening[410-411]
   x. Jornay PM[24] by Highland Therapeutics, Inc./Ironshore Pharmaceuticals Inc.
     a. "Has delayed-release and extended-release properties" due to a proprietary drug-delivery technology, called Delexis[®].
     b. Dosed in the evening from 6:30 to 9:30PM
     c. Onset in 8-10 hours with peak in 16-18 hours
     d. Effects can last up to 22-24 hours
   xi. Metadate CD / ER[27]
     a. CD - 70:30 ratio of IR to ER contents
       1. E.g., 10 mg = 3 mg IR + 7 mg ER
     b. ER - Duration of action of approx. 8 hours
     c. ER dose is equivalent to the total daily dose of regular-release and sustained-release
   xii. Methylin[®] / Methylin[®] chewable / Methylin oral solution (methylphenidate)[28,29]
     a. Caution Phenylketonurics (PKU): contains phenylalanine

b. Peak levels in 1.9 hours (range 0.3 to 4.4 hours)
xiii. Methylin® ER[28] (methylphenidate)
a. Peak levels in 4.7 hours (1.3-8.2)
b. Duration of action of approx. 8 hours
xiv. Quillichew ER®[23] (methylphenidate)
a. 20 & 30 mg cherry-flavored tablets are scored (40 mg tablet is not)
b. Contains ~30% uncoated (IR) microparticles & ~70% film-coated (ER) microparticles
c. Caution Phenylketonurics (PKU): contains phenylalanine
xv. Quillivant XR®[25] (methylphenidate)
a. Extended-release (once daily) oral suspension
1. Powder is ~20% uncoated (IR) microparticles & ~80% film-coated (ER) microparticles
b. Reconstitute with water prior to use
1. Good for 4 months after reconstitution
2. Vigorously shake bottle for at least 10 seconds before each dose
xvi. Relexxii™[26] (methylphenidate)
a. Must not be chewed, divided, or crushed
b. Contraindicated in those with marked anxiety or agitation, glaucoma, tics or Tourette's, and concomitant MAOI therapy
xvii. Ritalin / Ritalin SR / LA®[18] (methylphenidate)
a. Regular-release peak levels in 1.9 hours (range 0.3-4.4 hours) – dosed BID to TID
1. Onset in 30-45 minutes
b. SR peak levels in 4.7 hours (range 1.3-8.2 hours) - dosed QD to BID
c. SR duration of action of approx. 8-12 hours
d. LA produces a bi-modal peak plasma level approximately 4 hours apart
e. 1st peak is in 1-3 hours / 2nd is 4 hours later - dosed QD

6. **Non-stimulants**
i. Onset of effect may take 3-4 weeks
ii. Atomoxetine (Strattera™)[4] – approved for children $\geq$ 6-years-old
a. Shown to be less effective than stimulants, but has advantage of being non-abusable
b. MOA: Selective Norepinephrine reuptake inhibitor
c. Dosing: Start at 0.5 mg/kg/day and increase up to 1.2 mg/kg/day
1. Max. dose is 1.4 mg/kg/day or 100 mg/d
2. Give QAM or AM & late afternoon/early evening (no later, to reduce insomnia)
3. Dose adjustment recommended for patients with moderate or severe hepatic insufficiency
d. Side effects are much more prevalent in poor metabolizers of CYP2D6
1. Dyspepsia, constipation, dry mouth, nausea, vomiting, fatigue, decreased appetite, dizziness, irritability, and mood swings
2. Watch for increases in BP and heart rate, and allergic reactions
3. Extremely rare case of severe liver injury have been reported to the FDA
e. Supplied as 10, 18, 25, 40, 60, 80, and 100 mg capsules
f. Black Box warning: Potential increase in suicidal ideation/ behavior in pediatric patients
g. Requires a medication guide be given to patients when dispensed
h. Contraindicated in patients with narrow angle glaucoma
iii. NeuroSigma's Monarch® external trigeminal nerve stimulation system (eTNS®)[412]
a. Indicated for patients aged 7 to 12 years who are not taking prescription ADHD medication
b. Sends a low-level electrical pulse through a wire to a small patch adhered to the patient's forehead, just above the eyebrows during periods of sleep at home
1. Patient must be supervised, and may take up to 4 weeks to see effects
c. Common side effects:
1. HA, N&V, lightheadedness, trouble sleeping, nightmares, cutaneous reactions, tooth pain
d. Price for the starter kit is currently $980
1. Includes a 4-week supply of electric patches (7 refill patches are $70)

7. **Alpha$_{2A}$ agonists**
i. Can be used as monotherapy or adjunctively to psychostimulants[413]
a. Shown to be more effective as monotherapy vs. adjunctive therapy
b. Superior to placebo on decreasing hyperactivity, impulsivity, inattention and aggressiveness
ii. Useful for stimulant-induced insomnia
iii. Can take 1-3 weeks to see full effect
iv. MUST taper off over 3-7 days to prevent rebound hypertension
v. Side effects: Somnolence, fatigue, abdominal pain, dizziness, hypotension, upper respiratory tract infection (cough, rhinitis, sneezing, sore throat), irritability, insomnia, nightmares, constipation, nasal congestion, increased body temperature, dry mouth, and ear pain
a. Warning: May cause bradycardia and syncope
vi. Clonidine (Catapres®[5] and Kapvay™[6] - an extended-release formulation)
a. May be used for sleep
b. Dosed at 0.004-0.005 mg/kg/day (in 0.05 mg increments) up to 25 mcg/kg/day or maximum of 0.4 mg/d (divided BID, even for Kapvay™)
c. MUST taper off over 3-7 days to prevent rebound hypertension
d. Transdermal patch only lasts 5 days in children compared to 7 days in adults
e. Patch is available in 0.1, 0.2, or 0.3 mg/d for 7 days
vii. Guanfacine (Tenex®/Intuniv™)[14]

a. Dosing begins at 1 mg a day (not to exceed 7 mg/d)
b. Increase dose each 3-7 days (target weight based dose of 0.05-0.12 mg/kg)
c. Intuniv ™ is dosed QD in the AM or PM
d. Available in 1, 2, 3, & 4 mg extended-release tablets
e. Less likely to lower BP than clonidine

## 19. PSYCHOSTIMULANT COMPARISON CHART[414-417]
### (NOTE: ALL OF THESE ARE C-II CONTROLLED SUBSTANCES)

| Generic Name | Brand Name | Dosing (mg per day) | Dosage Strengths (mg) | T½ (hours) | Dosage forms[418] |
|---|---|---|---|---|---|
| Amphetamine sulfate Approved for children > 3y.o. | Evekeo® | 2.5 (3-5 y.o.) or 5 (>6 y.o.) QD/BID; ↑ by 5 every week as needed (Max 40) | 5, 10 | 10-11.7 | Tablets (can crush, cut or split) |
| Mixed levo- & dextro-amphetamine (racemic mix) +Approved for children > 6 y.o.  ++Only approved for children > 13 y.o. | Adzenys® ER+ | 6.3 (5 ml) (<17 y.o.) / 12.5 (>18 y.o.) Max 18.8 for 6-12 y.o. / 12.5 for >13 y.o. | 1.25 mg/ml | Also see Table on page 1 | ER suspension (orange) |
| | Adzenys® XR-ODT+ | 6.3 (5 ml) (<17 y.o.) / 12.5 (>18 y.o.) Max 18.8 for 6-12 y.o. / 12.5 for >13 y.o. | 3.1, 6.3, 9.4, 12.5, 15.7, 18.8 | | ER tablets (orange ODT) |
| | Dyanavel® XR+ | 2.5 QAM and adjust + 2.5/d every 4-7 days until response achieved (Max. 20) | 2.5 mg/ml | 12.36-15.12 | ER suspension (bubble-gum) |
| | Evekeo ODT™+ | 5 QD or BID; ↑ by 5 every week as needed (Max 40) | 5, 10, 15, 20 | 10-11.7 | Tablets (ODT) |
| | Mydayis®++ | 12.5-25 (Max adult dose is 50) | 12.5, 25, 37.5, 50 | 10-13 | ER capsules (sprinkles) |
| Mixed amphetamine salts Approved for children > 3y.o. | Adderall® | Initially 5 QAM or BID; Titrate by 5 every week; (Max 30) | 5, 7.5, 10, 12.5, 15, 20, 30 | 9-14 | Tablets (can crush, cut or split) |
| | Adderall XR® | | 5, 10, 15, 20, 25, 30 | | ER capsules (sprinkle) |
| Dextro-amphetamine[8] Approved for children > 3 y.o. | Dexedrine® | 2.5 (3-5 y.o.) or 5 (>6 y.o.) QAM + 1-2 doses 4-6 hours apart; ↑ by 5 every week as needed (Max 40) | 5, 10 | 11.75 | IR tablets |
| | Dexedrine Spansule® | | 5, 10, 15 QAM | 12 | ER capsules (sprinkle) |
| | Dextrostat® | | 5, 10 | 11.75 | IR tablets (can cut) |
| | ProCentra® | | 5 mg/5 ml | 11.75 | IR solution (bubble-gum) |
| | Zenzedi® | | 2.5, 5, 7.5, 10, 20, 30 | 12 | IR tablets |
| Lis-dexamfet-amine dimesylate Approved for children > 6y.o. | Vyvanse™ (a prodrug) and Chewable tablets | 30 QAM and adjust by 10-20 a day each week until response achieved (Max 70) | 10, 20, 30, 40, 50, 60, 70 (chewable not available in 70 mg) | 12 | Capsules (can open) & Chewable tablets (strawberry) |
| Meth-amphetamine Approved for children > 6y.o. | Desoxyn® | 5-25 QAM or divided BID | 5 | 4-5 | IR tablets (can cut) |
| Dexmethyl-phenidate Approved for children > 6y.o. | Focalin® | 2.5-5 QAM/BID; ↑ to a max of 20 (10 BID) | 2.5, 5, 10 | 2.2 | IR tablets (can cut) |
| | Focalin XR® | 5-40 QAM (Max 30 in children) | 5, 10, 15, 20, 25, 30, 35, 40 | 2-3 | ER capsules (sprinkles) |
| Methyl-phenidate[17] | Adhansia XR™ | 25-70 (<17 y.o.) / 25-85 (>18 y.o.) QAM | 25, 35, 45, 55, 70, 85 | 7 | Capsules (sprinkles) |
| | Aptensio XR™ | 10-60 QAM | 10, 20, 30, 40, 50, 60 | 5.1-5.4 | ER capsules (sprinkles) |

| Approved for children ≥ 6 y.o. | Concerta® | 18-54 QAM (6-12 y.o.) / 18-72 QD (≥13 y.o.) | 18, 27, 36, 54 | 3.6 | ER tablets with IR outer coat |
|---|---|---|---|---|---|
| | Cotempla XR ODT® | 17.3-51.8 (≤17 y.o.) QAM | 8.6, 17.3, 25.9 | 4 | ER tablets (grape ODT) |
| | Daytrana™ (patch) | 10-30 | 10, 15, 20, 30 | 1.4-4.5 | Transdermal patch |
| | Jornay PM™ | 20-100 *in the evening* | 20, 40, 60, 80 & 100 | 5.9 | ER capsules (sprinkles) |
| | Metadate CD® | 10-60 QAM | 10, 20, 30, 40, 50, 60 | 6.8 | Capsules (ER & IR sprinkles) |
| | Metadate ER® | 20-60 QAM or divided BID | 10, 20 | 3.6 | ER tablets |
| | Methylin® | 5-60 divided BID to TID | 5, 10, 20 | 2.5-3.5 | Tablets (can cut) |
| | Methylin® chewable | 5-60 divided BID to TID | 2.5, 5, 10 | 2.5-3.5 | Tablets (can cut) |
| | Methylin ER® | 20-60 QAM or divided BID | 10, 20 | | ER tablets |
| | Methylin® (oral solution) | 5-60 divided BID | 5, 10 mg/5 ml | 2.5-3.5 | Liquid (grape) |
| | Quillichew ER® | 20-60 QAM | 20, 30 scored, 40 | 5.2 | ER chew tabs (cherry) |
| | Quillivant XR® | 20-60 QAM | 25 mg/5 mL (5 mg/mL) | 5.6 (±0.8) | ER suspension (banana) |
| | Relexxii™ | 18-72 QAM | 18, 36, 54, 72 | 3.5 | ER tablets |
| | Ritalin® | Initially 5-60 divided BID to TID Max 2 mg/kg/d | 5, 10, 20 | 2.5-3.5 | Tablets (can cut) |
| | Ritalin SR® | 20-60 QAM or divided BID | 20 | | ER tablets |
| | Ritalin LA® | 20-60 QAM | 10, 20, 30, 40 | | ER capsules (sprinkles) |

y.o. = years old
NOTE: All sprinkle-filled caps can be opened, and the contents placed on food (i.e., applesauce)

## K. Non-FDA approved therapies
1. Bupropion (Wellbutrin®)[191,392]
   i. Antidepressant with stimulant-related properties which has been shown effective in both childhood and adult ADHD in several studies over placebo[419]
   ii. Average dose in children is 3-6 mg/kg/day, not to exceed 300 mg/d divided
   iii. Contraindicated in patients with an eating disorder or seizure disorder
   iv. Consider as a 3rd-line therapy
   v. See details in *Antidepressants* section
2. Memantine (Namenda®)[92]
   i. Small study in adults with ADHD showed osmotic release oral system-methylphenidate (OROS-MPH) + memantine improved executive function deficits (EFDs)[420]
3. Other Antidepressants (TCAs, MAOIs, and SSRIs) are 3rd-line agents
   i. Desipramine (Norpramin®) is most well-studied for ADHD
   ii. Imipramine (Tofranil®)[162] and nortriptyline (Pamelor®) also used
   iii. Sudden death reported
   iv. May take weeks to be effective
   v. Caution: cardiac side effects with TCAs and MAOIs
4. Modafinil (Provigil®) or Armodafinil (Nuvigil®)[52,62,421]
   i. Not FDA-approved for ADHD, but is approved for Narcolepsy
   ii. A study in adults failed
   iii. Positive results seen with children's inattention and hyperactivity, short-term
5. Antipsychotic medications[392]
   i. Useful in Autism Spectrum Disorder when disruptive aggression occurs
   ii. ***NOT*** recommended to treat the core symptoms of ADHD

## L. COMPLEMENTARY AND ALTERNATIVE THERAPIES (CAM) for ADHD
1. Bacopa monnieri/brahmi (water hysop)[360,422]
2. Passiflora incarnata (passionflower)
   i. Showed comparable effects to methylphenidate in study
   ii. Considered safe and nontoxic
   iii. Side effects include: nausea, vomiting, drowsiness, tachycardia and mental slowing

3. Melissa officinalis (lemon balm)
4. Valeriana officinalis (valerian) – Warning: natural *valeriana* smells horrible
5. Melatonin 1-5 mg HS for sleep
   i. Estimated 1 in 17 school-aged children take melatonin at least once a week[423]
M. POTENTIAL FUTURE TREATMENTS FOR ADHD IN STUDY [424]
1. Ampakine® (CX-717) by Cortex Pharmaceuticals, NIDA, and RespireRx Pharmaceuticals
   i. AMPA receptor modulators
   ii. Phase II clinical trials completed
2. AR-08 by Arbor Pharmaceuticals in Phase II clinical trials
   i. Adrenergic receptor agonist
3. Centanafadine (EB-1020) by Otsuka Pharmaceutical/Neurovance in Phase III trials
   i. DA > NE > 5HT uptake inhibitor (SNDRI - triple reuptake inhibitor)
4. **Dasotraline (SEP-225289)** by Sumitomo Dainippon Pharma Co., LTD / Sunovion
   i. Balanced reuptake inhibitor of serotonin, norepinephrine and dopamine (SNDRI)
   ii. In clinical trials for Adult and Pediatric ADHD (4 mg vs. 6 mg/d)
   iii. Also being studied for Binge eating disorder (BED)
   iv. FDA rejected its approval in August 2018, citing a need for more data
   v. More info at: http://www.ds-pharma.com/rd/clinical/pipeline.html or
      https://clinicaltrials.gov/ct2/show/study/NCT02276209
5. Dexamfetamine transdermal (ATS) by Noven Pharmaceuticals in Phase II trials
6. Edivoxetine (LY-2216684) by Eli Lilly and Company in Phase III clinical trials
   i. NE reuptake inhibitor
   ii. http://mentalhealthdaily.com/2015/09/14/new-adhd-medications-in-the-pipeline-2015/ 4/28/16.
   iii. ClinicalTrials.gov Identifier: NCT02477748
7. Eltoprazine by Amarantus Bioscience (Elto Pharma) in Phase III trials for adult ADHD
   i. MOA: $5HT_{1A}$ and $5HT_{1B}$ partial agonist, as well as a and $5HT_{2C}$ receptor antagonist
   ii. A phenylpiperazine, similar to aripiprazole, brexpiprazole, and cariprazine
   iii. Originally developed as an anti-aggressive (*serenic*) agent to ↓ aggressive behaviors and
       impulses
8. Mazindol controlled release (NLS-0, NLS-1, Nolazol) by NLS Pharmaceutics
   i. 5HT, DA, NE-predominant reuptake inhibitor (SNDRI) - norepinephrine
   ii. In Phase II for Adult Attention-Deficit Hyperactivity Disorder
9. Metadoxine ER by Alcobra and Arcturus Therapeutics in Phase III clinical trials
   i. Mechanism: $5HT_{2B}$ selective agonist / GABA modulator (prevents GABA degradation)
   ii. Comprised of an ion pair salt of pyridoxine (Vitamin B6) and L-pyroglutamate
   iii. Used in Europe to treat alcohol intoxication
   iv. ClinicalTrials.gov Identifier: NCT02547428
10. Molindone HCl (SPN-810) by Supernus Pharmaceuticals
    i. MOA: Selective $D_2$ receptor antagonist with a low affinity for $D_1$ receptors
    ii. Typical antipsychotic that may be helpful for conduct problems + ADHD
    iii. In Phase III (FDA fast track status) for Impulsive Aggression (IA) in ADHD
    iv. ClinicalTrials.gov Identifiers: NCT02618408, NCT02618434, and NCT02691182
11. OPC-64005 by Lundbeck A/S and Otsuka America Pharmaceuticals in Phase II clinical trials
    i. 5HT, NE, and DA reuptake inhibitor (triple reuptake inhibitor)
12. Serdexmethylphenidate chloride by KemPharm in Phase III clinical trials
    i. A prodrug of Dexmethylphenidate, so less potential for abuse
    ii. Same drug with 3 intended indications:
       a. **KP415** for ADHD in children & adolescents
       b. **KP484** for adult ADHD
       c. **KP879** for Stimulant Substance Use Disorder (abuse/misuse of cocaine, methamphetamines,
          Rx methylphenidate or amphetamine, and designer stimulants (Flakka/"bath salts")
    iii. https://kempharm.com/pipeline-products/
13. TRN-110 by Tris Pharma in clinical trials for adult and pediatric ADHD
    i. Current clinical phase is unknown, but Tris Pharma lists it as being in "advanced clinical" stage
14. Viloxazine (SPN-809/SPN-812) – by Supernus Pharmaceuticals
    i. NE reuptake inhibitor: Phase III trials for pediatric ADHD & Phase II for adult ADHD (completed)
    ii. Was approved in Europe as an antidepressant, but newer drugs have replaced it
    iii. SPN-809 is in Phase I/II trials for depression, even though it is an older drug
    iv. ClinicalTrials.gov Identifiers: NCT01107496, NCT02633527, and NCT02736656
IV. TREATMENT OF AGGRESSION (WITHOUT ADHD)[392]
A. Psychosocial interventions are first-line
B. Pharmacotherapy is second-line
C. Recommended (in order of quality of evidence for use (i.e., Evidence-based Medicine))
   1. Grade A: risperidone or aripiprazole (low dose)
   2. Grade B: psychostimulants, clonidine, guanfacine, atomoxetine, valproate (caution in females),
      or ziprasidone (with EKG)
   3. Grade C: carbamazepine or paliperidone
D. Not recommended due to negative side effect profile (in order of quality of evidence for use)
   1. Grade A: lithium, chlorpromazine, or haloperidol
   2. Grade B: olanzapine or quetiapine (because of metabolic side effects)

E. **POTENTIAL FUTURE TREATMENTS OF *INTERMITTENT EXPLOSIVE DISORDER* (PHASE II)**
  1. AVP-786/AVP-923 (deuterium-modified dextromethorphan + quinidine) by Otsuka/Avanir
    i. MOA: Sigma-1 (σ1) receptor agonist, SNRI, and NMDA receptor antagonist
  2. SRX246 by Azevan Pharmaceuticals
    i. MOA: Vasopressin $1_a$ receptor antagonist
    ii. Phase II trials have been completed for Intermittent Explosive Disorder
    iii. Also being studied for other behavioral disorders and PTSD
    iv. Vasopressin $1_a$ receptor antagonists are intended to reduce stress, fear, aggression,
      depression, and anxiety, as shown in preclinical tests

## V. DISRUPTIVE MOOD DYSREGULATION DISORDER (DMDD)
A. No treatment guidelines yet exist and no medications are yet approved
B. Diagnosis
  1. Severe recurrent temper outbursts that are grossly out of proportion to the situation
    i. Temper outbursts are inconsistent with developmental level
    ii. Temper outbursts occur, on average, three or more times per week
  2. Mood between temper outbursts is persistently irritable or angry most of the day, nearly every
    day, and is observable by others (e.g., parents, teachers, peers)
  3. Symptoms present for > 12 months, but not absent for > 3 months in between
  4. Present in > 2 of 3 settings (i.e., at home, at school, with peers) and are severe in > 1 of these
  5. Diagnosis should not be made for the first time before age 6 or after age 18
  6. Age at onset of symptoms is before 10-years-old
  7. Exclude if oppositional defiant, intermittent explosive or bipolar disorder present

## VI. AUTISM SPECTRUM DISORDER (ASD)
A. Heritability estimates range from 37 to 90%, based on twin concordance rates[245]
B. As many as 15% of cases appear to be associated with a known genetic mutation
C. Risperidone and aripiprazole are approved to treat irritability and aggression
  1. Clozapine, haloperidol, and other antipsychotics are also effective
D. Intranasal oxytocin improves social impairments, emotion recognition, & eye gaze in ASD pts[425]
E. Memantine (Namenda) and (Exelon) can increase cognition
F. Mirtazapine and SSRI/SNRI antidepressants can help with repetitive behaviors, self-injurious
  behaviors, sleep, and anxiety
G. Secretin hormone therapy is ineffective and should not be used
H. Melatonin can be used for sleep
I. Sulforaphane (50–150 μmol) derived from broccoli sprout extracts, for 18 weeks[426,427]
  1. Significant improvement on the Aberrant Behavior Checklist (ABC), Social Responsiveness
    Scale (SRS), and CGI-Improvement Scale vs. placebo
J. **POTENTIAL FUTURE TREATMENTS FOR AUTISM IN STUDY**
  1. Arbaclofen (r-baclofen / STX-209) by Seaside Therapeutics
    i. $GABA_B$ receptor agonist
    ii. In Phase 0 for Autistic Disorders, but has Orphan Drug Status by FDA for Fragile X syndrome
  2. Balovaptan (RG7314) by Roche Pharmaceuticals
    i. A selective small molecule antagonist of the vasopressin V receptor
    ii. On 1/29/2018, Roche announced that the FDA granted Breakthrough Therapy Designation for
      balovaptan in individuals with autism spectrum disorder (ASD)[428]
    iii. As of August 2019, it is in a Phase III clinical trial for adults and a Phase II trial for children
  3. Bumetanide (Bumex) by Servier Pharmaceutical Company
    i. Shown to significantly reduced the *Childhood Autism Rating Scale (CARS)* and improve *Clinical
      Global Improvement (CGI)* scores[429]
    ii. In Phase III study for Autistic Disorder & Phase III for Pervasive child development disorders
  4. D-cycloserine[357]
  5. Fatty acid amide hydrolase (FAAH) inhibitors (JNJ-42165279/JNJ-5279) by Janssen-Cilag
    i. Phase II completed for social anxiety and Pervasive child development disorders
  6. NBTX-001 (the noble gas xenon) by Nobilis Therapeutics[430]
    i. Antagonist of NMDA, AMPA, nicotinic ACh (α4β2), $5HT_3$, & plasma membrane $Ca^{2+}$ ATPase
    ii. Currently in Phase III trials using the Zephyrus™ inhalational Device
    iii. Also in Phase II for Irritable Bowel Syndrome (IBS), Alzheimer's and Parkinson's Disease
  7. Oxytocin (Syntocinon) nasal spray
    i. In Phase III trials for the treatment of social impairment in individuals with high functioning
      Autism Spectrum Disorder or Pervasive Developmental Disorder
      a. At Massachusetts General Hospital
    ii. Also in Phase II/III trials at the University of Sao Paulo General Hospital to evaluate the
      influence of oxytocin in some aspects of Autism Spectrum Disorder, such as repetitive and
      stereotyped behavior, social skills, quality of life and disruptive behaviors
      a. ClinicalTrials.gov Identifiers: NCT02007447 & NCT02985749
    iii. Other Phase III and IV trials for ASD: NCT03640156, NCT02940574
    iv. In Phase III study for Prader-Willi Syndrome (ClinicalTrials.gov Identifier: NCT03649477)
  8. Viloxazine and Viloxazine E.R. (SPN-809/SPN-812/ICI-588834) by Supernus Pharmaceuticals
    i. MOA: NE reuptake inhibitor
    ii. In Phase III trials for pediatric ADHD and Phase II for adult ADHD (completed)
    iii. Was approved in Europe as an antidepressant, but newer drugs have replaced it
    iv. SPN-809 was in Phase I/II trials for depression, even though it is an older drug, but recently

the trials for depression have been abandoned
  v. ClinicalTrials.gov Identifiers: NCT01107496, NCT02633527, and NCT02736656
VII. CHILD AND ADOLESCENT DEPRESSION AND ANTIDEPRESSANTS
  A. In 2017, 9.4% of the US population ages 12-17 experienced a major depressive episode[431]
    1. 70.77% had severe impairment / Only 39.9% received any treatment (60.1% did not)
  B. Most adults with anxiety or depression started in adolescence, with a peak at age 24[432]
    1. Less than half of adolescents with anxiety/depression had it in adulthood
    2. A 4-year study found for every extra hour per day an adolescent spends on the computer or on social media significantly increases depressive symptoms and reduces measures of self-esteem[433]
    3. Childhood bullying can more than double the risk of depression later in life[434]
  C. Rates of suicide and suicide attempts in 15-19-year-olds has risen sharply in the last 2 decades[263]
    1. 47% more suicides than in 2000 (currently at its highest level)[435]
    2. 2nd leading cause of death in 15-24 y.o.'s (after unintentional motor vehicle accidents)[436]
  D. ALL antidepressants carry a **Black Box Warning** about ↑ risk of suicidal ideation (up to age 24)
    1. 23 randomized trials revealed approx. 2 X increased risk vs. placebo[437]
    2. No completed suicides occurred in studies
    3. ALL children and young adults should be seen by a health-care practitioner <u>weekly</u> for the first month, and then <u>every 2 weeks</u> for a month, and then <u>monthly</u>
    4. Tennessee Medicaid study of youth on antidepressants revealed that risk of suicide was no different between any of the SSRIs or venlafaxine[438]
      i. Suicide attempts were 24 - 29.1 per 1000 person-years of exposure (very rare)
      ii. *Fast initial titration* and *shorter half-life antidepressants* are SIGNIFICANTLY (p<0.005) correlated with suicide-related events[439]
      iii. Starting at high doses doubles the risk of self-harm behaviors versus slow titration[440]
        a. *SLOW TITRATION* in children is HIGHLY recommended[441]
        b. Possible strategy to reduce suicidality studied: $5HT_{1A}$ antagonist + SSRI
    5. Large meta-analysis showed that antidepressants have a *high placebo-effect*, but <u>ARE</u> more effective than placebo overall (also for anxiety, OCD, and PTSD)[442]
    6. Caution: trazodone (partial $5HT_{1A}$ agonist) used for sleep reduced antidepressant response rates and ↑ suicidality and irritability, *significantly*[443]
  E. Fluoxetine (ages 8-17) and escitalopram (ages 12-17) are the <u>only</u> FDA-approved newer agents for depression
    1. Evidence-based support is lacking with other antidepressants for depression
    2. 2016 world-wide meta-analysis found that fluoxetine was the <u>only</u> effective antidepressant[444]
      i. Only venlafaxine was associated with suicidal ideation
  F. Doxepin[54] (ages >12) is FDA-approved, but TCAs have high cardiac risks
  G. Imipramine (ages >6) is FDA-approved for bedwetting; not effective for adolescent depression[445]
  H. Paroxetine should be <u>avoided</u>—suicidal ideation & "emotional lability" (2x as likely); short t½[445]
    1. FDA has issued a warning against its use in children & adolescents
  I. Venlafaxine should be <u>avoided</u>—short t½
  J. POTENTIAL FUTURE TREATMENTS FOR PEDIATRIC DEPRESSION IN STUDY
    1. Fetzima (Levomilnacipran extended-release) by Allergan in Phase III trials
    2. Trintellix (vortioxetine) by Lundbeck in Phase III trials
VIII. CHILD AND ADOLESCENT ANXIETY AND ANXIOLYTICS[305,446]
  A. Lifetime prevalence rates for any anxiety disorder in adolescents is 31.9% (Median onset is 6-y.o.)
  B. Always use psychotherapy / Cognitive Behavioral Therapy (CBT) as first-line treatment
  C. Predictors of treatment response
    1. Males, non-minority status, younger, no 1st degree relatives with anxiety, & good family functioning
  D. For GAD (Generalized Anxiety Disorder)
    1. Sertraline, fluoxetine, duloxetine, and buspirone have shown efficacy in studies
    2. SSRIs have shown earlier and greater efficacy than SNRIs in study
    3. Drizalma Sprinkle™ & Irenka™ (duloxetine) approved for GAD in patients > 7 y.o.
  E. For Social Anxiety Disorder and Social Phobia
    1. Venlafaxine ER and paroxetine (not recommended in children) are effective in studies
      i. Side effects of significance: suicidal ideation, vomiting, ↓ appetite, insomnia, asthenia
  F. For Panic Disorder, paroxetine may be effective, but has questionable safety in children
  G. For children with more than one ("mixed") anxiety disorder
    1. Sertraline + CBT was ≈ 81% effective vs. sertraline or CBT alone (55-60% effective)
    2. Fluoxetine or fluvoxamine were 61-76% effective vs. placebo (29-35% effective)
    3. Guanfacine is also effective (54% response vs. 31.6% placebo response)
  H. BZDs (e.g., clonazepam / alprazolam) were *no more effective than placebo* for anxiety disorders
    1. Studies show an increase in oppositional behavior and irritability
    2. BZDs are more likely to cause disinhibition and have more abuse potential in adolescents
    3. Avoid BZDs if at all possible
  I. In PTSD, psychotherapy is more effective than medication treatment
  J. In OCD, fluoxetine (ages >7), fluvoxamine (ages >8), clomipramine (ages >10), and sertraline (ages >6) are FDA-approved
    1. Usually in OCD, highest tolerable doses are used to treat symptoms

## IX. CHILD AND ADOLESCENT PSYCHOSIS, SCHIZOPHRENIA, AND ANTIPSYCHOTICS

A. < 25% of children receiving antipsychotics receive psychotherapy[447]
B. Many atypicals approved in pediatric Bipolar and/or Schizophrenia *(see chart on page 102)*
   1. Should be 1st-line treatment for childhood schizophrenia
C. Childhood onset schizophrenia must be diagnosed before age 13
   1. Associated with significant early cortical gray and white matter deficits[448]
   i. . High comorbidity with Depression (>50%), OCD (>20%), and Anxiety (15%)
   ii. Almost 1/3 have symptoms of comorbid autism spectrum disorder (e.g., echolalia and hand flapping)
   iii. An autoimmune response to D2 or NMDA glutamate receptors may be involved[449]
   2. Risperidone (ages 5-16) and Aripiprazole (ages >6) FDA-approved for irritability in Autism
   i. Risperidone significantly increases prolactin (may double)[450] and increases risk of EPS
   3. Haloperidol (ages >3), chlorpromazine (ages >6 months), thioridazine (ages >2), and Orap (pimozide) (ages >12 for Tourette's)
   4. Approx. 2.1% of U.S. children are prescribed antipsychotics[451]
   i. Boys prescribed at almost 2 times rate of girls (2.78% vs. 1.45%)
   ii. Most commonly prescribed for ADHD or Depression without psychosis
     a. 44-69% prescribed with a psychostimulant
     b. The APA advises against using antipsychotics for improper indications[452]
   iii. Less than 1/3 of prescriptions are by a Child & Adolescent Psychiatrist
   iv. Long-term effects of antipsychotics in children are not fully known
   5. Youth exposed to antipsychotics are at *significantly greater risk* of developing Type II Diabetes[453]
D. POTENTIAL FUTURE TREATMENTS FOR PEDIATRIC SCHIZOPHRENIA IN STUDY
   1. Brexpiprazole (Lu AF41156, OPC-34712; Rexulti) by Otsuka/Lundbeck
   i. In Phase III trials for adolescent schizophrenia
   2. NaBen® - Sodium benzoate (SND-11, SND-12, SND-13, SND-14; Clozaben) by SyneuRx
   i. In Phase II/III trials for adolescent schizophrenia
   ii. MOA: D-amino acid oxidase inhibitor

## X. CHILD AND ADOLESCENT BIPOLAR DISORDER & MOOD STABILIZERS

A. There is a similarity between ADHD and Bipolar disorder (symptoms appear alike)
   1. Bipolar → have very long temper tantrums, insomnia, and hallucinations
   2. If amphetamine use in "ADHD" has none or worse response, then may be Bipolar
B. Prodromal symptoms - *mood swings* (i.e. lability) a strong predictor of bipolar[454]
   1. Severe early depression and antidepressant use ↑ risk 2½ times (≈8.2%)
C. Cannabis use (>2-3 x a week) is an independent risk factor for developing future hypomania[455]
D. Randomized controlled trials show that risperidone and other atypical antipsychotics are highly effective and lithium or valproic acid are moderately effective[456,457]
E. Oxcarbazepine, omega-3 fatty acids, and amphetamines are NOT effective
F. Open-label trials for mania show a modest response with atypical antipsychotics, lithium, valproic acid, carbamazepine, topiramate and lamotrigine[456]
   1. Side effects: rash, weight gain, GI problems, ↓ platelets, and impaired cognition
G. Lithium approved for ages >12 – Not recommended for children < 12 yrs old
   1. Must monitor for side effects and hypothyroidism
   2. Meta-analysis of 12 DBPCts shows efficacy in mania of 50% of patients with long-term maintenance efficacy[458]
   i. Most common side effects seen were gastrointestinal, polyuria, or headache
H. Valproic acid – monitor LFTs, platelets, polycystic ovarian syndrome (PCOS) in females
   1. Approved for ages >2 for seizures
   2. Valproic acid + lithium achieved 89.5% remission rates over 18 months459
I. Lamotrigine – ↑ incidence of rash; can progress to Stevens-Johnson Syndrome
   1. *MUST titrate slowly!!!*
   2. Not approved for Bipolar in children
   3. Open-label study found 84% response and 58% remission by week 8 for Bipolar Depression[460]
   4. Beware of interactions affecting lamotrigine with birth control pills (↓ lamotrigine blood levels)
   i. Inform females to skip the placebo week (stay on continuous active medication) to keep lamotrigine levels stable
J. Carbamazepine – Drug interactions with oral contraceptives, causes hyponatremia, rash!!!
   1. Approved for any age for seizures
K. PEDIATRIC BIPOLAR DEPRESSION[461]
   1. Lurasidone and olanzapine/fluoxetine (Symbyax®) are FDA-approved
   i. Recommended doses are ½ that for adults
   2. Quetiapine was not effective in study
   3. Open-label lithium and lamotrigine were effective in studies (no placebo control used)[460]
L. POTENTIAL FUTURE TREATMENTS FOR PEDIATRIC BIPOLAR DISORDER IN STUDY
   1. Geodon (ziprasidone) by Pfizer is in Phase III study
   i. Because of potential QT-prolongation, baseline & follow-up EKGs are warranted
   2. Open-label Uridine 500 mg BID x 6 weeks showed efficacy in adolescent Bipolar Depression[462]

# 20. BIPOLAR AFFECTIVE DISORDER AND MOOD STABILIZERS[284-286,463-470]

## I. BACKGROUND
A. Bipolar spectrum disorders affect ~ 2.4% of the world's population[471] (US estimate is up to 4 - 6%)
  1. Prevalence of 0.6 to 1% for bipolar type I and 0.4 to 4% for bipolar type II[472,473]
  2. Up to 70% of patients may be initially misdiagnosed as having unipolar depression
B. High comorbidity with anxiety and panic disorder
  1. Half of patients have a comorbid substance use disorder (EtOH or other drugs)
  2. Common symptoms overlap with Cyclothymic Disorder and Borderline Personality Disorder[474,475]
    i. Abandonment fear and chronic emptiness are only in the DSM-5 Borderline criteria
C. Most prevalent state is depression (about 32% of a lifetime) with mania (about 15% of lifetime)[476]
  1. Euthymia (normal mood) is about 53% of a lifetime
  2. Over 50% of individuals with Bipolar Disorder attempt suicide over their lifetime[477]
D. Antidepressant treatment is associated with an ↑ risk of subsequent mania/bipolar disorder[478]
  1. In first 3 months of treatment, risk of switching is ↑ 2.83 x if on antidepressant monotherapy[479]
    i. Risk of switching into mania is higher with TCAs and SNRIs vs. SSRIs or bupropion
    ii. Switch rates are 4.3 x greater in juveniles than adults (esp. if diagnosed with MDD ≤ 25 y.o.)
  2. Antidepressants should NOT be used as monotherapy in bipolar patients[480]
  3. Discontinue antidepressant(s) if patient has any manic symptoms
  4. Use of antidepressants as adjuncts in bipolar is of questionable benefit[481-483]
  5. *Possibly* safe & effective as monotherapy in Bipolar II depression[484]
  6. NOTE: Approx. 6-8% of patients put on an antidepressant will develop bipolar later[485]
E. Large genetic influence
  1. 33-90% concordance in identical twins[486]
  2. 80-90% have a biological relative with a mood disorder
    i. 5-10% have a 1st degree relative with Bipolar (approx. 7 x more likely to develop Bipolar)
F. Influenza during pregnancy ↑ risk of bipolar with psychotic features in offspring by fourfold[487]
  1. Higher risk if influenza is during the 1st or 2nd trimester
G. 95% of patients have a comorbid psychiatric and/or medical condition (e.g., HTN, diabetes)[476]
H. Life expectancy is 10 years shorter
I. The earlier medication is started, the better the long-term outcomes[488]
J. All mood stabilizers have at least one BBW
K. Most are not safe in pregnancy - for women, *advise to use 2 methods of birth control*

## II. TYPES OF BIPOLAR DISORDER AND DIAGNOSES[245]
A. Bipolar I = depression with mania
  1. Symptoms present every day for at least *1 week*
B. Bipolar II = depression with hypomania
  1. Hypomania is similar to mania, but the person retains some of their function and judgement
  2. Symptoms are not severe enough to cause marked impairment in social or occupational functioning or to necessitate hospitalization
  3. Symptoms present every day for at least *4 days*
C. Cyclothymic Disorder
  1. Some symptoms of hypomania and depression, but not enough for a full diagnosis of either
  2. Duration of at least 2 years (at least 1 year in children and adolescents)
  3. Symptoms are never absent for > 2 months at a time
D. "with mixed features" = having symptoms of both mania/hypomania and some depression symptoms (but not enough for a full diagnosis)
  1. With mixed features can also be used for Bipolar Depression with some manic symptoms

## III. SYMPTOMS OF MANIA (DIG FAST) - an acronym of mania symptoms

| D = Distractibility and easy frustration | |
|---|---|
| I = Irresponsibility and erratic uninhibited behavior | |
| G = Grandiosity | NEED ≥ 3 |
| F = Flight of ideas | for diagnosis |
| A = Activity increased with weight loss and increased libido | |
| S = Sleep is decreased | |
| T = Talkativeness | |

## IV. UNDERLYING TRIGGERS OF MANIA

| A. Medications / Drugs | |
|---|---|
| ♦ α2-agonist withdrawal | ♦ Hallucinogens: LSD, phencyclidine |
| ♦ Anticonvulsants | ♦ Dopaminergic agents |
| ♦ Antidepressants | ♦ Interferon (withdrawal) |
| ♦ Baclofen (Lioresal®) | ♦ Isoniazid |
| ♦ BZDs and Alcohol | ♦ NSAIDs (e.g., Motrin®, Aleve®) |
| ♦ Bronchodilators | ♦ Procainamide / Quinacrine |
| ♦ Calcium replacement | ♦ Steroids (Anabolic, corticosteroids, ACTH) |
| ♦ Cimetidine (Tagamet®) | ♦ Stimulants |
| ♦ Decongestants /Sympathomimetics | ♦ Xanthines |
| ♦ Disulfiram (Antabuse®) | ♦ Yohimbine |

| B. **Medical Illnesses** | o Infections / Post-infection |
|---|---|
| o Traumatic brain injury | ▪ HIV / AIDS |
| ▪ CVA / stroke | ▪ Encephalitis, influenza, neurosyphilis |
| ▪ Subarachnoid hemorrhage | ▪ Hepatitis |
| ▪ Subcortical or right frontotemporal lobe lesions | ▪ Creutzfeldt-Jakob disease |
| ▪ Surgical trauma | o Neurologic Disorders |
| o Addison's disease | ▪ Epilepsy (temporal lobe) |
| o Carcinoid tumors | o Huntington's disease |
| o Cushing's disease | o Multiple sclerosis |
| o Hyperthyroidism | o Sleep deprivation |
| o Excessive bright light (e.g., summer in Alaska) | o Vitamin B12 deficiency |

## V. TREATMENT

A. To evaluate an agent's efficacy, allow up to 2 full weeks before changing to another medication[489]

B. Antipsychotic drugs (*refer to chapter on Schizophrenia and Antipsychotics*)

  1. *Antipsychotic drugs are more effective than mood stabilizers in treating & preventing mania*

  2. First-line agents: aripiprazole, asenapine, olanzapine, quetiapine, risperidone, ziprasidone, brexpiprazole, cariprazine[490-493]

    i. Potent $D_3$ and $D_2$ receptor partial agonist ($D_3 > D_2$ effects)

  3. Can be combined with lithium or valproate in acute mania for better & faster response

  4. In order of efficacy: risperidone > olanzapine > haloperidol (haloperidol not a first-line agent)[489]

    i. From 68 randomized controlled trials of 16,073 patients[494]

C. Benzodiazepines

  1. Useful in prn rapid sedation of manic patients (along with antipsychotics)

  2. Should not be continued, as they are associated with greater illness complexity[495]

D. Classic **"Mood Stabilizers"**

  1. The term "Mood Stabilizers" may not be as accurate as the term "Anti-manic agents"

    i. They are *more effective* for treating mania than depression, and don't prevent mood cycling

  2. **Lithium (Li⁺) (Eskalith®, Lithobid®)**[119,120] - approved for mixed episodes and maintenance therapy

    i. Works best for a classic manic episode (i.e., not mixed or rapid cycling)

    ii. Mechanism of action suspected to be as a glutamate stabilizer (affects glutamate reuptake)[496]

     a. Also increases the expression of BDNF and inhibits glycogen synthase kinase-3 (GSK-3)[497]

     b. A dozen other theoretical mechanisms make it difficult to be absolutely certain

    iii. Pre-treatment (and routine monitoring) work-up: SrCr, urinalysis, CBC w/diff, serum electrolytes, glucose, weight, EKG, pregnancy test (if applicable) and thyroid function tests (TFTs)

     a. QT-prolongation, t-wave inversion, sick sinus syndrome and Brugada Syndrome can occur

    iv. Using just 5 neural cells, scientists have found a way to determine if lithium will work for a person, with 92% accuracy[498]

     a. Possible hippocampal mitochondrial disorder[499]

    v. Available as: 150, 300, 450, & 600 mg lithium carbonate ($Li_2CO_3$) tablets/capsules and 8 mEq (300 mg)/5 mL raspberry-flavored liquid (lithium citrate)

    vi. Usual starting dose is 300 mg BID to TID with food (to ↓ GI upset, or use SR tabs)

    vii. Approx. 300 mg of $Li_2CO_3$ will raise the plasma Li⁺ concentration by 0.2-0.4 mEq/L in adults

    viii. Li⁺(daily dose) = 100.5 + [752.7 x L(ec)] − [3.6 x age] + [7.2 x wt (kg)] − [13.7 x BUN( mg/dl)] where - L(ec) is the expected lithium concentration in mmol/L (same as mEq/L)[500]

    ix. Li⁺(daily dose) = 486.8 + (746.83 x level desired) - (10.08 x age) + (5.95 x weight (kg)) + (147.8 x sex) + (92.01 x inpatient) - (74.73 x TCA)[501]

     a. Sex =1 for male, 0 for female; inpatient = 1 for yes, 0 for no; & TCA use = 1 for yes, 0 for no

     b. See http://www.russellcottrell.com/md/lithium.shtm for an on-line calculator

    x. 95-100% readily absorbed from the GI tract

    xi. > 95% renally excreted, so t½ depends on renal fx. ≈ 18-36 hrs (24 hrs avg.)

    xii. Not protein bound or metabolized

    xiii. CSF/Brain concentration is 40-50% that of plasma

    xiv. Steady state in 5 days of each dosage change

     a. Levels should be drawn 12 hours post dose (i.e., trough)

     b. Serum level range:

      1. 0.6 – 1.2 mEq/L (acute phase) – up to 1.5 mEq/L may be used

      2. 0.6 – 1.0 mEq/L (maintenance phase)

      3. QD dosing results in a **10-26%** ↑ level compared to BID or TID dosing

    xv. When discontinuing lithium, a slow taper is best[502]

     a. Bipolar recurrence is 63% for rapid discontinuation vs. 37% for gradual taper

    xvi. **Early side effects:** *GI disturbances (N/V/D)*, lethargy, sedation, ↓ memory & concentration, headache, *polyuria & polydipsia* (70%), *tremor*, dry mouth, leukocytosis (*may be beneficial*)

    xvii. **Maintenance side effects:** *fine hand tremor* (50%), *weight gain* (20%), goiter, EKG changes, ↓ libido & sexual fxn, metallic taste, hyperparathyroidism, hypercalcemia, ↓ *renal fxn*

     a. Tremor – Treat with *B*-blockers (may ↑ Li⁺ level up to 20%) or calcium channel blockers

     b. Sexual dysfunction – Treat with PDE5 inhibitors (e.g., sildenafil) or aspirin 240 mg/day[503]

     c. Cutaneous side effects have been observed in almost 40% of patients

      1. Psoriasis (1.8-6%), alopecia (mostly women), rash, acne (33%), urticaria, and more[504]

     d. Cardiac - AV block (avoid in 3°) & conduction abnormalities (28-40%)

1. May unmask Brugada
  e. **Hypothyroidism is usually *irreversible*!**
    1. Not dose-related, but auto-immune related - Can occur in 6-18 months
    2. Estimated to be approx. 3% in men and 17% in women from a New Zealand study[505]
    3. 5-10X more frequent in women and ↑ incidence with those > 50 yrs old after starting Lithium
    4. If baseline TSH is 2.5-3 mIU/L, patient is at higher risk
xviii. **Long-term effects:** hypercalcemia, nephrogenic diabetes insipidus, possibly renal tumors[506]
  a. Meta-analysis found: avg. GFR ↓ by 6.22 ml/min, a very small risk of renal failure
    1. Odds ratio of developing hypothyroidism of 5.78, ↑ TSH of 4.00 mIU/L, ↑ $Ca^{2+}$ 0.09 mmol/L,
       ↑ PTH 7.32 pg/ml, and a 1.89 odds ratio of weight gain[507]
xix. **Toxicity side effects can occur with** levels ≥ 1.5 mEq/L
  a. Diarrhea, severe nausea and vomiting, coarse hand tremor, hyperreflexia, drowsiness,
     lethargy, ataxia, blurred vision, dry mouth, large output of dilute urine, confusion, arrhythmias,
     hypotension, seizures, coma, death (*person may appear drunk*)
    1. Lavage (for acute ingestion) & intermittent dialysis if blood levels > 3.5mEq/L
      i. $Li^+$ is the only psychotropic that is dialyzable!
    2. Correct / maintain fluid and electrolyte balance
    3. Monitor cardiac & respiratory fxn, and $Li^+$ level q3-4 hours
    4. Seizure precautions
  b. Situations which may ↑ Lithium levels and cause toxicity
    1. Renal disease
    2. Low sodium diet (↓$Na^+$ = ↑$Li^+$) (Patients need to maintain a consistent salt intake)
    3. Dehydration (e.g., excess sweating and exercise, protracted diarrhea, or vomiting)
    4. Postpartum fluid changes
  c. Once tolerant to GI effects, QD dosing can ↓ urinary side effects
    1. Lower doses are needed[508]

xx. *FUN FACTS:* [535-522]

‖ Newspaper clipping from February 19, 1949.[521]

• It's only # 3 on periodic table of elements (Atomic weight = 7)
• Discovered thousands of years ago in natural spring water
  ▲ **2nd Century AD** - Soranus of Ephesus treated mania & melancholia with alkaline $Li^+$ waters
• $Li^+$ can ↓ uric acid levels and was used to treat gout and kidney stones since **1847** [509]
• **1870** - Philadelphia neurologist (Dr. Mitchell) recommended lithium bromide as an anticonvulsant and a hypnotic, then later prescribed it for "general nervousness" & "mania"
• **1929** - Charles Leiper Grigg of the Howdy Company invented **7UP**
  ▲ Lithium citrate in **7UP** ("Bib-Label Lithiated Lemon-Lime Soda" later called "**7UP** Lithiated Lemon Soda") from **1929** until **1948**
  ▲ **7UP** was launched just before the great stock market crash of **1929**
  ▲ In "Great Depression" times, was marketed to lift people's spirit up
  ▲ Also promoted as a hangover cure
  ▲ $Li^+$ just happened to be in natural St. Louis spring water being used
• Lithium Chloride (LiCl) used as a salt substitute in CHF patients
  ▲ Brand names "Westal", "Foodsal", and "Salti-salt"
  ▲ Removed from US market in **1949** because of several deaths
• **1949** - John Cade, an Australian psychiatrist published his $Li^+$ experiments with guinea pigs
  ▲ He was injecting guinea pigs with the urine of psychotic patients and found it to be toxic
  ▲ Lithium's use was incidental - he was actually studying toxicity of uric acid & used $Li^+$ urate
  ▲ In guinea pigs, lithium was found to cause lethargy and unresponsiveness to stimuli[522]
  ▲ His experiments went on to human trials, but ended when some became toxic
• **1952** - first double-blind, placebo-controlled trial of lithium in mania conducted in Denmark
• Around the world small amounts of $Li^+$ (70-160 mcg/l) found in natural drinking water sources[523]
• Just 1/1000th of the therapeutic dose (called a "microdose") is correlated with many benefits[524]
  ▲ Lower violent crime rates, homicides, burglaries, theft, narcotic arrests, and rapes
  ▲ Lower admissions to psychiatric hospitals and suicides
  ▲ Reduced incidence of developing Alzheimer's Disease

## Substitute for Salt Reported Cause Of 4 Fatalities

CHICAGO.—(P)—A common table salt substitute was blamed yesterday by the American Medical association for at least four recent deaths.

The U. S. food and drug administration ordered it withdrawn from the market and asked all persons who have purchased it to "stop using this dangerous poison at once."

The substance was described by the AMA as lithium chloride. The AMA said three of the deaths occurred in Cleveland, Ohio, and one in Ann Arbor, Mich.

In Cleveland, the physician reportedly handling the cases refused to identify the victims, saying that it would be difficult to be positive that lithium chloride caused their deaths because of other contributing factors.

The Ann Arbor city health officer, Dr. John A. Wessinger, said he did not know of any such death as the AMA reported in Ann Arbor.

Dr. Morris Fishbein, editor of the AMA Journal, said "we do not know how widely the product has been distributed. There must be many cases of poisoning that have not been reported. It is to be expected that many more cases will be reported within the next few weeks."

Dr. Fishbein said the substance "is highly poisonous if a person is on a salt restricted diet."

xxi. Drug interactions:
  a. *NSAIDs, thiazide diuretics, ACEIs & ARBs* ↑ $Li^+$ up to 3X
  b. Antipsychotics (e.g. *haloperidol*) ↑ neurotoxic effects
  c. Osmotic diuretics (e.g., mannitol, urea) and methyl xanthines
     (e.g., theophylline, aminophylline & caffeine) ↓ $Li^+$ levels
xxii. Contraindications: significant renal, cardiovascular, thyroid disease
  a. Pregnancy Category D[525-531] - teratogenic in the first trimester
    1. *Ebstein's cardiac anomaly,* caution in breastfeeding, dehydration

2. Can be used in the 2nd and 3rd trimesters if benefits outweigh risks

xxiii. Lithium benefits – highly effective (80-90%)
    a. Results of 33 studies revealed a 13 X ↓ risk of suicide/attempts with long-term Li+ use[532,533]
    b. Li+ with or without VPA have less relapses in 24 months vs. VPA alone[534]
    c. Meta-analysis of 48 studies shows long-term use (>12 weeks) significantly ↓ risk of suicide for unipolar & bipolar depression[535] (60% reduced risk of suicide compared with placebo)
       1. Li+ also ↓ risk of self-harm when compared to anticonvulsant use

3. **Valproic acid (VPA)/ divalproex / valproate (Depakote®/ER, Depacon®, Stavzor®, Depakene®)**[122]
    i. Best agent for a mixed manic episode, rapid cycling, or when other comorbities are present
    ii. > 50-90% effective for acute mania and maintenance therapy
    iii. Dosage forms: 125, 250, & 500 mg D.R. tablets, 250 & 500 mg ER tablets, 125 mg D.R. sprinkle caps, 250 mg RR caps (Depakene®), 100 mg/mL injection (Depacon®), 250 mg/5 mL syrup
    iv. MOA: inhibits GABA metabolism and ↑ synthesis and release of GABA
    v. Contraindications:
      a. Those who have (or may have) a mitochondrial disorder caused by mutations in mitochondrial DNA polymerase γ (POLG) or a POLG-related disorder (e.g., *Alpers-Huttenlocher Syndrome*)
      b. Patients with known urea cycle disorders, hepatic disease or significant hepatic dysfunction
    vi. Baseline assessment
      a. CBC w/diff, LFTs, TFTs, electrolytes, SrCr, BUN, urine pregnancy test, H&P, neuro workup, EKG
    vii. Dose is 10-30 mg/kg/day / maximum 60 mg/kg/day or 3000 mg total/day
      a. Quick dosing guideline: multiply weight (in lbs.) times 10 (i.e. 150lbs x 10 =1500 mg/d)
        1. Approximates 20 mg/kg/day dose
      b. If switching to Depakote ER given QD, *must* ↑ dose by 10-20% of divalproex DR or IR dosage
    viii. Half-life is 9-16 hours, so reaches steady state in 2-3 days
    ix. Serum level range: 50-125 µg/mL (acute tx); 50-100 µg/mL (maintenance - same as for seizures)
      a. Trough: draw level just before next dose, even if it means going to a lab in the evening[536]
    x. Adverse effects: *weight gain* (70% gain > 5% body weight), *tremors, GI effects* (give with food), thrombocytopenia, alopecia, PCOS (polycystic ovarian syndrome), hyperammonemia, dizziness, rash (incl. SJS), and DRESS (i.e. Multi-organ Hypersensitivity)
    xi. **Black Box Warnings:** pancreatitis, teratogenicity, hepatotoxicity
    xii. Pregnancy Category D[526-531] for bipolar mania/seizures & Category X for migraine prophylaxis
      a. Causes *neural tube defects, spina bifida,* ↓ child's IQ by ~ 10 points[537] and ↑ risk for autism[538]
      b. Caution with breastfeeding
    xiii. Drug interactions:
      a. VPA inhibits CYP2C9[539]
      b. Others: Lamotrigine (↑ LMT levels), topiramate (↑ risk of hyperammonemia), other highly protein bound drugs, aspirin (↑ risk of bleeding), carbapenem antibiotics (↓ VPA levels)
    xiv. Pooled analysis shows significant response on YMRS (Young Mania Rating Scale) when blood levels are > 71.4 ug/mL and highest response when levels are > 94.1 ug/mL[540]
      a. Tolerability was similar at all dosages
    xv. Off-label uses include: Aggression, agitation, impulsivity, adjunct in schizophrenia, alcoholism

4. **Carbamazepine (CBZ) (Tegretol®, Tegretol XR®, Equetro™, Epitol®, Carbatrol®)**[116]
    i. Dosage forms: 100 mg cherry-flavored chewable tablets, 200 mg tablet, 100 mg/200 mg/400 mg ER tablets (Tegretol XR), 100 mg/200 mg/300 mg ER capsules (Carbatrol/Equetro), 100 mg/5 mL citrus vanilla-flavored suspension
    ii. MOA: structurally similar to TCAs; ↓ kindling (rapid cycling), ↓ DA and GABA turnover
    iii. 60% effective for acute mania; 60-75% effective for prophylaxis
    iv. Baseline assessment: same as for valproic acid + EKG (TCA-like)
    v. Initiate dosing at 100-200 mg BID and ↑ by 200 mg every 3-5 days
      a. Up to 600-1600 mg/d in divided doses used
    vi. Half-life is 25-65 hours (12-17 hours after autoinduction occurs)
      a. Initial blood level in 5 to 7 days / Serum level range: 4-12 µg/mL (trough)
    vii. Auto-inducer of its own metabolism, so should re-check CBZ levels in 5 weeks because levels may go down and dose may have to be increased
    viii. Side effects: neurologic (60% - drowsiness, nystagmus, diplopia), photosensitivity, dry mouth, GI upset (15%), hematologic (25% - transient ↓ in WBCs), rash → (incl. SJS), *hyponatremia*/SIADH, hepatic changes, hypocalcemia, & rare **agranulocytosis** (*8 per 1 million patient-yrs exposure*)
    ix. **WARNINGS:** HLA-A*3101 and HLA-B*1502 genetic allele variants are at 3-5 x ↑ risk of **SJS/TEN**
      a. 90% of time it occurs in first few months
      b. Up to 15% of non-Caucasians may carry the gene
      c. Genetic testing should be done before starting on Asians, Native Americans, Indians, etc.
      d. Not an absolute contraindication if benefits outweigh risks
      e. 25-30% cross-reactivity with oxcarbazepine
      f. HLA-A*2402 allele is independent risk factor for rash (if with HLA-B*1502 = **25 x ↑ risk**)[541]
    x. Caution with breastfeeding; Pregnancy Category D
    xi. Metabolized by CYP3A4 to active metabolite - carbamazepine-10,11-epoxide (CBZ-E)
    xii. Drug interactions: other protein bound drugs
      a. Enzyme inducer of CYP1A2 & CYP3A4 (e.g., birth control, antibiotics, anticonvulsants, anticoagulants); Must counsel patients about birth control pills not being as effective
      b. CYP3A4 inhibitors ↑ CBZ levels (e.g., -azole antifungals, grapefruit, cimetidine, fluoxetine)

5. <u>Lamotrigine (LMT) (Lamictal® / Lamictal XR®)</u>[117,118]
  i. FDA-approved for maintenance of Bipolar I in adults (not children) -- (not for acute treatment)
  ii. <mark>BBW: Risk of life-threatening rash (possible **SJS** or **TEN** - toxic epidermal necrolysis)</mark>
    a. Incidence: 0.8% of pediatrics / 0.3% of adults
    b. Usually within 2-8 weeks of initiation
    c. Angioedema may also occur
    d. *Discontinue lamotrigine at the first sign of any rash*
    e. **MUST** <u>titrate</u> dosage <u>slowly</u> to avoid triggering a serious rash
  iii. Side effects: N&V (7-25%), diarrhea (5-11%), dizziness, insomnia, somnolence, vertigo, blurred vision, diplopia, anxiety, depression, dysmenorrhea, anemia, headache, back/abdominal pain, fatigue, DRESS
    a. Rare: aseptic meningitis & agranulocytosis (1/280,000 pt-yrs exposure), hepatic failure (without rash) -- Up to 10% get a benign rash (not related to an immune response)
    b. May get flu-like symptoms and fever weeks before rash occurs
    c. People with HLA-B*1502 genetic allele variants may be at higher risk of this serious rash[542]
    d. If patient develops any signs or symptoms of systemic inflammation, they should be evaluated for Hemophagocytic Lymphohistiocytosis (HLH) is a rare but potentially fatal disease of normal but overactive histiocytes and lymphocytes
  iv. Major interaction with valproic acid, as well as EIAEDs (enzyme-inducing antiepileptic drugs)
    a. Oral contraceptives ↓ lamotrigine blood levels by 50% (no effect on oral contraceptive levels)
  v. Half-life of 24-41 hours (with valproic acid, is up to 70 hours)
  vi. Pregnancy Category C
    a. Combined oral contraceptives can ↓ lamotrigine levels by 25-50% (UGT induction)[543]
  vii. Dosing depends on other drugs being given

| | With valproic acid | As monotherapy | With an EIAED* |
|---|---|---|---|
| **Weeks 1&2** | 25 mg QOD or 12.5 mg QD | 25 mg QD | 50 mg QD |
| **Weeks 3&4** | 25 mg QD | 25 mg BID or 50 mg QD | 50 mg BID |
| **↑ dose q1-2 weeks thereafter** | 25-50mg | 50mg | 100mg |
| **Avg maintenance dose** | 100-200 mg QD (or ÷ BID) | 225-375 mg ÷ BID | 300-500 mg ÷ BID |
| *EIAED = Enzyme-inducing Anti-Epileptic Drug, such as: carbamazepine, phenytoin, phenobarbital, primidone, rifampin, estrogen-containing oral contraceptives | | | |

    a. Use ½ usual dose of lamotrigine when giving with a glucuronidation *inhibitor* (i.e., valproate)
    b. Use a higher dose of lamotrigine when giving with a glucuronidation *inducer*
      1. e.g., estrogen-containing oral contraceptives, rifampin, protease inhibitors: lopinavir/ritonavir and atazanavir/ritonavir
      2. For women on birth control pills - during the placebo week, lamotrigine levels may rise quickly
        i. If patient experiences ↑ side effects during the placebo (pill-free) week, an overall dose adjustment may be necessary, or patients should consider changing to a progestin-only contraceptive or skipping the placebo week altogether
    c. Adjust dose every 1-2 weeks, depending on other drugs being used
  viii. Availability:
    a. Tablets (scored): 25, 100, 150, and 200 mg; / XR tablets: 25, 50, 100, 200, 250, and 300 mg
    b. Chewable Dispersible Tablets: 2, 5, and 25 mg
    c. Orally Disintegrating Tablets (blackcurrant-flavored ODT): 25, 50, 100, and 200 mg

## VI. FDA-APPROVED TREATMENTS FOR BIPOLAR DISORDER

| | MANIA | DEPRESSION | MAINTENANCE |
|---|---|---|---|
| Aripiprazole | 2004*+ | | 2005* / Abilify Maintena – 2019 |
| Asenapine | 2009*+ | | 2017 |
| Carbamazepine ER | 2004 | | |
| Cariprazine | 2015 | 2019 | |
| Chlorpromazine | 1973 | | |
| Divalproex | 1994 | | |
| Lamotrigine | | | 2003 |
| Lithium | 1970+ | | 1974+ |
| Lurasidone | | 2013*+ | |
| Maprotiline | | 1974 | |
| Olanzapine | 2000*+ | | 2004 |
| Quetiapine / XR | 2004*+ | 2006 | 2008 (adjunct only) |
| Risperidone | 2003*+ | | Risperdal Consta - 2009* |
| Symbyax (OLZ/FLX) | | 2003+ | |
| Ziprasidone | 2004 | | 2009 (adjunct only) |

* = Approved as monotherapy <u>OR</u> adjunctive to lithium/valproate
+ = Also approved in pediatric patients

## VII. ADJUSTMENTS FOR RENAL AND HEPATIC IMPAIRMENTS

| NAME | RENAL | HEPATIC |
|---|---|---|
| *Mood Stabilizers* | | |
| Carbamazepine (Tegretol®) | ----- | Reduce dose |
| Lamotrigine (Lamictal®) | Reduce dose | Reduce dose |
| Lithium (Eskalith®, Lithobid®) | CrCl 10-50: ↓ dose 20-25%<br>CrCl <10: ↓ dose 50-75%<br>Dialysis: give dose after; no supplement | ----- |
| Valproic acid (Depakote/ER®, Stavzor®) | ----- | Do not use |

## VIII. OTHER BIPOLAR TREATMENTS (CONSIDERED LAST-LINE THERAPIES)[544]

A. <u>Other anticonvulsants</u>
1. *May be potentially harmful because of physical and behavioral side effects*[545]
2. Oxcarbazepine (Trileptal®)
   i. Not FDA-approved for bipolar disorder or acute mania
   ii. Can be considered as a *third-line option* when all other options have failed
   iii. Randomized controlled trials have had poor results in adults, and in children found no significant improvement in mania symptoms as compared to placebo[142,546,547]
   iv. Watch for hyponatremia and rash
3. Topiramate (Topamax®) - Some evidence in acute mania and adjunctive therapy[548-550]
   i. Not recommended for acute mania
4. Zonisamide (Zonegran®) - Positive results from an open-label trial in mania[551]
5. Gabapentin (Neurontin®), levetiracetam (Keppra®), and tiagabine (Gabitril®)[552,553]
   i. Not effective therapy vs placebo in children or adults with Bipolar
6. Pregabalin (Lyrica®) - 1 open-label trial[554]
7. Eslicarbazepine (Aptiom®) - based on case reports[555]
B. Ramelteon (Rozerem®)
1. Norris *et al.* found that adding ramelteon 8 mg/day to mood stabilizers in euthymic bipolar disorder patients with sleep disturbances for 24 weeks reduced the rate of relapse by half vs. placebo[556]
C. Riluzole (Rilutek®) - glutamate modulator
1. Evidence from case reports and open-label trials[557]
2. >200 mg/d had 66% response[544]
D. Lisdexamfetamine (Vyvanse®)
E. Calcium Channel Blockers
1. Verapamil (Calan®, Isoptin®)[558-561]
F. Antihypertensives
1. Nimodipine (Nimotop®)[562,563]
   i. Better efficacy when combined with lithium[564]
   ii. Has anticonvulsant effects
   iii. May be safer in pregnancy
2. Clonidine
3. Propranolol

## IX. COMPLEMENTARY AND ALTERNATIVE THERAPIES (CAM)[544]

A. **Omega-3 Fatty Acids** (from fatty fish)
1. Mixed results in studies due to multiple variables[565]
2. Must be combination of >60% eicosapentaenoic acid (EPA) and docosahexanoic acid (DHA)[566]
3. May be better in preventing bipolar depression[567]
4. Also safe for use in children & adolescents with bipolar disorder
B. **Electroconvulsive Therapy** (ECT)[568]
C. **L-tryptophan** (5-hydroxy-L-tryptophan) – immediate precursor of serotonin synthesis
1. 200-300 mg/d
D. **Ketogenic diet**
E. **TMS** (transcranial magnetic stimulation) and **tDCS** (transcranial direct current stimulation)
F. **Curcumin**
1. Simple table pepper (or the extract piperine) dramatically increases GI absorption of curcumin
G. Amber-colored, blue-blocking glasses
1. Worn from 6 PM to 8 AM can dramatically reduce mania in less than a week[569]
2. More information available at https://cet.org
  a. Center for Environmental Therapeutics
H. **High-density negatively-charged ionized air**[570]
1. Used in the morning for 30-90 minutes each day
2. Studies in depression show it to be very effective, but limited evidence in bipolar depression
I. **N-acetylcysteine** (NAC) – 2 grams a day for at least 8 weeks[568]
1. Precursor of glutathione
J. **Light therapy** for bipolar depression
K. **Inositol** supplementation of 12,000 to 20,000 mg/d for bipolar depression[358]
1. More effective if used as adjunctive therapy
L. **Choline** 2000-7200 mg/d added to lithium for 12 weeks for rapid cycling and mania

# X. POTENTIAL FUTURE TREATMENTS FOR BIPOLAR DISORDER IN STUDY

A. **DLP-115** by Delpor in Phase I for Bipolar I Disorder
  1. Risperidone 6-12 month formulation injection
B. **Monoclonal antibody therapy**
  1. Infliximab was not effective in study[571]
C. **Rykindo® (LY03004)** - Risperidone ER microspheres by Luye Pharma Group
  1. New Drug Application has been submitted to the FDA for both Bipolar and Schizophrenia
D. **SEP-4199** (200 & 400 mg) Currently in Phase II trials (Sunovion Pharmaceuticals)
  1. https://clinicaltrials.gov/ct2/show/NCT03543410
E. **SPN-604** (oxcarbazepine) by Supernus Pharmaceuticals is in Phase II trials for bipolar disorder

# XI. TREATMENT OF BIPOLAR DEPRESSION[463-465,468]

A. All approved medications carry a BBW about suicidal thoughts in pediatric & young adult patients
B. Symbyax® (olanzapine + fluoxetine [OLZ/FLX]), quetiapine (Seroquel®), and lurasidone (Latuda®)[572] approved for bipolar depression
C. Quetiapine also approved for mania and bipolar maintenance
D. Antidepressants not recommended to be used alone; can induce mania and ↑ rate of cycling
  1. May be no more effective than placebo[481]
E. Bupropion (Wellbutrin®) has least likelihood of inducing mania (no 5HT effects)
  1. Not FDA-approved for use in bipolar disorder
F. Maprotiline (Ludiomil®)[169] is FDA-approved for depression from manic-depressive illness
G. Olanzapine [OLZ] and fluoxetine [FLX] HCl capsules (Symbyax®)[121]
  1. FDA-approved for bipolar depression and Treatment-Resistant Depression
    i. Approved in children >10 yrs old
  2. Available in 3/25 mg, 6/25 mg, 6/50 mg, 12/25 mg, and 12/50 mg capsules [OLZ/FLX]
  3. Start with lowest dose possible and titrate slowly
  4. Side effects: Drowsiness, weight gain, increased appetite, feeling weak, swelling, tremor, sore throat and difficulty concentrating
  5. Fluoxetine can increase QT-interval
  6. Caution when combining with QT-prolonging drugs
H. Quetiapine (Seroquel XR®)[227]
  1. FDA-approved as monotherapy for bipolar depression
  2. Average dose in study responders was approximately 300 mg/d
I. Cariprazine (Vraylar®)[215]
  1. FDA-approved as monotherapy for bipolar depression
  2. Average doses are 1.5-3 mg/d
  3. For bipolar depression, the maximum recommended dose is 3 mg/d
J. Lurasidone (Latuda®)[220]
  1. FDA-approved as monotherapy for bipolar depression in children ≥ 13 y.o. & adults
  2. Not yet approved for bipolar mania, although studies underway
  3. Low risk of metabolic effects
  4. In bipolar depression, dose is 20-80 mg/d
K. Thyroid hormone supplementation
  1. CANMAT 2018 Guidelines[573] and studies[574,575] found that supratherapeutic levels of thyroid hormone (e.g., 300 mcg/d) will help with bipolar depression without significant side effects
  2. Keep TSH around 2.6 mIU/L (especially in lithium-treated patients)

# XII. COMPARISON OF NNT TO NNH FOR BIPOLAR DEPRESSION TREATMENTS[576-578]

| Medication | NNT (lower is better) | NNH (higher is better) | LHH (Risk:benefit ratio) |
|---|---|---|---|
| Antidepressants (pooled data) | 29 | 200 (mania) | 6.9 |
| Lithium | 15 | 38 (tremor/nausea) | 2.5 |
| Valproic acid | 4.4 | 5 (nausea) | 1.1 |
| Carbamazepine | 3.4 (1 trial only) | 8.8 (dizziness) | 2.6 |
| Armodafinil (Nuvigil®) - *off-label* | 9 | 29 (anxiety) | 3.2 |
| Lamotrigine | 12 | 37 (sedation) | 3.1 |
| Olanzapine + fluoxetine combo | 4 | 6 (weight gain) | 1.5 |
| Quetiapine | 6 | 5 (sedation) | 0.8 |
| Lurasidone | 5 | 15 (akathisia/nausea) | 3 |
| Cariprazine | ? | ? | ? |

★ NNT (number needed to treat - how many patients to treat before getting one positive response)
★ NNH (number needed to harm - i.e., side effects)
★ LHH = NNH ÷ NNT (LHH > 1 means that treatment more likely to help than harm)
★ Based on table above, the agent with the best profile is lurasidone

**XII. OTHER BIPOLAR DEPRESSION TREATMENTS (LAST-LINE THERAPIES)[544]**
  A. Lamotrigine and antidepressants > 2 X as likely to yield benefit as harm
    1. Lamotrigine better in severely depressed patients and/or with adjunct lithium[579]
    2. Antidepressant efficacy is low (not superior to mood stabilizer alone)[481,495]
    3. *The International Society for Bipolar Disorders (ISBD) guidelines say that antidepressants may be used if there's a previous history of prior positive response*[480]
      i. *Antidepressants should be AVOIDED if history of rapid cycling, mixed bipolar, or previous antidepressant-induced mania*
      ii. *Never use as monotherapy (i.e., without a mood stabilizer)*
    4. Antidepressant + antipsychotic may be useful and supported by expert opinions[484]
  B. Lithium and valproic acid not overly effective. May be useful as adjuncts[580]
  C. Aripiprazole, ziprasidone, and risperidone not effective in trials

**XIV. POTENTIAL FUTURE TREATMENTS FOR BIPOLAR DEPRESSION IN STUDY**
  A. **ALKS 3831** - Alkermes plc developed combination product of olanzapine + samidorphan to mitigate the metabolic effects of olanzapine[581]
  B. **Armodafinil/modafinil**[582] adjunctive therapy
  C. **Brexpiprazole** (Lu AF41156, OPC-34712; Rexulti) by Otsuka in Phase III trials
  D. **Coenzyme Q10** (CoQ10) for bipolar depression
    1. Supported by a few studies, particularly in geriatric bipolar depression[583]
  E. **Cyclurad™** (NRX-101) by NeuroRx (Pharmaceutical company) in Phase II/III trials
    1. A combination of D-cycloserine (Seromycin®) and lurasidone (Latuda®) into one pill[584]
      i. D-cycloserine is a partial agonist/antagonist of the glycine site of the NMDA receptor
    2. Administered daily for 6 weeks following an initial, single infusion of NRX-100 (ketamine)
    3. Small open-label trial results with 4 patients show efficacy for up to 2 months[585]
    4. Also being studied in patients with Acute Suicidal Ideation & Behavior (ASIB)
  F. L-methylfolate, pioglitazone, and celecoxib -- Need further study
  G. **Lumateperone** (ITI-007, ITI-722)[586] – Intra-cellular Therapies
    1. Phase III for Behavioral disorders & Bipolar depression (finished 2 Phase III trials)
    2. An atypical antipsychotic with a complex mechanism of action
      i. Dopamine and NR2B glutamate receptor modulator, 5HT2A antagonist; 5HT plasma membrane transport protein inhibitor and 5HT reuptake inhibitor
  H. **Pramipexole**[587] (>60% response and a large effect size of 0.77-1.1)
  I. **Tamoxifen**[588], **ramelteon**, and **ketamine**
  J. **Zuranolone** (SAGE-217/S812217) - SAGE Therapeutics
    1. A synthetic, orally active, inhibitory pregnane neuro-steroid, that acts as a positive allosteric modulator of the $GABA_A$ receptor
    2. Developed as an improvement of allopregnanolone (brexanolone/Zulresso™) with high oral bioavailability and a biological half-life suitable for once-daily administration
    3. Currently in Phase III trials for Major depressive disorder, Postnatal depression, and Insomnia
    4. In Phase II trials for Bipolar Depression, Essential Tremors, and Parkinson's Disease

# 21. DEPRESSIVE DISORDERS AND ANTIDEPRESSANTS[589-597]

## I. MAJOR DEPRESSIVE DISORDER (MDD) BACKGROUND
A. In 2017, affected more than 17.3 million (7.1%) American adults[431]
   1. Highest among young adults aged 18-25 (13.1%)
   2. More prevalent among adult females (8.7%) compared to males (5.3%)[296]
   3. Median age at onset is 32.5-years-old, but can develop at any age
B. The leading cause of disability in the U.S. for ages 15 to 44
C. Heritability is approximately 40%[245,598]
D. About 65% of adults with MDD are receiving combined care of medication and therapy
E. In 2017, men died by suicide 3.54x more often than women[599]
   1. Women attempted suicide twice as often as men
   2. The rate of suicide is highest in middle-age white men (70%)
   3. Firearms account for > 50% of all suicide deaths
F. Recurrence rates of major depression[275,600,601]

|                          | After 1 year | After 2 years | After 5 years |
|--------------------------|--------------|---------------|---------------|
| After 1st episode        | 25%          | 42%           | 60%           |
| After 2nd episode        | 41%          | 59%           | 74%           |

G. **Persistent Depressive Disorder or PDD** (formerly called dysthymia)
   1. A consolidation of chronic MDD and dysthymic disorder from the DSM-IV-TR
   2. Affects around 3.3 million American adults (~ 1.5% of the U.S. adult population in a given year)

## II. DSM-5 DIAGNOSES
A. Major Depressive Disorder (MDD)
   1. Depressed Mood <u>or</u> loss of pleasure (i.e., anhedonia), most of the day (more days than not)
   2. With > 4 SIGECAPS (acronym for symptoms)[244]
   3. Sx must be present for > 2 weeks to diagnose
B. Disruptive Mood Dysregulation Disorder
   1. See Child & Adolescent Disorders chapter
C. Persistent Depressive Disorder
   1. Depressed mood, as with MDD
   2. For > 2 yrs (1 yr in children/adolescents)
   3. Symptoms absent no more than 2 months at a time
D. Premenstrual Dysphoric Disorder (PMDD)
   1. Symptoms present in the week before menses
   2. Symptoms improve a few days after menses
   3. Symptoms minimal or absent in weeks post-menses
   4. > 5 total symptoms from below
      i. > 1 symptom: Mood is labile, irritable, angry, anxious, and/or depressed
      ii. > 1 symptom from the indicated SIGECAPS, being overwhelmed, and/or physical symptoms (breast tenderness, joint/muscle pain, bloating, weight gain)

> **SIGECAPS**
> SUICIDE (or thoughts of death)
> INTERESTS (including SEX)
> GUILT
> ENERGY
> CONCENTRATION
> APPETITE (↓ or ↑)
> PSYCHOMOTOR
>   (agitation or retardation)
> SLEEP (↓ or ↑)

## III. SOME SUB-TYPES OF DEPRESSION[245,602]
A. Clinical content subtypes [and characteristics][603]
   1. Subtype 1: Depressed mood [sad, depressed, tearful, with recurrent thoughts of death/suicide]
   2. Subtype 2: Anhedonic depression [markedly diminished interests or pleasure in most everything]
   3. Subtype 3: Cognitive depression [diminished ability to concentrate, think, and make decisions]
   4. Subtype 4: Somatic depression [weight changes, sleep changes, low energy, and psychomotor agitation, irritability or retardation]
   5. Matching antidepressant therapy's effects/side-effects can improve tolerability of therapy and target symptoms directly
B. *Melancholic Depression's* hallmark characteristics:
   1. Also called "endogenous depression"
   2. Considered to be a severe form of depression that may be biologically-based[604]
   3. More associated with ↑ cortisol from a hyperactive HPA (hypothalamic-pituitary-adrenal) axis
   4. Higher prevalence in colder climates and low sunlight exposure[605]
   5. Anhedonia (loss of pleasure) in most or all activities
   6. Practically devoid of the capacity for pleasure
   7. Lack of reactivity to usually pleasurable stimuli (does not feel much better when circumstances around them are very good)
   8. Profound despondency, despair, moroseness, or empty mood
   9. Highly anxious / Increased sympathetic activity
   10. Mood is regularly worse in the morning
   11. Early-morning awakening (i.e., at least 2 hours before usual awakening)
   12. Significant anorexia or weight loss
   13. Risk of increased infections from immunosuppressed state
   14. Risk of premature osteoporosis
   15. Significant and observable psychomotor agitation or retardation
   16. May respond better to TCAs and SNRIs

C. *Atypical Depression's* hallmark characteristics:
  1. Occurs in approx. 16-37% of all depressed patients[606]
  2. Also called "exogenous depression"
  3. Associated with normal or reduced HPA (hypothalamic-pituitary-adrenal) axis activity
  4. May respond to a test dose of prednisone
  5. Mood improves when good things happen (i.e., positive mood reactivity)
  6. Significant weight gain or increase in appetite
  7. Hypersomnia (at least 2 more hours of sleep than when not depressed)
  8. "Leaden paralysis" (a feeling that the arms or legs are heavy and hard to move)
  9. Overly sensitivity to rejection by others that results in severe social or occupational impairment
  10. More common in younger patients and females
  11. Depression worse in the evening
  12. Strong link to bipolar
  13. Decreased sympathetic activity and low anxiety
  14. Increased inflammation from immuno-enhanced state
  15. Long ago, MAOIs were the drugs of choice for treatment
    i. SSRIs & bupropion considered first-line today
D. *Peri-partum's* hallmark characteristics:
  1. Can occur during pregnancy or within 4 weeks after giving birth
  2. 50% of women who develop depression will have depression start during their pregnancy
  3. High comorbidity with anxiety
  4. Depression with psychotic features very rare, but can pose risk to the infant by the mother
E. Other types of depression:
  1. Seasonal (previously called Seasonal Affective Disorder)
  2. With catatonia
  3. With psychotic features or symptoms

## IV. MEDICAL CONDITIONS FREQUENTLY ASSOCIATED WITH DEPRESSION[275,276]

| | |
|---|---|
| ★ Cardiovascular Disease | ★ Metabolic disorders |
| ★ Collagen disorders | ★ Neurologic disorders (e.g., Parkinson's, |
| ★ Endocrine disorders (i.e., hypothyroidism - |   Wilson's Disease, CVA - 30-50%)[609] |
|   40%)[607] | ★ Systemic Lupus Erythematosis (SLE) |
| ★ Infections (i.e. encephalitis, hepatitis, | ★ Vitamin and mineral deficiencies and |
|   tuberculosis) |   excesses [Vitamin D deficiency not |
| ★ Restless Leg Syndrome (2.6 - 4x ↑ risk)[608] |   proven[610]] |

## V. DRUGS THAT CAN CAUSE DEPRESSIVE REACTIONS[611]

| | |
|---|---|
| ★ Alcohol | ★ Hydralazine (Apresoline®) |
| ★ Amantadine (Symmetrel®) | ★ Levodopa (Larodopa®, Dopar®) |
| ★ Any CNS depressant | ★ Marijuana |
| ★ *Beta*-blockers (i.e., propranolol)[612] | ★ Methyldopa (Aldomet®) |
| ★ Clonidine (Catapres®) | ★ Non-aspirin NSAIDs or high dose Aspirin[615] |
| ★ Guanethidine (Ismelin®) | ★ Opiate analgesics |
| ★ Corticosteroids | ★ Oral contraceptives *(Treat with Vitamin B6* |
| ★ Gabapentin & Pregabalin[613] |   *50 mg/d* [616-620]*)* |
| ★ Efavirenz (Sustiva®) - risk of suicidal | ★ Reserpine from *Rauwolfia serpentina* (Indian |
|   ideation/attempt doubles[614] |   snakeroot) |

## VI. HISTORY OF ANTIDEPRESSANTS[621]

A. For > **5000 years**, Chinese physicians used stimulants to treat many depressive disorders
  1. Natural *ephedrine* was derived from its herbal source, *Ma-huang*[394]
B. **Mid-1800s**: cocaine was widely available
  1. Used as a stimulant, euphoriant, nasal decongestant, and anesthetic
C. **Circa 1870**: "Wine of Coca" - an alcoholic extract was marketed[622,623]
  1. Contained 6 mg cocaine per ounce of wine
D. **1886**: John Pemberton (pharmacist in Atlanta, Georgia) made *Coca-Cola* with cocaine laced syrup
  and *kola nut* (due to public pressure the cocaine content was dropped from *Coca-Cola* in **1903**)
E. **1887**: Case reports from Myerson in 1936 revealed amphetamines usefulness in depression,
  manic-depression, and "dementia praecox"[398]
  1. Mood-lifting effects of the stimulants were temporary
    i. Antidepressant effects did not last because of excessive release of CNS neurotransmitters
    ii. Once a majority of neurotransmitters released from pre-synaptic vesicles & used in neuro-
      transmission, they can't be remanufactured quickly enough to sustain the antidepressant effect
      a. The net effect is too much demand and not enough supply, hence the depression returns
    iii. Benzedrine marketed in 1935 for narcolepsy and depression
F. **1938**: Cerletti and Bini first experimented with Electroconvulsive Therapy (ECT) to treat
  schizophrenia, mood disorders, and other psychiatric conditions[624]
  1. Quickly became the standard treatment for mental illness as there were very few viable options[395]
  2. Deemed successful in 74-90% of severe depression cases while maintaining remission in 50%[625]
G. Late **1940s** and early **1950s**: *tuberculosis* was a widespread epidemic
  1. Patients were isolated from society in long-term hospitals called "*sanitariums*" for treatment
  2. Some patients became depressed because of their circumstances
H. **1951** and **1952**: two drugs were used to treat the tuberculosis infection: isoniazid and iproniazid[626]

1. *Iproniazid*, but not isoniazid, elevated the mood of the depressed patients
2. *Iproniazid* was discovered to inhibit the enzyme monoamine oxidase (MAO)
3. Marketed **1958** as a commercial antidepressant[627]
   i. Due to hepatotoxicity, it was withdrawn in the U.S. (but not in the United Kingdom) and replaced with a less toxic monoamine oxidase inhibitor (MAOI) medication, isocarboxazid[626]
I. **1931**: reserpine (Serpasil®) was extracted from Indian Snakeroot (*rauwolfia serpentina*)[628-631]
   1. Used in India (Ayurvedic medicine) for hundreds of years to treat "insanity"
      i. Called "pagla-ka-dacra" ("insanity herb"), which in Urdu, also means "crazy ass"
   2. Found to irreversibly inhibit the intracellular vesicular monoamine transporter (VMAT)
      i. Neurotransmitters couldn't be "packaged" into vesicles for presynaptic release
   3. In **1940's**, use grew as a psychotropic and sedative
   4. **1950's**: Use as an antihypertensive was associated with a 10-15% risk of severe depression
J. **Mid 1900s**, chemists were discovering antihistamines & sedatives to use as surgical anesthetics[395]
   1. **Late 1940s**: 40 derivatives of *iminodibenzyl* were discovered by Häflinger and Schindler[626]
      i. **1957**: found *Imipramine* (G22355) a promazine analogue - was the **first** TCA approved in **1959**
K. **1965** and **1969**: noradrenaline and serotonin molecules discovered, respectively[632]
   1. Antidepressants tested and discovered to ALL activate cyclic AMP within specific brain regions

**VII. ANTIDEPRESSANTS (ONCE CALLED THYMOANALEPTICS OR THYMOLEPTICS)**
A. Mechanisms of action (shared by most antidepressants)[633]
   1. Inhibit the pre-synaptic reuptake of 5HT, NE, and/or DA by impairing specific transporter proteins
      i. Serotonin (5HT) reuptake transporter (SERT)
      ii. Norepinephrine (NE) reuptake transporter (NET)
      iii. Dopamine (DA) reuptake transporter (DAT)
   2. Antidepressants ↑ brain-derived neurotrophic factor (BDNF)[634]
   3. They are neuroprotective, ↑ synaptogenesis, and ↑ neuroplasticity
      i. Neuroplasticity includes changes in gene regulation & intracellular signaling cascade, variations in neurotransmitter release, modifications of synaptic number & strength, modeling of dendritic & axonal architecture and, in some areas of the CNS, the generation of new neurons[635]
   4. They ↑ volume of the hippocampus (lost because of depression)
B. Length of antidepressant treatment[274]
   1. 1st time depressed → treat 6 months to 1 year
   2. 2nd time depressed → treat 2 years (have 70% chance of relapse)
   3. 3 or more times depressed → treat with lifetime therapy
      i. Have > 90% chance of relapse, which increases with each subsequent episode
C. 50-65% response rate / remission rates are lower ≈ 30-40%
   1. Placebo response decreases with more severe depression[636]
   2. Publication biases (i.e., only publishing positive trial results) may actually reveal a much lower response rate (avg. 32%)[637]
D. May take 2 to 6 weeks to work (sometimes even up to 12 weeks)
E. *Always start with the lowest possible dose and slowly titrate up for best tolerability to side effects*
F. All antidepressants lower seizure threshold!!
   1. Highest risk with bupropion, amoxapine, and maprotiline (B A M)
G. Antidepressants are not addictive
H. 55% of patients taking SSRIs (except fluoxetine), SNRIs, and mirtazapine may gain some weight in first 3 years of taking their antidepressant (40% gain ≥ 7% body weight)[638]
I. SSRIs may be associated with a small ↑ risk of bone fractures in peri-menopausal women[639]
J. An "umbrella" review (i.e., a meta-analysis of 45 meta-analyses of 4471 studies) found no convincing evidence of long-term negative side effects of antidepressant use[640]
K. Long-term SSRI use may actually *delay the progression* of mild cognitive impairment to dementia or Alzheimer's Disease[641]
L. Nortriptyline (and possibly other TCAs) may reduce progression of Parkinson's Disease
   1. Nortriptyline prevents the formation of intracellular inclusions comprised primarily of misfolded, fibrillar α-synuclein (α-syn), which cause neuronal cell death[642]
   2. The *Michael J. Fox Foundation* is currently funding a study to validate this[643]
M. **ALL** antidepressants carry a **Black Box Warning** about suicidal thoughts and behaviors in children, adolescents, and young adults (up to age 24)
   1. **March 2004** – FDA cautions prescribers to monitor for suicidal ideation (SI) and issues BBW[644]
      i. Based on 24 RCTs (n=4400 youth) showing new onset SI seen in 4% of antidepressant-treated vs. 2% of placebo-treated patients[645]
      ii. No deaths occurred in any trials reviewed
   2. Paroxetine & venlafaxine: ↑ suicidality more[646,647]
      i. FDA issued a warning not to use paroxetine in children/adolescents
   3. From 1998-2002: a 50% ↑ in antidepressant prescribing
   4. Completed suicides ↓ over 10 years (1992-2002) in youth
   5. After FDA warning in **2004**: 10-16% ↓ in antidepressant prescribing[648]
   6. U.S. teen & young adult suicide rates ↑ by 22-34%[649]
   7. Largest annual change since **1979** (when CDC started data collection)
   8. **2007**: Meta-analysis of RCT for antidepressants in youth show antidepressants more effective than placebo for MDD, OCD, and non-OCD anxiety disorders[650]
   9. Highest suicide risk in the first 9 days of treatment and with higher starting doses[440]

10. Patients should NEVER be started on an antidepressant without someone periodically monitoring their thoughts and mood
   i. For children and adults $\leq$ 24-years-old: *every week for the first month*, then every 2 weeks for a month, and then again in 1 month
N. Antidepressants are considered relatively safe in pregnancy (if benefits outweigh risks)
  1. A majority (up to 80%) of new mothers experience some depressive symptoms[651]
  2. Estimated 10 to 20% of new mothers have clinical postpartum depression (PPD)
    i. Risk is > 30% higher if there are previous episodes of depression or PDD
  3. 50% of women may began experiencing depressive symptoms during pregnancy
  4. National Pregnancy Registry for Antidepressants
    i. 1-844-405-6185 or online at https://womensmentalhealth.org/clinical-and-research-programs/pregnancyregistry/antidepressants/
O. **July 2014** - *Warning* added to <u>ALL</u> antidepressants for potential *angle closure glaucoma*[652]
P. Caution: SSRIs, SNRIs, and bupropion can trigger a first-time seizure in some patients
  1. Risk is double of those with no antidepressant exposure[653]
Q. *Hyponatremia* - more common with SSRIs and venlafaxine - less with mirtazapine and TCAs[654]
R. Diabetes doubles the risk of developing depression and vice-versa[655]
  1. SSRIs, SNRIs, and bupropion are preferred because of less weight gain vs. TCAs/MAOIs
S. Cognitive therapy enhances recovery rate with antidepressants in severe, non-chronic depression[656]
T. Cardiovascular diseases
  1. In Acute Coronary Syndrome, depression is a risk factor for poor prognosis[657]
  2. After a myocardial infarction - 6 x more likely to die within 6 months (risk $\uparrow$'ed for 18 mo.)[658]
  3. Receiving treatment for depression increases survival[659]
  4. Treatment of moderate to severe depression $\downarrow$ risk of CV death, CAD, and stroke[660]
U. Danish study: low-dose aspirin, statins, allopurinol and ACE/ARBs $\downarrow$ risk of incident depression[615]
  Canadian nested case-control study found risk of suicide was 1.6 x higher for ARBs than ACEIs[661]
V. Initial co-treatment with short-term prn BZD can reduce initial $\uparrow$ anxiety (est. in 10.6% of pts.)[662]
  1. Approx. 1 in 8 will continue on long-term BZD use, so caution advised to prevent future addiction
W. **Antidepressant Discontinuation Syndrome** (ADS)[663-666]

| | |
|---|---|
| 1. Antidepressant withdrawal associated with an antidepressant's side effects<br>2. Occurs mostly with short half-life antidepressants<br>3. TCA withdrawal may include cholinergic " rebound" such as abdominal cramping, diarrhea, Parkinsonism and other problems with movement | 4. Characterized by the "FINISH" syndrome<br>**F**lu-like symptoms<br>**I**nsomnia<br>**N**ausea<br>**I**mbalance<br>**S**ensory disturbances<br>**H**yperarousal (anxiety/agitation) |

## VIII. ANTIDEPRESSANTS' MECHANISM OF ACTION SIMPLIFIED

A. Once started, antidepressants $\uparrow$ quantity of neurotransmitters (5HT, NE, or DA) in the synaptic cleft
B. This begins a domino effect[302]
C. Chronic 5HT stimulation is believed to desensitize somatodendritic $5HT_{1A/1B/1D}$ & $5HT_7$ autoreceptors
D. This downregulates (desensitizes) presynaptic $\alpha2$ autoreceptors and postsynaptic $\beta1$ receptors
E. Theoretically, antidepressant response can be hastened by $5HT_{1A/1B/1D}$ & $5HT_7$ antagonists
F. $5HT_{1A}$ post-synaptic receptors inhibit neural firing in the limbic center, which may be hyperactive in depression[667]

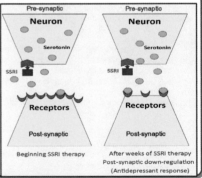

Beginning SSRI therapy — After weeks of SSRI therapy
Post-synaptic down-regulation
(Antidepressant response)

## IX. TCAs (HETEROCYCLIC / TRICYCLIC ANTIDEPRESSANTS)[161-169]

| Generic Name | Brand Name | Dosage range (mg/d) | Neurotransmitters affected | Amine class |
|---|---|---|---|---|
| Amitriptyline[161] | Elavil® | 25-300 | 5HT > NE | Tertiary (3°) |
| Amoxapine | Asendin® | 50-600 | NE > 5HT | Secondary (2°) |
| Clomipramine | Anafranil® | 25-250 | 5HT >> NE | Tertiary (3°) |
| Desipramine | Norpramin® | 25-300 | NE >> 5HT | Secondary (2°) |
| Doxepin | Sinequan® | 25-300 | 5HT = NE | Tertiary (3°) |
| Imipramine | Tofranil® | 25-300 | 5HT > NE | Tertiary (3°) |
| Maprotiline | Ludiomil® | 50-225 | NE >>>> 5HT | Secondary (2°) |
| Nortriptyline | Pamelor® | 25-150 | NE > 5HT | Secondary (2°) |
| Protriptyline | Vivactil® | 15-60 | NE > 5HT | Secondary (2°) |
| Trimipramine | Surmontil® | 25-300 | 5HT > NE | Tertiary (3°) |

A. MOA: 5HT/NE reuptake inhibitor (i.e., the first SNRIs)
B. Evaluate suicide potential because toxic doses (750-1500mg) can kill!!
C. Pregnancy category B or C
 1. Maprotiline (Ludiomil®) is pregnancy category B and FDA-approved for **Bipolar Depression**
D. Secondary (2°) amines inhibit the reuptake of NE more than 5HT
E. Tertiary (3°) amines inhibit the reuptake of 5HT more than NE
F. Amoxapine (metabolite of loxapine) also blocks $D_2$ receptors (watch for EPS)
G. Adverse reactions: drowsiness, CNS stimulation (2° amines), toxic psychosis
 1. Anticholinergic effects (dry mouth, constipation, tachycardia etc.)
 2. Autonomic side effects (nasal congestion, tremors, sexual dysfunction)
 3. Cardiac side effects (arrhythmias, *QT interval prolongation*, hypotension/orthostasis)
  i. ☻ Responsible for death in overdoses ☻
  ii. Do not use during the acute recovery period after a myocardial infarction
 4. Weight gain
 5. Rare: seizures, allergic reactions, agranulocytosis, cholestatic jaundice
H. Many are metabolized by CYP2D6, so dosage adjustments may be needed with CYP2D6 inhibitors or inducers, or those with polymorphisms of CYP2D6

## X. MAOIs (MONOAMINE OXIDASE INHIBITORS)
A. All are cautioned for use during pregnancy
B. MOA: non-selectively and irreversibly inhibit monoamine oxidase (MAO)
 1. Takes up to 2 weeks for the body to replenish MAO enzymes after drug discontinuation
 2. Medications are non-selective for MAO-A and MAO-B
  i. MAO-A breaks down 5HT, melatonin, NE, epinephrine, tyramine and dopamine
  ii. MAO-B breaks down dopamine and phenethylamine
C. Adverse reactions: postural hypotension, hepatic complications, anticholinergic effects (< TCAs), sedation (most with phenelzine), stimulation (most with tranylcypromine), sexual dysfunction
D. Phenelzine and isocarboxazid are labeled for use in those over 16 years of age[170,172]
E. ***SIGNIFICANT*** drug-drug and food-drug interactions – USE THESE DRUGS WITH CAUTION!!!
 1. Hypertensive crisis with tyramine-containing foods or sympathomimetic-containing drugs[171]
 2. Phentolamine 5 mg IV has been used in emergencies to lower BP
 3. Drugs to avoid:
  i. OTC decongestants, dextromethorphan
  ii. ALL other antidepressants, stimulants, cocaine
  iii. "Street drugs", herbal remedies
  iv. Buspirone, meperidine, cyclobenzaprine, carbamazepine, fenfluramine
  v. Dopamine agonists used in Parkinson's disease
  vi. Excessive caffeine intake
 4. Avoid tyramine-containing foods, in which aging is used to increase flavor
  i. Essentially anything pickled, canned, aged, or bottled for later
  ii. Cheese (particularly strong or aged varieties)
  iii. Cream, chocolate, soy sauce, sauerkraut, yeast extracts, yogurt
  iv. Chianti wine, sherry, beer (including non-alcoholic beer), liqueurs
  v. Pickled herring, anchovies, caviar, liver, meat extracts, or meat prepared with tenderizers
  vi. Canned figs, dried fruits (raisins, prunes, etc.), bananas, raspberries, avocados, overripe fruit, the pods of broad beans (e.g., fava beans)
F. Isocarboxazid (Marplan®)[172]
 1. Dose range 10-60 mg/d divided BID to QID
 2. Available in 10 mg tablets
 3. Pregnancy category C
G. Phenelzine (Nardil®)[170]
 1. Derived from isoniazid
 2. Dose range is 15-90 mg/d divided TID to QID
 3. Available in 15 mg tablets
H. Selegiline patch (EMSAM®) – supposedly no dietary restrictions necessary at 6 mg/d dose[103]
 1. Higher doses (9-12 mg/d) require dietary restrictions
 2. Available in 6, 9, and 12 mg/24h patches
 3. Pregnancy category C
 4. Contraindicated in children under 12 and not approved for use in 12-17 year-olds
  i. DBPC trial in adolescents showed no benefit[668]
 5. Contraindicated to be used along with carbamazepine
I. Tranylcypromine (Parnate®)[171]
 1. Dose range is 10-60 mg/d divided up to TID
 2. Available in 10 mg tablets

## XI. SSRIs (SELECTIVE SEROTONIN REUPTAKE INHIBITORS)
A. *Common adverse reactions:* weight loss, anorexia, anxiety, insomnia, headache, sweating, nausea, diarrhea, sexual dysfunction (very common, but under-reported by patients)
 1. ↑ risk of gastrointestinal bleeding, because of ↓ platelet aggregation[669]
B. *The best tolerated SSRIs are escitalopram and sertraline*[669]
C. Citalopram (Celexa®)[179] – Discovered in 1977
 1. Metabolized by CYP3A4 and CYP2C19

2. 80% protein bound
3. Half-life: 35 hours
4. Interacts with QT-prolonging drugs in congenital long QT syndrome (NOT RECOMMENDED!)
   i. 60 mg dose ↑QTc by about 18.5 ms (mostly due to R-enantiomer)
   ii. http://www.fda.gov/Drugs/DrugSafety/ucm269086.htm
5. Less adverse reactions than other SSRIs
6. Available in 10, 20, and 40 mg tablets, and 10 mg/5 mL peppermint-flavored oral solution
7. Adult Dosing: 10-40 mg/d (clinical trials showed 60 mg no more effective than 40mg)
   i. Elderly (over 60 y.o.) or patients receiving potent CYP2C9 inhibitors: Max dose of 20 mg/d
   ii. Known CYP2C19 poor metabolizers – Max dose of 20 mg/d
D. Escitalopram (Lexapro®)[180]
   1. S-optical isomer (enantiomer) of citalopram
   2. 2-4 times as potent as citalopram
   3. Half-life: 35 hours
   4. Little or non-significant drug interactions
   5. Available in 5, 10, and 20 mg tablets, and 1 mg/mL mint-flavored oral solution
   6. Dosing: 5-20 mg/d (max dose for geriatric patients is 10 mg/d)
E. Fluoxetine (Prozac®, Sarafem®)[173] – Discovered in 1974
   1. Active metabolite - norfluoxetine
   2. T½ = 4-16 days (VERY LONG!!!) – including active metabolite
   3. May be good for non-adherent patients
   4. 95% protein bound
   5. Metabolized by CYP2D6 (potent inhibitor)
   6. Dosing: 10-80 mg/d usually given in the AM (to reduce insomnia)
   7. Available in 10, 15, 20, 40 & 90 mg caplets/tablets, and 20 mg/5 mL mint-flavored oral solution
      i. Generic 60 mg scored tablet also available (Edgemont Pharmaceuticals)
   8. Drug interactions: MAOIs or Tryptophan (serotonin syndrome), other highly protein bound drugs, other drugs metabolized by CYP2D6
   9. Fluoxetine can increase QT-interval. Caution when combined with QT-prolonging drugs
      i. Can cause Torsades de Pointes (TdP)
   10. Not recommended for use if breastfeeding
   11. Recently discovered to inhibit the Hepatitis C virus[670]
F. Fluvoxamine (Luvox®/Luvox CR®)[178]
   1. Metabolized by CYP1A2 and CYP3A4 (potent inhibitor) > 9 metabolites (most inactive)
   2. 80% protein bound
   3. Half-life: 16 hours (26 hours in the elderly)
   4. ↓ clearance with hepatic impairment
   5. Should be given with food to decrease nausea
   6. Usually dosed in the PM (AM if insomnia occurs) or BID - Luvox CR® is QD
   7. Dosage range: 25-300 mg/d
   8. Available in 25, 50, & 100 mg tablets or 100 & 150 mg ER capsules
   9. Drug interactions: MAOIs, inhibits CYP1A2 and CYP3A4, propranolol and metoprolol (bradycardia/hypotension), triazolam and alprazolam (↑ levels), digoxin and warfarin (↑ levels), smoking ↑ clearance by 25%, lithium (seizures), tryptophan (vomiting)
G. Paroxetine (Paxil®/Paxil CR®/Pexeva®/Brisdelle™)[175-177] - Discovered in 1990
   1. NO active metabolites
   2. 95% protein bound
   3. Half-life: 21 hours
   4. CYP2D6 enzyme inhibitor > Prozac
   5. Dosing: 10-60 mg/d usually given at HS
      i. Above 40 mg/d, it potently inhibits NE reuptake
      ii. Max dose for depression: 50 mg/d
      iii. Max dose for OCD: 60 mg/d
      iv. Reduce dose by 50% in patients with CrCl < 50 ml/min
   6. Brisdelle™ (for vasomotor symptoms associated with menopause) available in 7.5 mg capsules
   7. Paxil® and Pexeva® (paroxetine mesylate): available in 10, 20, 30, and 40 mg tablets, and 10 mg/5 mL orange-flavored oral suspension
   8. Paxil CR®: available in 12.5, 25, and 37.5 mg tablets
   9. Most sedating, anticholinergic, and most likely to cause long-term weight gain of the SSRIs
   10. Pregnancy Category D!!![671]
   11. Not good for breastfeeding
   12. FDA has issued a warning against its use in children due to increased emotional lability!!!
H. Sertraline (Zoloft®)[174] – Discovered in 1983
   1. Active metabolite - desmethylsertraline
   2. ≥ 97% protein bound
   3. Half-life: 26 hours
   4. Minor inhibitor of CYP2D6 and CYP3A4 (not very significant)
   5. Dosing: 25-200 mg/d (avg. 100-150 mg/d) usually given in the AM (to reduce insomnia)
   6. Available in 25, 50, and 100 mg tablets, and 20 mg/mL menthol-flavored oral concentrate
      i. Must dilute oral concentrate prior to administration
   7. Slightly more GI side effects than Prozac

## XII. SNRIs (SEROTONIN NOREPINEPHRINE REUPTAKE INHIBITORS)

A. **Desvenlafaxine succinate (Pristiq™) / Desvenlafaxine** (*Khedezla™ was discontinued*)[185,672]
1. MOA: Major metabolite of venlafaxine in an extended-release tablet
2. 5HT reuptake is 10 x more than NE
3. Empty shell may be found in patient's stool
4. Dosing: 50 mg QD up to a max of 100 mg QD (no benefit of 100 mg dose seen in studies)
5. Available in 50 and 100 mg tablets
6. Administer every other day in severe renal impairment
7. Half-life of 11 hours
8. Mostly metabolized by conjugation by UGT isoforms
9. May have lower risk of sexual dysfunction (study revealed ≈ 50% incidence - same as placebo)[673]
10. Do not confuse with desvenlafaxine (base) ER tablets, which are not generically substitutable

B. **Duloxetine (Cymbalta® / Irenka™/ Drizalma Sprinkle™ (delayed-release capsules))**[186,187,188]
1. Also approved for chronic musculoskeletal pain, GAD (including children), Fibromyalgia, and Diabetic nerve pain
2. A serotonin and norepinephrine reuptake inhibitor
3. >90% plasma protein binding
4. Elimination half-life of 12 hours
5. Metabolized by CYP1A2 and 2D6 (inhibitor)
6. Dosing: Begin with 20 mg QD, Max dose is 120 mg a day (QD or divided BID)
   i. Reduce dose if using in CYP2D6 poor metabolizers or with CYP2D6 inhibitors
   ii. **Avoid** using along with a potent CYP1A2 inhibitor
7. Availability: Cymbalta & generics - 20, 30, and 60 mg enteric-coated capsules
   i. Drizalma Sprinkle™ - 20, 30, 40 & 60 mg delayed-release capsules (can open & sprinkle on food)
   ii. Irenka™ - <u>only</u> available in 40 mg delayed-release capsules
8. Contraindications: Narrow-angle glaucoma
   i. Avoid use in patients with chronic liver disease or cirrhosis, or renal failure (CrCl < 30 ml/min)
9. Side effects: Anticholinergic, drowsiness, nausea, ↓ appetite, sweating, sexual dysfunction, ↑ BP
   i. Watch for rare hepatotoxicity (*not recommended to use in alcoholics*)
   ii. FDA WARNING: orthostatic hypotension, falls and syncope[674]

C. **Levomilnacipran (Fetzima®)**[189]
1. Dosing: 20-120 mg QD (extended-release capsules)
2. Available in 20, 40, 80, and 120 mg capsules
3. Half-life of 11 hours
4. Side effects similar to SSRIs and other SNRIs; can ↑ BP
5. Inhibits reuptake of NE > 5HT[675]
6. Lower the dose with strong inhibitors of CYP3A4
7. Shown positive benefits on measures of attention, cognition, and reaction time, with MDD[676]
8. May reduce the progression of Alzheimer's by inhibiting β-amyloid plaque formation (inhibits β-amyloid precursor protein cleaving enzyme-1 (BACE-1)[677]

D. **Venlafaxine (Effexor®)**[184] – Discovered in 1981
1. Was originally developed to be as an analgesic[678]
2. Also approved for GAD, Panic disorder (with/without agoraphobia) and social phobia
3. MOA: 5HT > NE and weak DA reuptake inhibitor
4. 27% protein bound
5. Half-life of 11 hours
6. Metabolized by CYP2D6 to 3 active metabolites
7. Adverse reactions similar to SSRIs (More nausea / may ↑ BP)
   i. Caution in patients with uncontrolled BP
8. Give with food to ↓ nausea
9. Dosing: 75-375 mg/d
10. RR (tablets): 25 mg, 37.5 mg, 50 mg, 75 mg & 100 mg tablets
    i. Max dose: 375 mg divided BID-TID
11. XR (capsules): 37.5 mg, 75 mg and 150 mg capsules (max dose: 225 mg QD)
12. May be beneficial to those with neuropathic pain syndromes
13. Drug interactions: drugs that inhibit CYP2D6 ↑ venlafaxine levels, MAOIs
14. Reduce dose by 50% in patients with CrCl < 50 ml/min
15. Package insert contains a warning not to use with phentermine or other weight loss agents

## XIII. SARIs (SEROTONIN RECEPTORS ANTAGONIST WITH SEROTONIN REUPTAKE INHIBITION)

A. **Nefazodone (Serzone®)**[181] – Brand name withdrawn from US market due to rare hepatotoxicity
1. MOA: NE and 5HT reuptake inhibitor and 5HT$_2$ blocker
2. 5HT$_2$ blockade = ↓ anxiety and ↓ sexual dysfunction
3. Food delays and decreases absorption by 20%
4. Half-life of 11-24 hours
   i. Active metabolite (mCPP) can cause migraine headache, as with trazodone
5. > 99% protein bound
6. Metabolized by CYP3A4 (potent inhibitor) to 2 active metabolites
7. Dosing: 50-600 mg/d divided BID
8. Available in 50, 100, 150, 200, and 250 mg tablets
9. Adverse reactions: anticholinergic effects, nausea, drowsiness, weakness, orthostasis

10. Drug interactions: ↑s levels of triazolam, alprazolam, theophylline; MAOIs; protein bound drugs
B. **Trazodone (Desyrel® / Oleptro™)**[69,182] - Discovered in 1975
  1. MOA: less potent SSRI, $5HT_{1A}$ partial agonist, $5HT_{2A}$ and $5HT_{2C}$ antagonist
  2. Also blocks $H_1$ and $α_1$ receptors
  3. Half-life of 9 hours
    i. Caution: Its active metabolite (mCPP) via CYP3A4 metabolism can trigger a migraine headache when mCPP's vasoconstricting properties wear off (usually morning after taking it)
    ii. mCPP is a $5HT_{2C}$ agonist
  4. Dosing: 25-400 mg/d given at HS (used for sleep) or divided
    i. Up to 600 mg/d can be used in hospitalized patients
  5. Desyrel® available in 50, 100, 150, and 300 mg tablets
  6. Oleptro™ available as 150 and 300 mg scored extended-release tablets
    i. Contramid® technology, so tablets can be broken in half
  7. 92% protein bound
  8. 65% bioavailable with peak concentrations in 1-2 hours
  9. Caution with CYP3A4 inducers or inhibitors (will affect trazodone blood levels)
  10. Adverse reactions: priapism (very rare), drowsiness, orthostasis, anticholinergic effects
    i. Low risk of male sexual dysfunction
    ii. May help with male erectile dysfunction[679-681]
C. **Vortioxetine (Trintellix®)**[183] - Distributed by Lundbeck for Takeda Pharmaceuticals
  1. MOA: $5HT_3$ antagonist > SSRI > $5HT_{1A}$ receptor agonist > $5HT_7$ antagonist > $5HT_{1B}$ receptor partial agonist > $5HT_{1D}$ receptor antagonist (relative to binding affinity constants)
    i. Theoretically, has the ideal MOA for a rapid-acting antidepressant
  2. Dosage: 5 to 20 mg a day
    i. Maximum recommended dose is 10 mg/day in known CYP2D6 poor metabolizers
    ii. Reduce to ½ usual dose when patients are receiving a CYP2D6 strong inhibitor concomitantly
    ii. Increase dose up to 3 x original dose in those on CYP inducers (e.g., rifampin, carbamazepine)
  3. Available in 5, 10, 15, and 20 mg tablets
  4. Pregnancy Category C
  5. 98% plasma protein bound
  6. Metabolized mostly by CYP2D6
    i. Also by CYP3A4/5, CYP2C19, CYP2C9, CYP2A6, CYP2C8 and CYP2B6
    ii. No active metabolites
  7. Half-life is approximately 66 hours
  8. Common adverse reactions: nausea, constipation, vomiting
  9. Low risk of sexual dysfunction[682]
    i. Treatment-emergent sexual dysfunction (TESD) improved when switched from an SSRI
  10. Trial data supports improvements in cognitive complaints associated with depression (difficulty concentrating, indecisiveness, trouble thinking, and forgetfulness)[683]
  11. *In vitro* evidence shows it has anti-inflammatory & immunomodulatory effects in humans[684]
XIV. SPARI (5HT_{1A} AUTORECEPTOR PARTIAL AGONIST WITH SEROTONIN REUPTAKE INHIBITION)
A. **Vilazodone (Viibryd™)**[182192] - Distributed by Trovis Pharmaceuticals LLC
  1. MOA - SSRI + $5HT_{1A}$ receptor partial agonist (like buspirone)
  2. Onset of antidepressant action may be as soon as 1 week[633]
  3. Dosing is 10 mg/d x7d, then 20 mg/d x7d, then 40 mg/d thereafter (WITH FOOD)
  4. Food ↑ AUC and bioavailability up to 150%
  5. Available in 10 mg, 20 mg, and 40 mg tablets
    i. 30 day starter kits are available
  6. Side effects: diarrhea (28%), nausea (23%), vomiting (5%), insomnia (6%)
    i. Low risk of sexual dysfunction
  7. No significant effects on weight or BP
  8. Rare symptoms of serotonin syndrome were noted in 0.1% of trial patients[685]
  9. Metabolized by Cytochrome CYP3A4 mostly (minor by CYP2C19 and CYP2D6)
  10. Any inhibitors or inducers of CYP3A4 will affect vilazodone blood levels
  11. May inhibit CYP2C8 substrates
  12. Half-life is 25 hours
  13. 96-99% protein bound
  14. Pregnancy Category C
XV. NDRI (NOREPINEPHRINE-DOPAMINE REUPTAKE INHIBITOR)
A. **Bupropion (Zyban®/ Wellbutrin®, SR/XL /Aplenzin® [HBr salt] /Forfivo™ XL /Budeprion®)**[191]
  1. Also approved for the *prevention of Seasonal Affective Disorder (SAD)*
  2. A derivative of the weight loss medication *diethylpropion* (Tenuate®)
    i. Also a synthetic cathinone (chloro-α-t-butylaminopropiophenone)
  3. Half-life is approximately 21 (±9) hours
  4. Metabolized by CYP2B6, but an inhibitor of CYP2D6
  5. MOA: DA reuptake inhibitor, which also stimulates the release of DA and NE
    i. Also a non-competitive antagonist at nicotinic acetylcholine receptors (nAChRs)
    ii. Specifically blocks α3β2 and α4β2 nAChRs; weak α7 blocker
    iii. Good choice for depressed smokers wanting to quit
    a. Zyban® indicated in smoking cessation

6. Usual dosage: begin with 150 mg SR/XL and after 3-7 days, increase to 150 mg SR BID or 300 mg XL QD
   i. Usually dosed in the AM and mid-afternoon (6 hrs apart, but not too late because of insomnia)
   ii. Not to exceed 450 mg/d XL (150 mg TID regular release) and 400 mg/d SR due to seizure risk
   iii. Moderate to severe hepatic impairment - 150 mg XL QOD
   iv. Renal impairment - reduce dose or increase frequency of dosing
7. Availability:
   i. Bupropion regular-release: 75 mg and 100 mg tablets
   ii. Bupropion SR / Zyban: 100 mg, 150 mg, and 200 mg tablets
   iii. Bupropion XL: 150 mg and 300 mg OROS tablets (ghost shell may be in patient's stool)
   iv. Aplenzin®: 174 mg, 348 mg, and 522 mg extended-release tablets
8. Adverse reactions: nausea, vomiting, constipation, dry mouth, headache, nervousness, dermatologic reactions (rare delayed urticaria[686]), little sexual dysfunction
9. Anaphylactic reactions and Stevens-Johnson Syndrome have been reported
10. CONTRAINDICATED in those with seizures or eating disorders, or abruptly discontinuing alcohol, benzodiazepines, barbiturates, or antiepileptic drugs
11. WARNING: because of its amphetamine-like properties, abuse by inhaling or injecting crushed tablets has been reported, along with seizures and deaths
12. May be as effective as Ritalin® for ADD/ADHD in adults
13. Lesser risk of inducing mania in bipolar patients compared to SSRIs
14. Drug interactions:[687]
    i. Ritonavir may induce bupropion's metabolism (i.e., need more bupropion)
    ii. Bupropion may increase levels of citalopram by 30-40%

## XVI. NOVEL ANTIDEPRESSANTS
A. Mitrazapine (Remeron® / SolTabs®)[190]
   1. MOA: $alpha_2$ antagonist, blocks post-synaptic $5HT_{2A/2C}$ and $5HT_3$ receptors, high $H_1$ blockade, weak antagonist of muscarinic and $alpha_1$ receptors
      i. $5HT_3$ blockade = anti-emetic effects
      ii. $5HT_2$ blockade = ↓ anxiety and ↓ *sexual dysfunction*
   2. 85% protein bound
   3. Metabolized by CYP2D6, 1A2, 3A4
   4. Half-life of approximately 20-40 hours[688]
   5. Dosing: 15-45 mg/d usually given at HS
   6. Available in 15, 30, and 45 mg tablets and orange-flavored orally disintegrating tablets
   7. Most common adverse reactions: somnolence, ↑ appetite, weight gain, dizziness
   8. Has been shown in studies to work faster than other antidepressants, but proof is lacking
   9. Drug interactions: MAOIs
      i. Maybe clonidine because of opposing mechanisms of action
         a. Cases have been reported of hypertensive urgency from the combination[689,690]
B. Esketamine (Spravato™)[193] C-III controlled-substance by Janssen Pharmaceuticals, Inc.
   1. Nasal Spray indicated for Treatment-Resistant Depression (TRD)
      i. Must have tried and failed 2 other antidepressants, but must be used with an oral antidepressant
   2. Non-competitive N-methyl-D-aspartate (NMDAR) antagonist & possible DA reuptake inhibitor
   3. Dosage Forms and Strengths
      i. Nasal Spray: 28 mg of esketamine per device
      ii. Each nasal spray device delivers two sprays containing a total of 28 mg of esketamine
         a. One spray per nostril
   4. Dosage and administration
      i. Self-administered intranasally under the supervision of a healthcare provider
         a. Monitoring required for 2 hours after due to risk of sedation
      ii. The spray cannot be taken home
      iii. Check BP before & after administration (BP peaks ≈ 40 minutes after administration)
      iv. Induction Phase:
         a. Week 1-4: twice a week treatment
            1. Day 1 starting dose: 56 mg (2 devices)
            2. Subsequent doses 56 mg or 84 mg (3 devices)
         b. Evaluate at the end of the induction phase to determine need for continued treatment
      v. Maintenance Phase: 56 mg or 84 mg
         a. Weeks 5-8: once a week
         b. Week 9 and after: Q 2 weeks or once weekly
      vi. Patient should recline and wait 5 minutes between each device used
   5. Pharmacokinetics
      i. Absorption: Tmax (intranasal): 20 to 40 minutes
      ii. Metabolized by CYP3A4, CYP2B6, CYP2C9/19 to noresketamine (major active metabolite)
      iii. Half-life: 7-12 hours
   6. BBWs: Sedation, Disassociation, Abuse and misuse, and Suicidal thoughts & behaviors
   7. Contraindications:
      i. History of psychosis, intracerebral hemorrhage or aneurism, or arteriovenous malformation
   8. Other Warnings and Precautions
      i. Increased BP, cognitive impairment, impaired ability to drive and operate machinery, embryo-fetal toxicity, and difficulty with attention, judgement & thinking

    ii. Females should not get pregnant or breast feed
      a. Animal studies revealed fetal & neonatal neurotoxicity
  9. Adverse Effects
    i. Dissociation, dizziness, nausea, sedation, vertigo, hypoesthesia, anxiety, lethargy, hypertension, vomiting, feeling drunk
      a. Patients should not eat or drink for 30 to 120 minutes prior to treatment to reduce vomiting
    ii. Due to risk of ulcerative or interstitial cystitis with illicit ketamine, monitor for bladder issues
  10. Drug Interactions
    i. Other nasal sprays should be used 1 hour before esketamine
    ii. Other CNS depressants can increase risk of sedation
    iii. Modest induction effects on CYP2B6 and CYP3A4
  11. Pharmacies must be certified in the REMS and must only dispense SPRAVATO to healthcare settings that are certified in the program
    i. See www.SPRAVATOREMS.com for REMS & Pharmacy information
  12. Spravato™ was fast-tracked by the FDA using "modest evidence it worked and then only in limited trials" with no long-term safety data[691]
    i. Unlike ketamine studies, esketamine's antidepressant effects were not proven "rapidly acting"
  13. A longer-term follow up study of patients with >16 week antidepressant + esketamine *response* or *remission* revealed a significantly longer time to relapse (70% & 51%, respectively) than those on only an antidepressant[692]
    i. Average times to relapse for each group was not disclosed
C. **Brexanolone (Zulresso™)**[194] – C-IV controlled-substance by Sage Therapeutics, Inc.
  1. The first and only treatment specifically indicated for Postpartum Depression
  2. Made from progesterone and chemically identical to endogenous allopregnanolone
  3. M.O.A. - neuroactive steroid gamma-aminobutyric acid (GABA) A receptor positive modulator
  4. Pharmacokinetics
    i. Metabolized through *keto-reduction (AKRs), glucuronidation (UGTs), & sulfation (SULTs)*
    ii. Excreted via feces: 47%; Urine: 42%; 1% unchanged
    iii. Avoid use in patients with end stage renal disease (ESRD)
    iv. Half-life: 9 hours
  5. Drug interactions: other CNS depressants can ↑ risk of sedation
  6. Dosage and availability
    i. It is only available through the restricted Zulresso™ REMS program
    ii. Administered via continuous IV infusion over *60 hours* (2½ days) with dose titration up & then tapered off
      a. Dosing is weight-based and time-dependent
  7. Available in single-dose vials: 100 mg/20 mL (5 mg/mL)
    i. Must be diluted in sterile water for inj. & normal saline
    ii. Immediately refrigerate IV bag(s) (stable up to 96 hrs)
    iii. Prepared IV is stable for 12 hrs at room temperature
      a. 5 IV bags will be required (more if pt. weighs ≥ 90kg)

| Timing | Dosing |
|---|---|
| 0 to 4 hours | 30 mcg/kg/hour |
| 4 to 24 hours | 60 mcg/kg/hour |
| 24 to 52 hours | 90 mcg/kg/hour |
| 52 to 56 hours | 60 mcg/kg/hour |
| 56 to 60 hours | 30 mcg/kg/hour |

  8. Common adverse reactions
    i. Sedation/somnolence, dry mouth, loss of consciousness, sinus tachycardia, & flushing/hot flush
    ii. **BBW:** Zulresso™ can cause serious sedation and loss of consciousness (L.O.C.)
      a. Brexanolone can only be administered in a REMS-registered Certified Health Care facility
        i. See www.zulressorems.com for more information
      b. L.O.C. reported in 4% of brexanolone-treated patients vs. 0% of placebo-treated patients
      c. Requires continuous observation & monitoring during the 60-hour infusion
      d. Immediately stop the infusion if pulse oximetry reveals hypoxia, and do not resume
      e. Patients must be accompanied during interactions with their child(ren)
  9. Pregnancy and lactation risks
    i. It is transferred to breast milk in nursing mothers, but there is no data on the effects to the infant
    ii. May cause harm to the fetus, but regardless, it should not be used pre-partum

# XVII. NON-ORAL ANTIDEPRESSANT OPTIONS[693,698,699]
A. Options are limited when a patient is NPO and cannot swallow pills
B. Some formulations (below) must be compounded or obtained directly from the manufacturer
C. Liquid antidepressants can be put down nasogastric and PEG tubes
D. Injectables:
  1. Amitriptyline (10 mg/mL IM or 25-100 mg/250 mL IV)
  2. Clomipramine (25 mg/2 mL IM or 25-250 mg/500 mL IV) - used for OCD
  3. Citalopram (40 mg/mL in 250 mL IV) - also used for OCD
  4. Mirtazapine (6 mg/2 mL IV and 15 mg/5 mL IV)
E. Rectal administration:
  1. Amitriptyline suppositories (50 mg QD to 50 mg BID)
  2. Clomipramine - plasma levels = oral route
  3. Dexedrine suppositories (5 mg QD)
  4. Imipramine - plasma levels = oral route
  5. Doxepin capsules (25-50 mg QD) - can be used for cancer pain control
  6. Fluoxetine capsules (20 mg QD) - only 15% bioavailable
  7. Trazodone suppositories - can be used for post-operative cancer pain control

F. Sublingual:
   1. Fluoxetine liquid (up to 60 mg/d) - plasma levels lower than oral dosing
G. Topical:
   1. Selegiline (EMSAM) patch[103] (6 mg, 9 mg, and 12 mg/24h)
   2. Doxepin (3.3-5% cream) and amitriptyline - not studied for depression - only for nerve pain
H. Nasal:
   1. Esketamine (Spravato™)

## XVIII. TREATMENT OF ANTIDEPRESSANT-INDUCED SEXUAL DYSFUNCTION[700-702]

A. Up to 70% of patients on antidepressants experience sexual dysfunction and stop treatment
B. Might be caused by $5HT_{2C}$ agonism
C. Methods of reducing risk of sexual dysfunction
   1. Switching agents to one with low risk
   2. Antidepressants with lowest risk of sexual dysfunction
      i. Trazodone, bupropion, mirtazapine, nefazodone, vilazodone
      ii. Possibly: vortioxetine, vilazodone, and desvenlafaxine
   3. Lower dose to lowest effective dose
   4. Adjuvant medications
      i. Buspirone 20-60 mg/d
      ii. Bupropion 75-150 mg/d
      iii. Phosphodiesterase inhibitors (e.g., sildenafil, tadalafil, vardenafil)
      iv. Ginkgo Biloba 60-240 mg/d ($α_2$ antagonist)
      v. Amantadine 100-300 mg/d (increases dopamine release)
      vi. Cyproheptadine (Periactin®) 4-12 mg as needed (antihistamine + $5HT_{2C}$ antagonist)
      vii. Yohimbine 5.4 mg TID ($α_2$ antagonist)

## XIX. TREATMENT-RESISTANT DEPRESSION (TRD)[600,601,703]

A. Approx. 30% of all patients treated for a mood disorder
B. Predictors of patient TRD[704]
   1. Longer episode of depression
      i. Causes more neurodegeneration of brain regions (e.g., hippocampus)
   2. Increased severity of the depressive episode
   3. Presence of melancholic features (see Subtypes of Depression at beginning of this chapter)
   4. Little to no improvement on an antidepressant within the first 2-3 weeks
   5. Having comorbidities, such as anxiety or a personality disorder (e.g., Borderline Personality or Avoidant Personality)
C. Occurs when a patient does not respond to an adequate course of 2 antidepressants
D. At least 6-12 weeks on each antidepressant at the maximally tolerated dose
E. Biomarkers of inflammation and inflammatory cytokines in the CNS correlate with TRD[705]
F. Combinations of antidepressants with differing mechanisms should be tried first[706,707]
G. Consider metabolic consequences of adjunctive atypical antipsychotics before use
H. **FDA-approved therapies:**
   1. Esketamine (Spravato™)
   2. Olanzapine + fluoxetine (Symbyax®)
   3. Aripiprazole (Abilify®) – Adjunctly, is associated with lower medical costs and rehospitalizations[708]
   4. Brexpiprazole (Rexulti®) - a "serotonin-dopamine activity modulator (SDAM)"
   5. Quetiapine (Seroquel®)
   6. Vagal nerve stimulation (pacemaker-like implant)
   7. Repetitive Transcranial Magnetic Stimulation (rTMS)[709]
      i. In medication-resistant patients, response is 58%, with a 37% remission rate[710]
      ii. Safe option for pregnant patients
   8. **Electroconvulsive Therapy (ECT)** - (6 to 12 exposures)[395,624,625,711]
      i. An underutilized therapy that can reduce depression in as little as 48 hours
         a. Shown to reduce 30-day recidivism rates by half[712]
      ii. 74-90% response rate and 50% rate of remission (if continued on an antidepressant)
         a. Large 2016 multisite study in geriatric depression resulted in a 62% remission rate
      iii. Modern "ultrabrief" pulse stimulation ↓ side effects (e.g., amnesia & recovery time) significantly
      iv. Right-sided unilateral ECT has fewer side effects than bilateral ECT
   9. Deplin® (L-methylfolate calcium)[195] – a "medical food" - 7.5-15 mg/d
      i. A methyl group donator to the synthesis of neurotransmitters
I. Non-FDA-approved therapies with evidence-based support:[713,714]
   1. Risperidone (Risperdal®)[715]
   2. Lithium
   3. Liothyronine (Cytomel®) - 25-50 µg/day
   4. Carbamazepine (Tegretol®)
   5. Buspirone (BuSpar®)
   6. Monoamine Oxidase Inhibitor + another Antidepressant [Caution!]
   7. Transcranial Direct Current Stimulation (tDCS)[716]
      i. 1-2 mA of current applied BID for 5 days or QD for 10 days (or up to 6 weeks)
      ii. Anode (-) applied to L dorsolateral prefrontal cortex (DLPC)
      iii. Cathode (+) applied to R dorsolateral prefrontal cortex
      iv. Side effects of headaches, itching, and redness at site of connectors
   8. Deep Brain Stimulation of the Subcallosal Cingulate of the brain[717]

## XX. COMPLEMENTARY AND ALTERNATIVE THERAPIES (CAM)[359-360,718-722]

A. *Should only be used as third-line therapy or adjunctive treatment*
   1. Some of these have poor quality evidence-based therapies
   i. Likely are effective, but have insufficient or poor quality studies
B. 5-MeO-DMT (5-methocy-N,-N-dimethyltryptamine)
   1. Naturally found in the venom of Bufo Alvarius toads
   2. Effects last approximately 30-90 minutes
   3. 80% of people who underwent a ceremony using 5-MeO-DMT were surveyed and reported rapid improvements in depression and anxiety[723]
C. Acupuncture (very safe & effective, but evidence is limited)
D. Borage / Weevil head[362] (Echium amoenum)
E. Brahmi / Bacopa monnieri (Water hysop)[360] - contains bacoside A and bacoside P
   1. Acts as a cholinesterase inhibitor, antioxidant, and protects β-amyloid
F. Bright white light therapy - also used for seasonal depression[569,724]
   1. A single photopigment in the retino-hypothalamic tract is activated by blue light[725]
   i. Decreases secretion of melatonin from the pineal gland
   2. 10,000-lux light therapy for 30 minutes a day upon awakening (full-spectrum 4000k)
   3. An 8-week DBPCT showed that light therapy and the combination of light therapy + an antidepressant were superior to the antidepressant alone by a large margin[726]
G. Chamomile[360]
H. Chronotherapy (sleep deprivation, sleep phase shifting and/or the use of bright light)
   1. Sleep deprivation - Stay awake for 36 hours, then sleep. Depression subsides in ~ 50% when awakened. Relapse usually occurs in 80-90% of patients after next night's sleep
   2. Generally superior to other therapies such as psychotherapy, antidepressants, exercise or light therapy alone after 5-7 days[727]
I. DHEA (dehydroepiandrosterone)[358]
   1. Precursor steroid hormone of androgen and estrogen, and possible CNS neurosteroid
   2. 90 to 450 mg/d showed significant reductions in depression vs. placebo in trials
J. Eschium amoenum[363] - ("ox-tongue") – an herb from Iran
   1. Flowers are brewed into a tea and used for mood enhancing & anxiolytic effects
   2. 375 mg in a DBPCT showed significance at week 4, but not at week 6
K. Exercise & Yoga [728,729]
   1. Increases BDNF (brain-derived neurotrophic factor)
   2. 30-45 minutes of moderate exercise 3-4 times a week significantly ↓ depression & recurrence
L. Free and Easy Wanderer Plus[730,731] (FEWP), an 11-herb Chinese compound
M. Ginseng (Panax / Korean / Siberian) - Eleutherococcus senticosus
   1. Active compounds: eleutherosides (phenolic glycosides), fitosterols, lignans, saponin glycosides, oleanolic acid derivatives
   2. Has anti-inflammatory and antioxidant + inhibits nitric oxide synthase
   3. Dose studied: ~400 mg QD
N. Griffonia (griffonia simplicifolia)
   1. Griffonia produces black fruits with seeds that are a source serotonin in the CNS
O. Kanna or Channa (sceletium tortuosum)
P. Kava-Kava (Piper methysticum)
   1. Contains kavain, dihydrokavain and dihydromethisticine, which are weak MAO inhibitors in vitro
   2. Should not be used with other monoaminergic drugs or MAO inhibitors such as ephedrine, oenothera oil, fenugreek, ginkgo biloba, lupulus, St John's Wort, tyrosine, valeriana, 5HTP, DHEA (dehydroepiandrosterone), DLPA (phenylalanine dl), SAM-e, vitamin B6, or chromium
   3. Reported to inhibit many CYP isozymes (i.e., CYP1A2, 2C9, 2C19, 2D6, 3A4, and 4A9/11)
   4. Can cause liver toxicity
Q. Lavender (Lavandula augustifolia)
   1. Proven to be better adjunctively to standard antidepressants vs. antidepressants alone
R. Mimosa (albizia julibrissin) - contains julibrosides
   1. Has receptor affinities for $5HT_{1A}$ and $5HT_{2C}$
S. Negatively-charged ionized air[570]
   1. Studies date back 80 years[732]
   2. Only high-density ions (e.g., 450 trillion ions/sec) within a 3-foot radius of the person are effective
   i. Device should not produce ozone byproduct at > 0.05 ppm (the FDA safety cut-off)
   3. Sessions should last 30-90 minutes, and can be done at night while sleeping
T. Nutraceuticals:
   1. Evidence is weak in supporting their use, and too much may have the opposite effect
   i. Omega-3 Fatty Acids[733] (from fatty fish)
   ii. L-Tryptophan - Precursor to serotonin in the CNS
   iii. N-acetylcysteine (NAC) - potent anti-oxidant and modulator of glutamate and dopamine
   iv. Dehydroepiandrosterone (DHEA), Folate, and Inositol
U. Rhodiola rosea (roseroot, rosewort, golden root, or arctic root, Hongjingtian, King's Crown)
   1. Side effects: headache, GI upset, drowsiness, dizziness, vivid dreams and insomnia
   2. Doses studied: 100-700 mg QD
   3. Active compounds: *salidroside* glycosides, rosarin, rosavin, rosin, flavonoids, phenolic acid: gallic acid and chlorogenic acid (an antioxidant), organic acids (succinic, citric, malic, oxalic), tannins, anthraquinones

4. Inhibits Monoamine Oxidase A and affects the neuroendocrine system
5. Significant ↓ in depression seen in a 6-week placebo-controlled trial using 340 & 680 mg/d
6. Shown in study not to be as effective as sertraline, but it had significantly less side effects[734]

V. S-adenosylmethionine (SAMe)[735,736]
1. SAM-e levels are dependent on the vitamin's folate and B12
   i. Peak in 3-5 hours / Half-life is 100 minutes
   ii. Recommended doses of SAM-e based on the literature are between 400 & 3200 mg a day
2. Side effects reported: insomnia, loss of appetite or anorexia, constipation, nausea, dry mouth, sweating, dizziness, and anxiety
   i. Cases of mania or hypomania in individuals with bipolar depression

W. Saffron (Crocus sativus)[360,360,737]
1. Active compounds: Safranal, crocin, and crocetin
2. Based on several 6-week RCTs, may be as effective as imipramine 100 mg/d or fluoxetine 20-40 mg/d (Grade A evidence)
3. Found to activate BDNF and acts as a GABA$_A$ agonist & post-synaptic NMDA antagonist
4. Dose studied: 30-90 mg QD
5. Other plants with safranal are Aspalathus linearis (Rooibos), Camellia sinensis (Tea leaf), Ficus carica (Fig leaf), Lycium chinense (Wolfberry), Cuminum cyminum (Cumin Seed)
6. Risk of miscarriage, so should not be used by pregnant women
7. Saffron overdose can be fatal - vomiting, diarrhea, urogenital & GI bleeding
8. In a small open-label, observational study, a combination of rhodiola 308 mg and saffron 30 mg dosed BID showed significant improvements in mild to moderate depression in > 85% of patients after only 2 weeks[738]

X. St. John's Wort (hypericum perforatum) - for mild to moderate depression
1. The most documented herb used in depression
2. Taken up to TID - causes photosensitivity and has CYP3A4 inducing drug interactions - can be toxic in overdose[739]
3. Hyperforin inhibits reuptake of 5HT, adrenaline, NE, GABA and L-glutamate
4. Contains natural melatonin & kynurenic acid (acts as an excitatory amino acid antagonist)
5. Lack of standards in production of this herb have resulted in mixed study results[358]

Y. Turmeric (curcuma longa)[740,741]
1. Also acts as an antispasmodic and as a relaxant intoxicant
2. Effects may be due to mesembrine – an SSRI and Phosphodiesterase-4 inhibitor

Z. Zinc and Magnesium supplements[742]
1. Required minerals for key functions related to mood and neuroplasticity
2. Zinc 25 to 50 mg a day
3. Magnesium used in depression since **1921**
   i. 248 mg of elemental magnesium as four 500 mg tablets of $MgCl_2$ per day found to be very effective in a 12-week randomized, cross-over trial[743]

AA. Others with much less evidence to support their use:
1. Aspalathus linearis (Rooibos), Camellia sinensis (Tea leaf), Ficus carica (Fig leaf), Lycium chinense (Wolfberry), Cuminum cyminum (Cumin Seed), Schisandra chinensis
2. Anthranilic acid (vitamin L1)
   i. May decrease the risk of depression development

XXI. POTENTIAL FUTURE TREATMENTS FOR DEPRESSION IN STUDY[744]
A. Ademetionine (SAMe [S-Adenosyl methionine], **Strada™**) by MSI Methylation Sciences Inc.
1. A methyl group donor and cofactor in monoamine neurotransmitter biosynthesis
2. Mediates cytokine effects on the CNS
3. May act as an indirect dopaminergic agent, impacting membrane fluidity and ↓ neuroinflammation
4. In Phase II study for the adjunctive treatment of MDD
5. May be the safest option for pregnant and breast-feeding depressed women[358]

B. Agomelatine [302,368] (AGO-178, Valdoxan®, Thymanax) by Novartis and Servier Pharmaceuticals
1. Melatonin MT$_1$ and MT$_2$ receptor agonist, & 5HT$_{2B}$/5HT$_{2C}$ receptor antagonist
2. In Phase III & IV trials in the US
3. Already approved as an antidepressant in Europe and Australia[368]
   i. European brand names: "Alodil", "Melitor" and "Vestin"
4. Substrate of CYP1A2 (90%), CYP2C9 and CYP2C19
   i. Contraindicated with potent CYP1A2 inhibitors
   ii. Short t½ of 140 minutes
5. Recommended dose is 25 mg at bedtime
   i. Can increase to 50 mg at bedtime after 2 weeks
6. Liver function tests are required in all patients
   i. Contraindicated in patients with hepatic impairment
7. Studies for insomnia and Generalized Anxiety Disorder have been discontinued

C. ALKS-5461 by Alkermes plc (Dublin, Ireland) and Allergan
1. Combination of buprenorphine and samidorphan (potent mu-opioid antagonist) as adjunct to antidepressants in treatment-resistant depression (TRD)[745]
   i. Short-term, low dose buprenorphine (0.1 mg/d) shown to reduce suicidal ideation in 2 weeks[746]
2. Feb. 2019 - FDA rejected the NDA (New Drug Application) filed in 2018
3. Alkermes has another Phase III trial of ALKS 5461 underway but, according to ClinicalTrials.gov, it is still around 30 months from completion (FORWARD 1 to 5 trials)

    i. Two of Alkermes' earlier Phase III studies lasted roughly 18 months
   4. https://www.fiercebiotech.com/biotech/fda-rejects-alkermes-depression-drug-alks-5461
   5. Current status is unknown
D. Ansofaxine (LY03005) by Luye Pharma (http://www.luye.cn/lvye_en/)
   1. An extended release serotonin-norepinephrine-dopamine triple reuptake inhibitor (SNDRI)
   2. A prodrug to desvenlafaxine with greater reuptake for all 3 neurotransmitters (5HT=NE, but < DA)
   3. Currently in Phase III trials in China, but Phase I in the U.S.
E. Apimostinel (AGN 241660, AGN 241751, NRX-1074) by Allergan and Naurex
   1. Small molecule N-methyl-D-aspartate receptor (NMDAR) modulator
   2. Phase II trials completed successfully in August 2019
F. Arketamine by ATAI Life Sciences (Germany-based biotech company)
   1. The R-optical isomer of ketamine
   2. An AMPA receptor agonist
   3. Possesses 4 - 5 times lower affinity for the PCP (phencyclidine) site of the NMDA receptor
   4. May be a more rapid-acting antidepressant than esketamine
   5. Still in pre-clinical trials
G. Aticaprant (CERC-501, LY-2456302) by Eli Lilly and Company/Janssen Pharmaceuticals
   1. A selective antagonist of the κ-opioid receptor (KOR) in Phase II trials
H. AV-101 (4-Cl-KYN, L-4-chlorokyurenine) by Vistagen Pharmaceutics
   1. An NMDA antagonist shown to have rapid, persistent, AMPA-dependent antidepressive effects
   2. In Phase II study as an <u>add-on</u> treatment for MDD in adults (has FDA fast track status)
I. AXS-05 (bupropion + dextromethorphan fixed-dose combination) by Axsome Therapeutics
   1. Currently in Phase III trials for TRD, Phase II/III for agitation, and Phase II for smoking cessation
J. Basimglurant (RG-7090) by Roche, currently in Phase II trials
   1. A metabotropic glutamate receptor 5 (mGluR$_5$) antagonist
   2. Initial study endpoints failed to meet primary objectives as adjunctive therapy for MDD[747]
K. BLI-1005 (PDC-1421) by BioLite Inc. (Taiwan), currently in Phase II study
   1. A norepinephrine reuptake inhibitor based on traditional Chinese medicine
L. Brexpiprazole (Lu AF41156/OPC-34712/Rexulti) by Otsuka/Lundbeck, currently in Phase III study
M. BTRX-246040 (LY-2940094) by BlackThorn Therapeutics & Eli Lilly and Company
   1. Nociceptin receptor antagonist (Phase II trial completed)
   2. Also being studied in Parkinson's Disease
N. Cariprazine (Vraylar) by Allergan, currently in Phase III trials
O. D-Cycloserine[357]
P. Deudextromethorphan (AVP-786, AVP-923, deuterium-modified dextromethorphan + quinidine)
   1. By Otsuka/Avanir Pharmaceuticals
   2. Sigma-1 (σ1) receptor agonist, SNRI, and NMDA receptor antagonist
   3. In Phase II/III study for the Negative symptoms of schizophrenia
Q. Dextromethadone (REL-1017) by Relmada Therapeutics, currently in Phase II study
   1. NMDA receptor antagonist open channel blocker
R. EVT-101 (ENS-101, RO-631908) by Evotec SE and Janssen Pharmaceuticals
   1. NR2B N-Methyl-D-Aspartate antagonist in Phase II study
   2. Trials for Alzheimer's and Pain have been discontinued
S. FKB01MD by Fabre-Kramer Pharmaceuticals (currently in Phase II study)
   1. 5HT reuptake inhibitor, 5HT$_2$ & 5HT$_{1A}$ agonist, and acts on central 5HT$_{1D}$ receptors
   2. Shown to down-regulate 5HT$_2$ receptors in animals overnight
   3. Doses of 10-30 mg BID were well tolerated by depressed patients
   4. Half-life of 4 hours
T. Ganaxolone - (CCD-1042) by Marinus Pharmaceuticals, Inc. (www.marinuspharma.com)
   1. A positive allosteric modulator of GABA$_A$,
   2. In Phase II trials for Postpartum Depression
   3. May also have antiepileptic, anxiolytic, and general antidepressant effects
U. Gepirone ER (Travivo™) by Fabre-Kramer Pharmaceuticals[370]
   1. A 5HT$_{1A}$ partial agonist (like buspirone, but stronger)
   2. Phase III trials completed, but FDA rejected the New Drug Application. In 2016, approved it.
   3. Mission Pharmacal will pursue its future commercial manufacture
   4. Common adverse effects: transient lightheadedness, nausea, and headache (no weight gain)
    i. Found to improve symptoms of sexual dysfunction in men and women
   5. Also in Phase II trials for hypoactive sexual desire disorder
   6. Status: Pre-registration to the FDA for MDD completed
V. JNJ-39393406 by Janssen Pharmaceutica, National Institutes of Health, & University of Pittsburgh
   1. An α nicotinic acetylcholine receptor positive allosteric modulator
   2. In Phase II study for MDD & smoking cessation
W. JNJ-42165279 by Janssen-Cilag
   1. Fatty acid amide hydrolase (FAAH) inhibitor
   2. Phase II study of "MDD with anxious distress" completed (ClinicalTrials.gov ID: NCT02498392)
   3. Also in Phase II for social anxiety disorders and Pervasive child developmental disorders
X. JNJ-67953964 (JNJ-3964) by Janssen Research & Development
   1. Opioid kappa receptor antagonist in Phase II study
Y. Ketamine[748,749] - NMDA receptor antagonist
   1. Produces a rapid antidepressant response (64% vs. 28% with placebo)

2. IV infusion - 0.5 mg/kg infused over 40 minutes - 2 or 3 times a week up to 4 weeks[750]
  i. Sub-anesthetic doses can ↓ anhedonia in 40 minutes[302]
  ii. Works much faster than ECT (24 hours vs. 48 hours for ECT)
3. Long-term use linked to irreversible bladder damage
Z. Liafensine (DB104) by Denovo Biopharma (originally by Bristol-Myers Squibb)
  1. Adrenergic receptor antagonists and 5HT & DA reuptake inhibitor
  2. Phase II trials completed, but now in unknown phase for treatment-resistant depression
AA. Lumateperone (ITI-007)[586] by Intra-cellular Therapies
  1. $5HT_{2A}$ receptor antagonist (60 x more affinity than to dopamine)
    i. Dopamine receptor phosphoprotein modulation (DPPM)
      a. A partial agonist of presynaptic $D_2$ receptors and an antagonist of postsynaptic $D_2$ receptors
    ii. A serotonin reuptake inhibitor with some affinity for the $D_1$ receptor
    iii. Also, indirect glutamatergic modulation
  2. An NDA (new drug application) was submitted to the FDA in the Fall of 2018
  3. Other possible future indications: bipolar depression (Phase III), schizophrenia (Fast Track status), autism, and sleep
  4. Phase III trial for behavioral disturbances in dementia was terminated because of inefficacy
AB. Memantine (Namenda®) adjunctive therapy for moderate-to-severe depression
  1. When added to sertraline (200 mg/d) or placebo, a more rapid response seen with memantine[751]
AC. MIJ821 (CAD-9271) by Novartis Pharmaceuticals and Cadent Therapeutics
  1. Negative allosteric modulator of NR2B subtype of NMDA receptors
  2. In Phase II study for treatment-resistant depression (TRD)
AD. MIN-117 by Minerva Neurosciences is currently in Phase IIb study
  1. $5HT_{1A}$ & $5HT_{2A}$ antagonist, 5HT & DA reuptake inhibitor
  2. Also modulates the levels of $alpha_{1a}$ and $alpha_{1b}$, which further modulates 5HT and DA
AE. Minocycline – in Phase III and IV study for adjunctive and monotherapy of depression
  1. Found to decrease pro-inflammatory cytokines
  2. Produced highly significant improvements vs. placebo when 200 mg/d given for 12 weeks[752]
AF. NSI-189 by Neuralstem, Inc.
  1. Specifically stimulates neurogenesis on in the hippocampus and subventricular zone in the CNS
  2. May treat MDD by promoting synaptogenesis or neurogenesis in the hippocampus
  3. Also being studied for cognitive impairment indications associated with hippocampal atrophy
  4. Currently in Phase II study
AG. NV-5138 by Navitor Pharmaceuticals, Inc. is still in Phase I trials
  1. Direct, post-synaptic activation of the mammalian target of rapamycin complex 1 (mTORC1) signaling pathway
    i. Selective mTORC1 activation has broad potential to treat neurological conditions such as depression and cognitive impairment
  2. Single oral dose of NV-5138 found to increase mTORC1 signaling and produce synaptogenesis in the mPFC (medial prefrontal cortex) and induce rapid antidepressant effects[753]
AH. Pimavanserin (Nuplazid, ACP-103, BVF-048) by ACADIA Pharmaceuticals
  1. $5HT_{2A}$ receptor inverse agonist
  2. In Phase III for MDD as adjunctive therapy (https://www.acadia-pharm.com/pipeline)
AI. Pramipexole dihydrochloride (Mirapex®) by Chase Therapeutics, currently in Phase II study
  1. Potent $D_3$ agonist, as well as a lesser $D_2$ & $D_4$ agonist
AJ. Pregnenolone methyl ether (3-methoxy-pregnenolone/MAP-4343) by Mapreg (France)
  1. Selective microtubule-associated protein 2 (MAP2) stimulant
  2. Promotes tubulin polymerization
  3. In Phase II for TRD, but has Orphan Drug Status for treating Spinal Cord Injuries
AK. Psilocybin by COMPASS Pathways & Yale University
  1. $5HT_{2A}$ receptor partial agonist
  2. In Phase II/III study for Depressive disorders and in Phase II study for Headaches
AL. Rislenemdaz (CERC-301, MK-0657) by Merck & Cerecor in Phase II study for depression
  1. Subunit GluNR2B-specific NMDA (N-Methyl-D-Aspartate) receptor antagonist
AM. Sarcosine (N-Methylglycine) - a dietary supplement in Phase II
AN. Seltorexant (MIN-202, JNJ-922, JNJ-42847922) - Janssen & Minerva Neurosciences
  1. A selective, small-molecule antagonist of the Orexin receptor type 2 (Ox2R or OX2)
    i. Also known as hypocretin receptor type 2 (HcrtR2)
  2. Phase II clinical trials have completed
  3. Also being studied for insomnia (Phase II) and sleep apnea (Phase I)
AO. Sirukumab (CNTO-136) by Janssen Research & Development
  1. Monoclonal antibody against interleukin-6 (Phase II study completed for MDD)
AP. SPN-604 by Supernus Pharmaceuticals
  1. Sodium channel blocker to start Phase III clinical testing in the second half of 2019
AQ. Statin medications[754-756] (e.g., atorvastatin, simvastatin, rosuvastatin, etc.)
  1. 3 short randomized trials used a statin as adjunctive to antidepressants & saw significant results
AR. SUVN-911 by Suven Life Sciences
  1. α4β2 nicotinic receptor antagonist in Phase I trials for MDD
AS. Tianeptine oxalate (TNX-601) by Servier and Vela Pharmaceuticals
  1. Atypical μ-opioid receptor agonist and AMPA receptor modulator

i. Already marketed in Europe for Alcoholism, Anxiety disorders, and Major Depressive Disorder under the brand names "Coaxil", Stablon" and "Tatinol"
2. Not currently in study in the U.S. – Phase I for PTSD planned for 2020
AT. Tramadol ER (ETS6103, Viotra) by E-Therapeutics
  1. μ-opioid receptor agonist and SNRI
  2. Completed Phase II for Major depressive disorder in March 2016 – no further development noted
AU. TS-121 (in Phase II clinical trials) & TS-161 (in Phase I clinical trials) by Taisho Pharmaceutical
  1. Vasopressin $1_B$ receptor antagonists (https://www.taisho-holdings.co.jp/en/ir/finance/development)
AV. Tulrampator (Ampakine-CX-1632, S47445) by RespireRx Pharmaceuticals and Servier
  1. AMPA receptor modulator and Nerve growth factor stimulant
  2. In Phase II for Alzheimer's disease & Major depressive disorder
AW. Viloxazine & Viloxazine E.R. (SPN-809, SPN-812, ICI-588834) by Supernus Pharmaceuticals
  1. NE reuptake inhibitor in Phase III trials for pediatric ADHD & Phase II for adult ADHD (completed)
  2. Was approved in Europe as an antidepressant, but newer drugs have replaced it
  3. SPN-809 was in Phase I/II trials for depression, even though it is an older drug, but recently the trials for depression have been abandoned
  4. ClinicalTrials.gov Identifiers: NCT01107496, NCT02633527, and NCT02736656
AX. Zuranolone (SAGE-217, S812217) by SAGE Therapeutics
  1. A synthetic, orally active, inhibitory pregnane neuro-steroid, that acts as a positive allosteric modulator of the GABA$_A$ receptor
  2. Developed as an improvement of allopregnanolone (brexanolone/Zulresso™) with high oral bioavailability and a biological half-life suitable for once-daily administration
  3. Currently in Phase III trials for Major depressive disorder, Postnatal depression, and Insomnia
  4. In Phase II trials for Bipolar Depression, Essential Tremors, and Parkinson's Disease
AY. Other potential future therapies' mechanisms of action
  1. Glutamate receptor modulators with direct affinity for cognate receptors[757]
    i. Non-competitive NMDA antagonists (e.g., ketamine, memantine, dextromethorphan)
    ii. NMDA receptor glycine-site partial agonists (e.g., rapastinel – no longer in study)
    iii. Metabotropic glutamate receptor (mGluR) modulators (e.g., basimglurant)
    iv. Other theoretical glutamate receptor targets
      a. α-amino-3-hydroxyl-5-methyl-4-isoxazoleproprionic acid (AMPA) agonists
      b. mGluR2/3 negative allosteric modulators
  2. Cholinergic (e.g., scopolamine) and opioid (e.g., samidorphan [ALKS-5461]) system antagonists
  3. Corticotropin releasing factor (CRF) receptor antagonists

---

# XXII. ANTIDEPRESSANT PEARLS

A. Bupropion - Not good for anxious patients – very stimulating – low sexual dysfx. – CYP2D6 inhibitor - ADD/ADHD – smokers – May ↑ BP & seizures – not for use in BZD or EtOH w/d pts.

B. Citalopram and escitalopram - Less activating – no significant interactions
  1. Dose-related QTc issue with Celexa

C. Duloxetine - Also used for neuropathy – anticholinergic – May ↑ BP – not for alcoholics

D. Fluoxetine - Stimulating - long t½ - CYP2D6 inhibition

E. Fluvoxamine - Short t½ - CYP1A2 and CYP3A4 inhibition – smoking induces metabolism

F. Mirtazapine - Much drowsiness and weight gain – low sexual dysfx. - blocks nausea

G. Nefazodone - CYP3A4 inhibitor – BID dosing – low sexual dysfx. – rare liver failure

H. Paroxetine - Anticholinergic – long-term weight gain - CYP2D6 inhibition – contraindicated in children/adolescents & pregnancy

I. Sertraline - Stimulating - some DA reuptake inhibition - food ↑'s absorption – more diarrhea

J. Trazodone - Best for prn use - sleep and daytime anxiety - may help male erectile dysfunction

K. Venlafaxine and levomilnacipran - SSRI-like (more nausea) – Useful for SSRI resistance – May ↑ BP

L. Vilazodone - Take with food - GI side effects - early antidepressant response possible - buspirone mechanism too - low sexual dysfx.

M. Vortioxetine - Long t½ - affects many 5HT receptor effects - low sexual dysfx.

## XXIII. SSRI/SNRI INDICATIONS (ASIDE FROM ADULT DEPRESSION)

| Generic name | Brand name | Pediatric Depression | Pediatric OCD* | Adult OCD | Bulimia Nervosa | PTSD ** | PMDD *** | GAD **** | Social Anxiety Disorder | Panic Disorder |
|---|---|---|---|---|---|---|---|---|---|---|
| Citalopram | Celexa® | | | | | | | | | |
| Des-venlafaxine | Pristiq™ | | | | | | | | | |
| Duloxetine | Cymbalta®△ / Drizalma Sprinkle™ / Irenka™ | | | | | | | X (≥7 y.o.) | | |
| Escitalopram | Lexapro® | X (≥12 y.o.) | | | | | | X | | |
| Fluoxetine | Prozac® | X (≥8 y.o.) | X (≥7 y.o.) | X | X | | Sarafem | | | X |
| Fluvoxamine | Luvox® | | X† | X | | | | | Luvox CR | |
| Levo-milnacipran | Fetzima® | | | | | | | | | |
| Paroxetine | Paxil® | (FDA warning against use) | | X | | X | Paxil CR | X | X | X |
| Sertraline | Zoloft® | | X† | X | | X | X | | X | X |
| Venlafaxine | Effexor® | | | | | | | X | X | X |
| Vilazodone | Viibryd™ | | | | | | | | | |
| Vortioxetine | Trintellix® | | | | | | | | | |

*OCD = Obsessive-Compulsive Disorder  **PTSD = Post-traumatic Stress Disorder
***PMDD = Premenstrual Dysphoric Disorder  ****GAD = Generalized Anxiety Disorder
†Pediatric age is not specified, however, children as young as 6 y.o. were in clinical trials
△Also approved for Diabetic peripheral neuropathy, fibromyalgia, and chronic musculoskeletal pain

## XXIV. APPROXIMATE DOSE EQUIVALENTS & KINETICS OF ANTIDEPRESSANTS

| Generic | Brand | Equivalent dose (mg)[758] | Avg. dose (mg) | Half-life (hr) | CYP substrate* | CYP inhibitor** |
|---|---|---|---|---|---|---|
| Bupropion | Wellbutrin® | 174 | 300 | 21 | 2B6 | 2D6 |
| Citalopram | Celexa® | Not studied | 20 | 35 | 3A4, 2C19 | Minor 2D6 |
| Desvenlafaxine | Pristiq™ | Not studied | 50 | 11 | Minor 3A4 | ------ |
| Duloxetine | Cymbalta® | Not studied | 60 | 12.5-19.1 | 2D6 | Minor 2D6 |
| Escitalopram | Lexapro® | 9 | 10 | 27-32 | 3A4, 2C19, minor 2D6 | ------ |
| Fluoxetine | Prozac® | 20 | 20 | >4-6 days | Partly 2D6 | *POTENT 2D6* |
| Fluvoxamine | Luvox® | 72 | 150 | 22-30 | Partly 2D6 | 2C9/19, 3A4, 1A2 |
| Levo-milnacipran | Fetzima® | Not studied | 40-80 | 12 | 3A4 | ------ |
| Mirtazapine | Remeron® | 25 | 15-30 | 20-40 | 2D6, 1A2, 3A4 | ------ |
| Nefazodone | Serzone® | 268 | 300-400 | 11-24 | ------ | 3A4 |
| Paroxetine | Paxil® | 17 | 20 | 21 | 2D6, 3A4 rarely | *POTENT 2D6* |
| Sertraline | Zoloft® | 49 | 100-125 | 26 | 2B6/D6, 2C9/19, 3A4 | Minor 2D6 |
| Trazodone | Desyrel® | 200 | 300-400 | 10 | 3A4 | ------ |
| Venlafaxine | Effexor® | 75 | 150 | 5 & 11 | 2D6 | Minor 2D6 |
| Vilazodone | Viibryd™ | Not studied | 20-40 | 25 | 3A4, 2D6, minor 2C19 | 2C8 |
| Vortioxetine | Trintellix® | Not studied | 10-20 | 66 | 2D6 | ------ |

*Substrate = antidepressant is metabolized through this CYP450 enzyme pathway
**Inhibitor = antidepressant inhibits these CYP450 enzymes, which can ↑ other drugs' blood levels

## XXV. ADJUSTMENTS FOR ANTIDEPRESSANTS FOR RENAL AND HEPATIC IMPAIRMENTS

| NAME | RENAL | HEPATIC |
|------|-------|---------|
| Amitriptyline (Elavil®) | ----- | Start low and ↑ dose as needed |
| Brexanolone (Zulresso™) | Avoid use in ESRD (CrCl<15 ml/min) | ----- |
| Bupropion (Wellbutrin®, Aplenzin®, Forfivo™ XL) | Reduce dose and/or frequency | Max dose: 50 mg every other day |
| Citalopram (Celexa®) | Use with caution | Max dose: 20 mg/d |
| Desvenlafaxine (Pristiq™) | ↓ dose to 50 mg every other day | Max dose: 100 mg/d |
| Duloxetine (Cymbalta®) | Avoid use if CrCl < 30 ml/min | Avoid in chronic disease or cirrhosis |
| Escitalopram (Lexapro®) | Use with caution | Max dose: 10 mg/d |
| Esketamine (Spravato™) | ----- | Severe: not recommended |
| Fluoxetine (Prozac®) | ----- | Lower or less frequent dosing |
| Fluvoxamine (Luvox®/CR) | ----- | Start low and ↑ dose as needed |
| Levomilnacipran (Fetzima®) | Max 40 mg for severe impairment | |
| Isocarboxazid (Marplan®) | Contraindicated | Contraindicated |
| Mirtazapine (Remeron®) | Slow titration recommended | Slow titration recommended |
| Nefazodone (Serzone®) | ----- | Avoid use |
| Paroxetine (Paxil®) | Max dose: 40 mg/d | Max dose: 40 mg/d |
| Sertraline (Zoloft®) | ----- | Lower or less frequent dosing |
| Venlafaxine (Effexor®/XR) | Mild to moderate: ↓ dose by 25-50% | Mild to moderate: ↓ dose by >50% |
| Vilazodone (Viibryd™) | ----- | ----- |
| Vortioxetine (Trintellix®) | ----- | Severe: not recommended |

## XXVI. CELEBRATE THE GLUTAMATE....[302]

*Glutamate is the most important excitatory neurotransmitter in the brain, and plays a key role in memory, neuronal development and plasticity, but excess release has been implicated in neuronal cell death*

➢ **2 Types**: A ligand-gated ionic channel (metabotropic) and a receptor
❖ *Ligand gated ion channels* (ionotropic or iGluRs) stimulate fast excitatory neurotransmission
  ♦ Effects from NMDA receptors (NMDARs) are a down-regulation of strychnine-insensitive glycine receptors, regulation of $Ca^{2+}$ influx, and nitric oxide synthesis and blocking Substance P receptors (NK1 receptors)[635]
  ♦ Glutamate + glycine or d-serine must bind to NMDAR to "activate" it and open the ion channel
  ♦ iGluRs: *NMDA, AMPA* (amino-3-hydroxy-5-methyl-4-isoxazolepropionic acid) & *kainate* receptors
    ★AMPA & NMDA channels are composed of many glutamate receptor subunits
    ★AMPA: GluA1, GluA2, GluA3, & GluA4
    ★3 NMDARs:
      ⊙ GluN1 (NR1) has 8 isoform variants (NR1-1a, 1b, 2b, 3a, 3b, 4a & 4b) – stimulatory effects
      ⊙ GluN2 (NR2) has 4 isoform variants (NR2a, 2b, 2c & 2d)
      ⊙ GluN3 (NR3) has 2 isoform variants (NR3a [works in the CNS] & NR3b [works on motor neurons])
        ○ GluN3 has inhibitory (antagonistic) effects on the NMDAR
  ♦ Glutamate reuptake is done by EAAT-2 (Excitatory Amino Acid Transporter-2)
    ⊙ Riluzole is a reuptake enhancer and terminal release inhibitors
  ♦ Some drugs targeting iGluRs have failed due to side effects, including cognitive & motor impairment
  ♦ Drugs can be Positive (PAM) or Negative (NAM) Allosteric Modulators
    ★NMDARs can be antagonized with:
      ⊙ 1) competitive antagonists (bind to & block glutamate);
      ⊙ 2) glycine antagonists;
      ⊙ 3) noncompetitive antagonists (bind to allosteric sites - e.g., ketamine [blocks NR2 and binds to the PCP site inside the ion channel, like $Mg^{2+}$]);
      ⊙ 4) uncompetitive antagonists (block ion channel by binding to a site within it)
❖ *G-protein coupled receptors* (metabotropic or mGluRs)
  ♦ mGluRs exert control over glutamate activity by stimulating several cell-signaling pathways via the activation of G-protein coupled receptors (GPCRs)
  ♦ mGluRs can be divided into 8 subtypes and 3 subgroups based on homology sequence
    ★**Group I** includes mGluR1 and mGluR5 (normally stimulatory and associated with phospholipase C activation and second messengers such as inositol and diacylglycerol production)
      ⊙ Located on the postsynaptic neuron and coupled to Gq/G11 subunits
    ★**Group II** includes mGluR2 & mGluR3 (presynaptic and coupled to Gi/Go subunits)
    ★**Group III** includes mGluR4, mGluR6, mGluR7 & mGluR8 (located presynaptically)
    ★**Groups II & III** inhibit glutamate transmission and are negatively coupled to adenylyl cyclase

## XXVII. COMMON ANTIDEPRESSANT SIDE EFFECTS

### A. TCAs - TRICYCLIC ANTIDEPRESSANTS

| ANTICHOLINERGIC SIDE EFFECTS | CARDIAC SIDE EFFECTS | OTHER: |
|---|---|---|
| • Toxic Psychosis | • Heart Block - 1° or 2° is contraindicated | • Weight gain |
| **CNS EFFECTS:** | • Arrhythmias - prolonged QT interval | • Allergic reactions |
| • Drowsiness (very common) | | • Rash, urticaria, fever, photosensitivity |
| • Stimulation (more with 2° amines) | • Hypotension / orthostasis | • Agranulocytosis (rare) |
| **SEIZURES** | • Tachycardia (direct, anticholinergic, and reflex) | • Hepatic obstructive jaundice (very rare) |
| • Highest with amoxapine and maprotiline | **AUTONOMIC SIDE EFFECTS** | • Endocrinologic (i.e. SIADH) |
| • All antidepressants lower seizure threshold!!! | • Nasal congestion | • Caution in pregnancy and breastfeeding! |
| | • Tremors | |
| | • Sexual dysfunction (<SSRIs) | |

### B. MAOIs - MONOAMINE OXIDASE INHIBITORS

| | | |
|---|---|---|
| • Postural hypotension | | • Sexual dysfunction |
| • Hepatic complications hydrazine > non-hydrazine | • Sedation (most with phenelzine) | • **Hypertensive crisis** with *tyramine*-containing foods or sympathomimetic |
| • Anticholinergic (< TCAs) | • Stimulation (most with tranylcypromine) | |

### C. SSRIs - SELECTIVE SEROTONIN REUPTAKE INHIBITORS

| | | |
|---|---|---|
| • Sexual dysfunction | • Nausea | |
| • Anxiety | • Diarrhea | • Hyponatremia |
| • Insomnia | • Weight loss | • Rare abnormal bleeding[759] |
| • Headache | • Weight gain (long-term) | • 1 in 250 patients if combined with NSAID |
| • Sweating | | |

### D. SNRIs - SEROTONIN NOREPINEPHRINE REUPTAKE INHIBITORS

| | | |
|---|---|---|
| • Similar to SSRIs | • Dry mouth | • Hypertension |
| • Somnolence (drowsiness) | • Dizziness | • Orthostatic hypotension |

### E. NOVEL ANTIDEPRESSANTS - MIRTAZAPINE / ESKETAMINE / BREXANOLONE

| | | |
|---|---|---|
| • Somnolence | • ↑ appetite with weight gain | • Dizziness |

### F. NDRI - BUPROPION

| | | |
|---|---|---|
| • Anxiety | • Seizures | |
| • Weight loss | • Insomnia | • Hypertension |

### G. SPARI & SARIs – VILAZODONE / TRAZODONE / NEFAZODONE / VORTIOXETINE

| | | |
|---|---|---|
| • Nausea | • Constipation | |
| • Vomiting | • Drowsiness or Insomnia | • Low sexual dysfunction |

---

## 22. SEROTONIN RECEPTOR PHARMACOLOGY

I. In mammals there are at least 14 known specific receptors in 7 major serotonin families
  A. Families: $5HT_1$, $5HT_2$, $5HT_3$, $5HT_4$, $5HT_5$, $5HT_6$, $5HT_7$
   1. 5HT families 1 & 5 are inhibitory
   2. 5HT families 2, 3, 4, 6 & 7 are excitatory
  B. Specific receptors: $5HT_{1A}$, $5HT_{1B}$, $5HT_{1D}$, $5-T_{1E}$, $5HT_{1F}$, $5HT_{2A}$, $5HT_{2B}$, $5HT_{2C}$ (formerly $5HT_{1C}$), $5HT_3$, $5HT_4$, $5HT_{5A}$, $5HT_{5B}$, $5HT_6$, and $5HT_7$
II. Agonists or antagonists at 5HT receptors can affect specific parts of the body or the entire body
  A. Can affect the CNS (e.g., depression, anxiety, migraines, psychosis, sleep, memory, appetite)
  B. Can affect the periphery (e.g., platelet aggregation, GI motility, vasoconstriction, temperature)
III. Receptors can be pre-synaptic (e.g., auto-receptor) or post-synaptic
IV. Pre-synaptic $5HT_{1A}$ autoreceptors can inhibit 5HT release initially, and therefore increase anxiety
  A. In pediatric patients, this correlates with impulsive and aggressive behavior
  B. Studies of adding $5HT_{1A}$ antagonists to antidepressants are under way
V. 90% of serotonin receptors are in the GI tract / 10% are in the brain and on platelets
  A. $5HT_{2B}$ receptors found on blood vessels and heart valves
VI. Antagonists of $5HT_{1A}$ autoreceptors + an antidepressant can quickly increase synaptic 5HT levels[760]

| Receptor/Role | Agonist (green) / Antagonist (red) / Unknown (purple) | | Function(s) |
|---|---|---|---|
| 5HT$_{1A}$ autoreceptor | ◆ Decreases memory<br>◆ Decreases cravings<br>◆ Decreases learning<br>◆ Decreases anxiety<br>◆ Decreases depression<br>◆ Increases analgesia<br>◆ Decreases emesis<br>◆ Thermoregulations<br>◆ Decreases aggression | ◆ Decreases positive, negative and cognitive symptoms of schizophrenia (partial agonists)<br>◆ ↑ DA release in the prefrontal cortex<br>◆ ↓ 5HT release and synthesis<br>◆ Modulates neurotransmitter release<br>◆ Neuroprotective properties<br>◆ Modulates cardiovascular function | ◆ Inhibitory presynaptic and postsynaptic receptor<br>◆ Linked to the inhibition of adenylate cyclase<br>◆ 5HT-1-like receptor functions are less clear, but 5HT1E receptor might be linked to cognition and memory. |
| 5HT$_{1B}$ autoreceptor | ◆ Decreases aggression<br>◆ Regulates locomotion<br>◆ Decreases appetite<br>◆ Decreases anxiety<br>◆ Decreases appetite<br>◆ Thermoregulation<br>◆ Controls appetite | ◆ Decreases bone mass<br>◆ Controls sexual behavior<br>◆ Induce antidepressant-like behavior<br>◆ Regulations sleep and sensorimotor inhibition<br>◆ Increases vasoconstriction | |
| 5HT$_{1C}$ . The 5HT$_{1C}$ receptor was reclassified as a 5HT$_2$ receptor based on its operation, transduction, and structure. It was renamed 5HT$_{2C}$. | | | |
| 5HT$_{1D\alpha}$ autoreceptor | ◆ ↑vasoconstriction<br>◆ Involved neurogenic inflammation | ◆ Speculative role in depression, anxiety, and other neuropsychiatric disorders<br>◆ Decreases migraine | |
| 5HT$_{1D\beta}$ | ◆ Vasoconstriction | ◆ Decreases migraine | |
| 5HT$_{1E}$ | ◆ Unknown | | |
| 5HT$_{1F}$ | ◆ Speculative role in visual and cognitive function<br>◆ Speculative role in migraines | | |
| 5HT$_{2A}$ | ◆ Antidepressant effects<br>◆ Hallucinogenic effects | ◆ Antidepressant effects<br>◆ Anxiolytic properties | ◆ Excitatory<br>◆ Coupled to Gq/11 to increase inositol phosphates and cytosolic Calcium |
| 5HT$_{2B}$ autoreceptor | ◆ Antidepressant effects | ◆ Cardiovascular functioning (agonists ↑ risk of pulmonary HTN) | |
| 5HT$_{2C}$ | ◆ Antidepressant effects<br>◆ Appetite<br>◆ Antipsychotic | ◆ Modulation of Dopamine<br>◆ Antidepressant effects | |
| 5HT$_3$ | ◆ Increases emesis<br>◆ Causes vasodilation<br>◆ May decrease depression<br>◆ Increases cognition<br><br>◆ May decrease anxiety<br>◆ May reverse helpless behavior<br>◆ Controls dopamine release<br>◆ ↓ gastrointestinal side effects<br><br>◆ Decreases chemotherapy-induced or radiation-induced emesis (ineffective against motion sickness and apomorphine-induced emesis)<br>◆ Abolishes the emotion-potentiated startle effect<br>◆ May be effective in the treatment of migraine pain<br>◆ May suppress the behavioral consequences of withdrawing chronic treatment with drugs of abuse, including alcohol, nicotine, cocaine, and amphetamine | | ◆ Ligand-gated ion channel superfamily<br>◆ Directly gates an ion channel-inducing rapid depolarization<br>◆ Causes release of neurotransmitter and/or peptides<br>◆ Controls DA & Ach release |
| 5HT$_4$ | ◆ Antidepressant effects<br>◆ Memory & Learning | ◆ Rapid anxiolytic effects[770]<br>◆ Movement of food across the GI tract | ◆ Signaling via Gαq activation of adenylyl cyclase |
| 5HT$_{5A}$ In rats | ◆ The clinical significance of 5HT$_5$ is unknown<br>◆ Based on location it may be involved in: | | ◆ Memory consolidation<br>◆ Signals via Gi/o inhibition of adenylyl cyclase |
| 5HT$_{5B}$ In humans | ◆ Exploratory behavior<br>◆ Locomotion<br>◆ Anxiety<br>◆ Depression | ◆ Learning<br>◆ Memory consolidation<br>◆ Adaptive behavior<br>◆ Brain development | |
| 5HT$_6$ | ◆ Memory & learning<br>◆ Feeding behavior<br>◆ cognitive enhancement | ◆ Antidepressant effects<br>◆ Antidepressant effects | ◆ Gs signaling via activating adenylyl cyclase |
| 5HT$_7$ | ◆ Analgesia<br>◆ Antipsychotic<br>◆ Antidepressant effects | ◆ Anxiolytic properties<br>◆ Cognition<br>◆ Analgesia | ◆ Gs signaling via activating adenylyl cyclase<br>◆ Regulates circadian rhythm, sleep & mood |

I. Characterized by rapid development of hyperthermia, HTN, myoclonus (involuntary muscle twitching), rigidity, autonomic instability, mental status changes (e.g., delirium or coma), and rarely, death

II. **Hunter Serotonin Toxicity Criteria**[771]
  A. A serotonergic agent + 1 of the following symptoms:
    1. Spontaneous clonus
    2. Inducible clonus **and** agitation **or** diaphoresis
    3. Ocular myoclonus **and** agitation **or** diaphoresis
    4. Ocular myoclonus **or** inducible clonus
    5. Tremor **and** hyperreflexia **or** hypertonia
    6. Temperature >38°C **and** ocular myoclonus **or** inducible clonus

III. **Sternbach Criteria for Serotonin Syndrome**[772]
  A. Recent addition or increase in a known serotonergic agent
  B. Absence of other possible etiologies (e.g., infection, substance abuse, withdrawal, etc.)
  C. No recent addition or increase of a neuroleptic agent
  D. At least 3 of the following symptoms: Mental status changes (confusion, hypomania), agitation, myoclonus, hyperreflexia, diaphoresis, shivering, tremor, diarrhea, incoordination, or fever

IV. **Clinical Presentation**
  A. Symptoms as above in Hunter/Sternbach criteria
    1. Symptoms may not all be present and can resemble Neuroleptic Malignant Syndrome (NMS)[773]
  B. May also include hallucinations, headache, coma, hypertension, tachycardia, nausea, ↑ CPK, ↑ WBCs, ↑ transaminase enzymes, and ↓ serum bicarbonate[774]

V. First-line treatment - withdraw the offending drugs and provide supportive care
VI. Can treat with benzodiazepines or cyproheptadine, an antihistamine with 5HT antagonist[775]
  A. Cyproheptadine: Give 12 mg po, then +/- 2 mg Q2h until improvement seen
  B. Dexmedetomidine ($\alpha_2$ agonist) has also been used successfully[776]

VII. **Real-world application**
  A. Activation of $5HT_{2A}$ receptors required for SS[777-782]
  B. $5HT_{1A}$ receptors are not involved
  C. FDA alert - based on 10 out of 29 reported cases meeting the Sternbach Criteria for diagnosis
    1. None met the Hunter Criteria
  D. Use of SSRIs with other serotonergic drugs is unlikely to cause SS
    1. SSRIs + triptans unlikely
    2. SSRIs + cyclobenzaprine may cause SS, as it's structurally similar to TCAs[783]
    3. **Black box warning** with methylene blue and serotonergic drugs causing SS[784]
    4. SSRIs + tramadol - caution advised - especially with CYP2D6 inhibitors (e.g., paroxetine & fluoxetine)

## 24. INSOMNIA, NARCOLEPSY AND OTHER SLEEP DISORDERS[785,786]

I. The American Academy of Sleep Medicine's (*AASM*) Clinical Guideline for the Evaluation and Management of Chronic Insomnia in Adults
  A. 1/3 to 1/2 of adults experience insomnia symptoms in their lifetime
    1. Significant insomnia occurs in 10-15% of the population
    2. Women twice as likely as men
    3. Up to 75% of mental health and/or chronic pain patients experience insomnia (most are chronic)
    4. Most acute incidences of insomnia are secondary to a known cause (drugs/stress/medical condition)

II. **DSM-5 Diagnosis**[244]
  A. Insomnia
    1. Either difficulty initiating sleep, difficulty maintaining sleep, or early-morning awakenings
    2. Causes distress and reduces ability to function
    3. Not associated with drugs or other mental/medical conditions
      i. *A list of these can be found in Anxiety chapter*
    4. Chronic Insomnia: Happens at least 3 times a week for more than 3 months
  B. Insomnia can take different forms
    1. Sleep onset latency (SOL - difficulty falling asleep)
    2. Wake time after sleep onset (WASO - premature awakening)
    3. Number of awakenings throughout the night
    4. Total sleep time (TST) or efficiency
    5. Acute or transient insomnia may last days to weeks
    6. Primary insomnia (with no underlying cause)

       7. Secondary insomnia - due to an underlying condition (e.g., stimulating medication side effect, hallucinations, depression, mania, anxiety, stress)
         i. Removal of the causative agent is usually curative
    C. Note: Kids who have childhood nightmares and night terrors are statistically more likely to report psychosis around age 12 [787]
       1. Medications are not recommended for childhood insomnia per the *AASM* [788]
III. Treatment[789-791]
    A. 1st line therapy is **Cognitive Behavioral Therapy** ± short-term treatment with sedative hypnotics
IV. Pharmacotherapy[792]
    A. Intermittent use of medication (i.e., not daily) is recommended in chronic insomnia to maximize the sedative properties of a medication
    B. Benzodiazepines
       1. Recommended only for short-term use (< 2-4 weeks)
         i. Sleep continuity is initially improved (e.g. sleep latency, total sleep time) but deep sleep is ↓
           a. Overall, a negative effect on sleep architecture[793,794]
         ii. Tolerance to the sedative effects implies that the original dose has progressively less effect, and higher doses are needed to obtain the desired effect[336]
       2. Caution of interaction with alcohol (added sedation and psychomotor impairment)
       3. See Anxiety chapter for more details
       4. Should not discontinue abruptly
         i. Can lead to rebound insomnia, anxiety, and seizures
    C. "*Z-drugs*" (e.g., eszopiclone, zaleplon, and zolpidem)
       1. All now have BBW about Complex Sleep Behaviors (sleep-walking, sleep-driving, and engaging in other activities while not fully awake)[795]
         i. Z-drugs are contraindicated for those who have already had a Complex Sleep Behavior
       2. Sleep-inducing effects from non-BZD receptor agonists (NBRA's) is slightly > than placebo[796]
       3. Decreased sleep latency (time to fall asleep) by approx. 22 minutes
       4. Advantage of Z-drugs - relatively non-addictive compared to BZDs at prescribed doses (very large doses can be abused and addictive)[797]
         i. Caution of interaction with alcohol (added sedation and psychomotor impairment)
       5. Selectively bind to the $BZD_1$ receptor, also called omega ($\omega$) receptor
         i. $BZD_1$ receptor is the *alpha* ($\alpha$) subunit of $GABA_A$ receptor
       6. In chronic insomnia, Z-drugs studied up to 12 months and showed continued efficacy[798]
       7. Z-drugs are known to cause psychosis, hallucinations, sleep walking, etc.
         i. More so in children/adolescents and the elderly (up to 7% incidence)
       8. All Z-drugs should be *taken on an empty stomach*
       9. No dose adjustments needed in renally impaired patients
       10. Zolpidem provides approx. 4-5 hours of sedation
       11. Zaleplon is good for middle of the night awakenings
       12. Eszopiclone is longest acting and provides approx. 7-8 hours of sedation
    D. **Eszopiclone (Lunesta™)[56]** - C-IV Controlled Substance
       1. Recommended dose: 1 mg to 3mg
         i. Those with severe hepatic impairment, taking potent CYP3A4 inhibitors, or geriatric patients
           a. Dose should not exceed 2mg
         ii. Available in 1 mg, 2 mg, and 3 mg tablets
       2. Peak level in 1 hour, with half-life of 6 hours
       3. Primarily metabolized by CYP3A4 and CYP2E1 enzymes
    E. **Zaleplon (Sonata®)[70]** - C-IV Controlled Substance
       1. Recommended dose: 10 mg, with 5-20 mg range
         i. Available in 5 mg and 10 mg capsules
       2. Peak level in 1 hour, with half-life of 1 hour
         i. A high-fat or heavy meal can delay the onset of effect up to 2 hours
       3. Primarily metabolism by aldehyde oxidase; also lesser by CYP3A4 - inactive metabolites
         i. Not recommended in those with severe hepatic impairment
    F. **Zolpidem (Ambien® / Zolpimist® oral spray / Edluar & Intermezzo® sublingual)[71]** - C-IV
       1. Available in 5 and 10 mg tablets, and 6.25 and 12.5 mg CR (controlled-release) tablets
       2. Recommended dose for men: 5 mg to 10mg
         i. **Geriatric** patients (men & women), adult **women**, and those with severe hepatic impairment metabolize zolpidem slower, so max dose should not exceed **5 mg** (6.25 mg for CR formulation)[799]
       3. Peak level in 96 minutes, with half-life of 2.5 hours
         i. CR peak level in 90 minutes, with half-life of 2.8 hours
         ii. Food can delay onset of effect up to 2-4 hours
       4. Metabolized mainly by CYP3A4
       5. Higher doses have been associated with an ↑ incidence of benign brain tumors[800,801]
         i. Highest risk when cumulatively taking ≥ 520 mg/year
       6. **Intermezzo® sublingual tablets[72]**
         i. Recommended dose (and available in) 1.75 mg for women & 3.5 mg for men
         ii. Peak level in 35-75 minutes

       7. **Edluar® sublingual tablets**[71]
         i. Available in 5 mg and 10 mg tablets
         ii. Peak level in 82 minutes (range: 30-180 min)
       8. **Zolpimist® spray**[73] (cherry flavored) contains 5 mg per actuation of the pump
       9. Recent review found that zolpidem may help in coma recovery, dystonias, Parkinson's disease, and with other motor, auditory, and verbal problems[802]
G. **Suvorexant (Belsomra®)**[66] - C-IV Controlled Substance
    1. Orexin receptor (OX1R and OX2R) antagonist with low abuse liability
    2. Recommended dose: 10mg
    3. Available in 5, 10, 15, and 20 mg tablets
    4. Peak level in 2 hours (range 30 min to 6 hours), with half-life of 12 hours
       i. Onset of effect is delayed by approx. 1.5 hours if taken with food
    5. Reduce dosage to a maximum of 5 mg if taken with *moderate* CYP3A4 inhibitors
       i. Not recommended for use with a *strong* CYP3A4 inhibitor
    6. Precautions/Warnings:
       i. CNS depressant effects and daytime impairment (e.g., driving)
       ii. Abnormal thinking and behavioral changes
       iii. Worsening of depression / suicidal ideation
       iv. Sleep paralysis, hypnagogic / hypnopompic hallucinations, cataplexy-like symptoms
       v. Respiratory impairment / COPD patients
    7. Studies show continued efficacy up to 3 months with no withdrawal or rebound effects[803,804]
       i. Improves sleep latency, sleep maintenance, and total sleep time
H. **Melatonin agonists** (e.g., rameiteon, tasimelteon)
    1. Full agonist of melatonin ($M_1$ and $M_2$) receptors, but not $M_3$ receptors
    2. May increase prolactin in women and lower testosterone in men
    3. May be used up to 6 months
    4. May require a few weeks of dosing before maximal effects are seen
    5. *Should be taken on an empty stomach*
    6. Not recommended in pregnancy or breastfeeding
I. **Ramelteon (Rozerem®)**[64]
    1. Recommended dose is 8 mg at HS (available in 8 mg tablets)
    2. Onset in 30-90 minutes, with half-life of 1-2.6 hours [weak metabolite (M-II) is 2-5 hours]
    3. Metabolized by CYP1A2 and CYP3A4
       i. Contraindicated in combination with fluvoxamine (Luvox®)
       ii. Affected by drugs which inhibit or induce these enzymes
    4. Severe allergic reactions have occurred (anaphylaxis and angioedema)
    5. Reduce dose in hepatic impairment / not recommended if severe
J. **Tasimelteon (Hetlioz®)**[68]
    1. Recommended dose is 20 mg at HS
    2. Available in 20 mg capsules
    3. Onset in ½ to 3 hours, with half-life of 1.3 to 3.7 hours
    4. Metabolized by CYP1A2 and CYP3A4
       i. Affected by drugs which inhibit or induce these enzymes
    5. Not studied in hepatic impairment, so use is not recommended
K. Antihistamines
    1. OTC sleep aids (i.e., antihistamines) are not recommended, due to lack of efficacy data
       i. They are usually first-line agents because of their easy accessibility
    2. **Doxepin (Silenor®)**[55,805] - tricyclic antidepressant originally FDA-approved in 1969
       i. At low doses, doxepin has a high affinity for the histamine $H_1$ receptor (Ki <1 nM)
       ii. Silenor® does not have a **BBW** about suicidal ideation
       iii. Recommended dose is 6 mg (3 mg in elderly)
          a. Max dose of 3 mg if taken with cimetidine (Tagamet®)
          b. Available in 3 mg and 6 mg tablets (not scored)
       iv. Take on an empty stomach
          a. Peak in 3.5 hours (food delays onset by an additional 3 hours)
       v. Metabolized by CYP2C19 and CYP2D6, and to a lesser extent by CYP1A2 and CYP2C9
          a. Affected by drugs which inhibit or induce these enzymes
          b. Half-life of 15.3 hours for doxepin and 31 hours for nordoxepin (main metabolite)
       vi. Efficacy maintained up to 12 weeks in trials (i.e., no tolerance develops)
       vii. Not recommended for patients with severe sleep apnea, glaucoma, or urinary retention
       viii. Not recommended in pregnancy or breastfeeding (although it is a Category C)
    3. **Diphenhydramine (Benadryl®)**[53]
       i. Usual dose of 25-50 mg at HS
       ii. Absolute maximum dose of 300 mg a day
       iii. Peak levels in 1-3 hours, with half-life of 2.4-9.3 hours
       iv. Metabolized by CYP2D6 (also an inhibitor)
       v. Also metabolized by CYP1A2, CYP2C9, and CYP2C19
       vi. Has anticholinergic side effects, so not recommended in the elderly
       vii. Tolerance develops quickly to sedation[806]
       viii. Should not use consecutively for more than 7-10 days
       ix. Pregnancy Category B / Contraindicated in breastfeeding

4. **Doxylamine (Unisom®)**
   i. Usual dose of 25 mg at HS (available OTC as a 25 mg tablet)
   ii. Peak levels in 2-3 hours, with half-life of 10-12 hours
   iii. Half-life in elderly women is 12.2 hours and in elderly men is 15.5 hours
   iv. Has anticholinergic side effects
   v. Available as a 12.5 mg/5 mL liquid, 12.5 mg chewable tablet, 25 & 50 mg capsule/softgel/tablet
   vi. Tolerance develops quickly to sedation[806]
   vii. Should not use consecutively for more than 7-10 days
   viii. Safety in pregnancy and breastfeeding are unknown
L. Antidepressants (very low abuse potential)[807]
  1. Used mainly if co-morbid depression exists, but can also be used if patient not depressed
  2. For detailed information, see Antidepressants chapter
  3. **Trazodone (Desyrel®)**[69]
   i. Usual dose is 25-150 mg at HS
   ii. Mechanism of sedation is believed to be due to $5HT_{2A}$ and $H_1$ blockade
   iii. Peak levels in 1-2 hours, with half-life of 9 hours
  4. **Mirtazapine (Remeron®)**[190]
   i. Sedation is reduced as doses are increased, so low doses are better for treating insomnia
   ii. Recommended dose of 7.5-15 mg at HS
   iii. May cause next-day sedation due to 20-40 hour half-life
M. *Alpha$_1$* adrenergic blocker prazosin is useful in PTSD-related nightmares[808]
N. For **specific sleep disturbances**, the **AASM guidelines recommend**:[790]

| | Recommended | Not recommended |
|---|---|---|
| **Sleep onset insomnia** | Eszopiclone<br>Ramelteon<br>Temazepam<br>Triazolam<br>Zaleplon<br>Zolpidem | |
| **Sleep maintenance insomnia** | Doxepin<br>Eszopiclone<br>Suvorexant<br>Temazepam | |
| **Sleep onset and sleep maintenance insomnia** | Eszopiclone<br>Temazepam<br>Zolpidem | Diphenhydramine<br>Melatonin<br>Tiagabine<br>Trazodone<br>Tryptophan<br>Valerian |

O. Other medications generally not recommended:
  1. Barbiturates, due to toxicity in overdose
  2. Chloral hydrate (Noctec®)
  3. Long-acting BZDs (e.g., flurazepam, diazepam)
  4. Anticonvulsants (e.g., gabapentin) unless there's a comorbid indication
  5. Atypical antipsychotics should <u>not</u> be used as hypnotic agents (unless patient has a psychiatric condition that could benefit from an antipsychotic)[809]
   i. Sedation is from antihistamine effects
   ii. American Psychiatric Association discourages such use as benefits do not outweigh risks[810]
P. COMPLEMENTARY AND ALTERNATIVE MEDICATIONS (CAM)[359-362,811,812]
  1. **California poppy** (eschscholzia californica)
   i. Binds to GABA receptors and has shown effects in animal studies
  2. **Chamomile** (Matricaria recutita/chamaemelum nobile)[813]
   i. More effective in the elderly
  3. **Chaste tree** (vitex agnus castus)
   i. Contains vitexin and casticin
   ii. Modulates circadian rhythm via increased melatonin secretion
  4. **Hops** (humulus lupulus)
   i. Contains humulone, lupulone, and xanthohumol
   ii. Binds to Melatonin-1 and -2 ($MT_1$ & $MT_2$) receptors
  5. **Kava-Kava** (not recommended due to hepatotoxicity)
  6. **Lavender oil**/Silexan [814]
   i. Patients in studies report an improvement in the overall quality of life and significantly less daytime fatigue compared to other sedatives
  7. **Lemonbalm**★ (melissa officinalis)
   i. Contains citranellal and geraniol
   ii. Inhibits MAO-A and GABA transaminase
   iii. Shown to reduce human stress levels acutely after dosing

8. **Melatonin** (and **Valerian root**) have shown effects on reducing sleep onset latency, but no effects on wake time after sleep onset or total sleep time
   i. Children, however, do have increased total sleep time
   ii. Melatonin (0.5-3 mg at HS) used mostly for insomnia from jet lag or for shift workers
9. **Passionflower** ★ (passiflora incarnata, maypop, purple passionflower)
   i. Contains harman and chrysin
   ii. BZD receptor partial agonist shown in animals to reduce anxiety without sedation
10. **Rosemary** ★ (Rosmarinus officinalis)[815]
11. **Sour date** (zizyphus jujuba)
   i. Contains jujuboside A & B which inhibit glutamate pathways in the hippocampus
   ii. In rats, was found to increase total sleep time
12. **Withania** (withania somnifera)
   i. Active compounds: withanolide and withaferin
   ii. Has GABA binding activity similar to lorazepam in animal models
13. **Valerian** ★ (valeriana officinalis)
   i. Contains valepotriate and valerenic acid
   ii. Various proposed MOAs include GABA modulation, interaction with adenosine-1 (A1) receptors, $GABA_A$ (β3 subunit) receptor agonism, and 5HT5A partial agonism
   iii. Systematic reviews and meta-analyses showed mostly no positive outcomes and < 1 minute reduction in sleep latency
   iv. Valerian Root 300-600 mg at HS
   ★ = Recommended by the European Medicine Agency (EMA), which is responsible for the evaluation and monitoring of medicines in the European Union

Q. Non-medication options
1. Warm milk and toast with jelly
2. Bananas, juice, and graham crackers (low-protein, high carbohydrate)
3. Turkey sandwich (contains tryptophan)
4. Hot bath or shower
5. Exercise
6. Reading a book or magazine
7. Relaxation techniques & tapes with deep breathing exercises
8. Expressing yourself to peers or loved ones
9. Avoid caffeine, soda, and other stimulating substances late in the day
10. Transcutaneous electrical stimulation to induce lucid dreaming[816]
11. Reducing exposure to blue light in the afternoon and evening[569]
   i. Blue light suppresses natural melatonin
   ii. On electronic devices, use "night mode" or change color mode to warmer

R. Combinations of drug classes can improve efficacy if monotherapy fails
1. Combination of a Z-drug with a BZD is **not** logical since they work on the same receptors
2. Long-term use (> 10 days) may be associated with rebound insomnia upon discontinuation
   i. BZDs are inherently psychologically reinforcing, because of rebound effects
      a. It may fool the patient in to thinking that they absolutely need the drug to sleep, when in reality, the BZD withdrawal caused the problem
   ii. Minimize withdrawal effects by tapering BZD off over weeks to months
   iii. Cognitive and behavioral therapy can increase the success of tapering
3. Caution with use of BZDs in the elderly
4. Risk of motor vehicle accidents is increased with BZDs and Z-drugs
5. Patient should be re-evaluated in 2-4 weeks to assess efficacy and side effects

# V. POTENTIAL FUTURE TREATMENTS FOR INSOMNIA / OTHER SLEEP DISORDERS IN STUDY
A. Various $5HT_2$ inverse-agonists/antagonists[817]
B. Various *orexin type 2 receptor (Ox2R or OX2) antagonists*
1. Orexin receptor is also known as hypocretin receptor type 2 (HcrtR2)
2. Lemborexant[818] (E-2006, LEM-10, LEM-5) – orexin receptor antagonist
   i. NDA filed with FDA in early 2019 based on SUNRISE-1 and SUNRISE-2 studies
3. Daridorexant (Nemorexant) (ACT-541468) by Idorsia Pharmaceuticals
   i. OX1 and OX2 antagonist In Phase III for insomnia
4. Seltorexant (MIN-202, JNJ-42847922, JNJ-922)
   i. By Janssen Pharmaceuticals & Minerva Neurosciences
   ii. A selective, small-molecule antagonist of the OX2 receptor
   iii. Phase II clinical trials for insomnia and sleep apnea (Phase I) are underway
5. Filorexant (MK-6096) by Merck & Co
C. JZP-507 by Jazz Pharmaceuticals Inc.
1. A dopamine receptor agonist in Phase II for Cataplexy & Narcolepsy
D. Lorediplon (GF-015535-00) by Ergomed & Ferrer
1. GABA receptor positive allosteric modulator (in Phase II study in Croatia and Poland)
E. Piromelatine (Neu-P11) by Neurim Pharmaceuticals
1. A melatonin receptor agonist and $5HT_{1A/1D}$ agonist and $5HT_{2B}$ receptor antagonist
2. In Phase II trials for Alzheimer's, Insomnia, Ocular hypertension and Open-angle glaucoma
F. Remimazolam (HR-7056) by Jiangsu Hengrui Medicine Co.
1. BZD in Phase III clinical trials in China for anaesthesia and sedation

G. S-117957 (V-117957) by Purdue Pharma – in Phase II for Insomnia
H. TS-142 by Taisho Pharmaceutical in Phase II study (in Japan) for insomnia as of Sept. 2019
I. Zuranolone (SAGE-217/S812217) - SAGE Therapeutics
  1. A synthetic, orally active, inhibitory pregnane neuro-steroid, that acts as a positive allosteric modulator of the GABA$_A$ receptor
  2. Developed as an improvement of allopregnanolone (brexanolone/Zulresso™) with high oral bioavailability and a biological half-life suitable for once-daily administration
  3. Currently in Phase III trials for Major depressive disorder, Postnatal depression, and Insomnia
  4. In Phase II trials for Bipolar Depression, Essential Tremors, and Parkinson's Disease

## VI. NARCOLEPSY[245]
A. Reoccurring periods of insatiable need to sleep, lapsing into sleep, or napping within same day
  1. Happens at least 3 times a week over > 3 month period of time
  2. Plus at least one of the following:
    i. Episodes of cataplexy at least a few times a month
      a. E.g., brief episodes of bilateral loss of muscle tone with maintained consciousness, precipitated by laughter or joking
      b. In children, it may present as spontaneous facial grimacing or episodes of jaw-opening with tongue thrusting or global hypotonia, without any obvious emotional triggers
    ii. Hypocretin deficiency, as measured in cerebrospinal fluid
    iii. Sleep polysomnography showing rapid eye movement (REM) sleep latency
  3. Narcolepsy may also be diagnosed with or without cataplexy or hypocretin deficiency
  4. May also present with just excessive daytime sleepiness (**EDS**), cataplexy, hypnagogic hallucinations, or sleep paralysis
B. Pharmacotherapy[819]
  1. FDA-approved medications: Stimulants, Wake-promoting agents, and sodium oxybate
  2. Stimulants (*See chapter on Child & Adolescent Disorders - ADHD*):
    i. Mixed amphetamine salts (Adderall XR®)
    ii. Amphetamine sulfate (Evekeo®) – also approved for Obesity
    iii. Dextroamphetamine (Dexedrine®, Zenzedi®, Dextrostat®, ProCentra®)
    iv. Methylphenidate (Ritalin®, Ritalin SR®, Concerta®, Methylin® / Methylin® ER)
  3. Wake-promoting agents:
    i. Modafinil (Provigil®)[62] and Armodafinil (Nuvigil®)[52]
    ii. Both have same indication, interactions, warnings, and side effects
      a. C-IV controlled substance (may also cause euphoria, similar to amphetamines)
      b. MOA: Unknown, but may have involvement with the dopamine transporter (DAT) system
      c. Indications: to improve wakefulness in adult patients with excessive sleepiness associated with narcolepsy, obstructive sleep apnea (OSA), or shift work disorder (SWD)
      d. Common side effects: headache, nausea, nervousness, rhinitis, diarrhea, back pain, anxiety, insomnia, dizziness, and dyspepsia
      e. Reduce dose in patients with severe hepatic impairment and geriatric patients
      f. **Significant warnings**:
        1. Serious rash, including Stevens-Johnson Syndrome
        2. DRESS/Multi-organ Hypersensitivity Reactions
        3. Angioedema and anaphylaxis reactions
        4. Persistent sleepiness
        5. Various psychiatric symptoms
        6. Known cardiovascular disease
        7. Effects on ability to drive and use machinery
      g. CYP3A4/5, CYP2C19 and P-glycoprotein substrate
      h. Drug interactions:
        1. CYP3A4/5 inducer
        2. CYP2C19 inhibitor
        3. May reduce effectiveness of estrogen-based oral contraceptives
          a. Use other methods of birth control
    iii. Modafinil (Provigil®)
      a. Dosing: 200 mg to 400 mg once a day in the morning
      b. Available in 100 & 200 mg capsule-shaped tablets
      c. Half-life is approximately 15 hours
    iv. Armodafinil (Nuvigil®)
      a. Dosing: 150 mg to 250 mg once a day in the morning
      b. Available in 50, 150, 200, and 250 mg tablets
      c. Half-life of approximately 4 hours
  4. Sodium oxybate (Xyrem®)[67]
    i. C-III controlled substance
    ii. Approved for EDS and cataplexy in children (over 7-years-old) and adults
    iii. GHB (gamma-hydroxybutyrate) – a "club drug"
      a. **Black Box Warnings** about Abuse Potential and CNS depression
      b. Additional warnings about suicidal ideation, driving, sleepwalking, and sodium overload
      c. GHB is the metabolite of GABA – GABA$_B$ is likely involved in its mechanism
    iv. Dosing: Pediatric doses are weight-based and described in the package insert

      a. Adults: 2.25 grams at bedtime and repeated again 2½ to 4 hours later (=4.5 g total)

      b. Increase by 1.5 grams (divided at night) each week (0.75 g per dose)

      c. Recommended dose: 6-9 grams (divided) each night (3-4.5 g per dose)

      d. Available as an oral solution – 0.5 grams per mL

      e. Take more than 2 hours after eating (i.e., empty stomach)

      f. Reduce dose by 50% with hepatic impairment

    v. Common side effects: nausea, dizziness, vomiting, somnolence, enuresis, and tremor

      a. Dependence and withdrawal can occur

    vi. Interactions – Reduce Xyrem dose by 20% if taken with Divalproex

      a. Contraindicated with sedative hypnotics and alcohol

    vii. Not safe in pregnancy

    viii. Metabolism

      a. Metabolic pathway involves a cytosolic $NADP^+$-linked enzyme called GHB dehydrogenase

      b. Final metabolic byproducts are carbon dioxide and water

      c. Half-life of 0.5 to 1 hour

    ix. Availability is restricted through a program called Xyrem REMS (www.XYREMREMS.com)

  5. Solriamfetol (Sunosi™)[65]

    i. Approved for EDS in patients associated with narcolepsy or obstructive sleep apnea (OSA)

    ii. Dual-acting dopamine and norepinephrine reuptake inhibitor (DNRI)

      a. Contraindicated with MAOIs and any drugs that increase BP or heart rate

    iii. Dosing – in the morning (at least 9 hours before bedtime)

      a. For Narcolepsy: 75 mg QAM

      b. For OSA: 37.5 mg QAM

      c. Doses can be increased every 3 days or more

      d. Maximum dose: 150 mg QAM

      e. Reduce dose in moderate renal impairment

        1. In severe renal impairment (CrCl $\leq$ 30), max. dose is 37.5 mg

        2. Not recommended in End Stage Renal Disease (ESRD) – CrCl $\leq$ 15

      f. Available in 75 mg (functionally scored) and 150 mg tablets

    iv. Not highly metabolized or protein bound

      a. Half-life is about 7.1 hours

    v. Most common adverse effects are headache, nausea, decreased appetite and anxiety

      a. Serious side effects include ↑ BP & HR, insomnia, irritability, and agitation

  6. Pitolisant (Wakix®)[63]

    i. Approved for EDS in adults with narcolepsy

    ii. Acts as an antagonist/inverse agonist at histamine-3 ($H_3$) receptors

    iii. Dosing – doses can be increased weekly

      a. 8.9 mg QAM x 1 week, then 17.8 mg QAM x 1 week, then 35.6 mg QAM (max dose)

      b. Poor metabolizers of CYP2D6 or moderate hepatic/renal to severe renal impairment

        1. Only titrate to 17.8 mg QAM after 1 or 2 weeks (max dose)

        2. Not recommended in End stage renal disease (ESRD)

      c. Available in 4.45 mg and 17.8 mg tablets

    iv. Pitolisant is highly protein bound (91-96%)

      a. Primarily metabolized by CYP2D6 and to a lesser extent by CYP3A4

      b. Half-life is approximately 20 hours (7.5-24.2 hours)

    v. Common side effects:

    vi. Levels are affected by strong CYP2D6 inhibitors and CYP3A4 inducers

      a. Patients should avoid H1 blockers (common antihistamines) and drugs that prolong QTc

      b. May reduce effectiveness of estrogen-based oral contraceptives

        1. Use other methods of birth control

  7. Useful agents if above not tolerated or ineffective

    i. Dexmethylphenidate (Focalin)

    ii. Lisdexamfetamine (Vyvanse)

    iii. TCAs / SSRIs / SNRIs


## VII. POTENTIAL FUTURE TREATMENTS FOR INSOMNIA AND OTHER SLEEP DISORDERS IN STUDY

A. Various **Trace Amine-Associated Receptor 1** (TAAR1) agonists

B. **Hypocretin-based** therapies, including administration of hypocretin-1, hypocretin peptide agonists, cell transplantation, and gene therapy

  1. Due to the blood-brain barrier's impermeability to hypocretin-1, only very high doses of hypocretin administered peripherally have produced some therapeutic effects

C. **Thyrotropin-Releasing Hormone** (TRH) direct or indirect agonists

D. **AXS-12** (reboxetine) by Axsome Therapeutics, Inc. (https://axsome.com/axs-pipeline/about-axs-12)

  1. Already marketed in other countries for depression (brand names: Davedax, Edronax, Irenor, Narebox, Norebox, Prolift, Solvex, Vestra)

  2. A highly selective and potent norepinephrine reuptake inhibitor

  3. Received Orphan Drug status by the FDA, but Phase II trial for Narcolepsy planned in the US

E. **Flecainide/modafinil** (THN-102) by Theranexus

  1. Combination of modafinil (dopamine reuptake inhibitor) and flecainide (antiarrhythmic)

  2. *Alpha*1 receptor agonist, CNS stimulants, and Na+ channel antagonist

      3. Has Orphan Drug Status Narcolepsy
- F. **FT-218** (sodium oxybate controlled release) by Avadel Pharmaceuticals
    1. GHB and GABA$_B$ receptor agonist
    2. Micropump® sodium oxybate in Phase III for narcolepsy
    3. Has Orphan Drug Status by the FDA for Narcolepsy
    4. 11/25/19 - Avadel Pharmaceuticals announced intention to submit NDA to FDA for Narcolepsy
- G. **Golexanolone** (GR-3027) by Umecrine Cognition
    1. GABA$_A$ receptor antagonist in Phase II for Hypersomnia
- H. **JZP-258** (oxybate mixed salt solution) by Jazz Pharmaceuticals
    1. GHB and GABA receptor agonist
    2. Has Orphan Drug Status by the FDA for Hypersomnia
    3. Jazz Pharmaceuticals intends to submit NDA to the FDA for Cataplexy & Narcolepsy in January 2020
    4. In Phase III study for Cataplexy, Hypersomnia and Narcolepsy
- I. **Mazindol** controlled-release (NLS-1001, NLS 0, NLS 1, NLS-10, NLS-13, Nolazol, Quilience)
    1. By NLS Pharmaceutics
    2. In Phase II for Hypersomnia & Narcolepsy, as well as for ADHD
    3. NE-predominant 5HT-NE-DA reuptake inhibitor (SNDRI)
- J. **Pentylenetetrazole** (BTD-001) by Balance Therapeutics
    1. GABA$_A$ receptor antagonist in Phase II for Narcolepsy and Hypersomnia
- K. **SUVN-G3031** by Suven Life Sciences
    1. An H$_3$ inverse agonist in Phase II for Narcolepsy
    2. At the end of Phase I trials for Cognitive Disorders and Sleep Disorders
- L. **TAK-925** and **TAK-994** by Takeda Pharmaceutical in Phase Ib studies
    1. Both agents are Orexin-2 receptor *agonists* for Narcolepsy
- M. **TS-091** (TS-0911) – by Taisho Pharmaceutical
    1. In Phase II for Hypersomnia & Narcolepsy (incl. adolescents)

## VIII. OTHER SLEEP-WAKE DISORDERS
- A. Delayed sleep phase
- B. Advanced sleep phase
- C. Irregular sleep-wake
- D. Non-24-hour sleep-wake
- E. Shift work
    1. All involve disrupted patterners of normal sleep

# 25. OBSESSIVE-COMPULSIVE DISORDER (OCD)[245]

## I. BACKGROUND
A. Obsessive-Compulsive Disorder
   1. Related disorders not included in the OCD diagnostic spectrum: body dysmorphic disorder, hoarding disorder, trichotillomania (hair-pulling disorder), excoriation (skin-picking) disorder, and others
B. OCD rarely remits without treatment
C. May be from overactive neural transmission from the midbrain raphe nuclei to the basal ganglia[302]
D. Patients may suffer lifelong disability
E. Not to be confused with Obsessive-Compulsive <u>Personality Disorder</u>
   1. Perfectionists; rigidly inflexible; preoccupied with rules, details, procedures

## II. EPIDEMIOLOGY
A. Affects 2.2 million adults, or 1.0% of the U.S. population[296]
   1. Average age of onset is 19, with 25 percent of cases occurring by age 14
      i. One-third of affected adults first experienced symptoms in childhood
   2. 12-month prevalence of 1.2% (1.1-1.8% world-wide) for adults[245]
B. 4th most common psychiatric disorder
C. High comorbidity with anxiety disorders, depression, and bipolar disorder
D. Large % do not seek treatment
E. Average age of onset: late adolescence to early 20's
F. Men slightly less than women, but boys more commonly affected in childhood vs. girls
G. Role of genetics
   1. A person with OCD is twice as likely to have a 1st degree relative with OCD
   2. A person with childhood OCD is 10 times as likely to have a 1st degree relative with OCD
   3. More common in monozygotic twins (57% concordance vs. 22% in fraternal twins)
   4. 30% of patients have a tic disorder
H. *If new and sudden onset, examine for subclinical infections and treat*
   1. Especially group A streptococcus
   2. Data from >1 million children in Denmark showed that the risk of any mental disorder was ↑ 1.18 times for individuals with a positive streptococcal test compared to those without a strep test[820]
   3. OCD (1.51 times ↑ risk) and tic disorders (1.35 times ↑ risk) were highest correlated disorders
   4. Risk of any mental disorder, OCD, and tic disorders was also increased among individuals with a non-streptococcal throat infection (1.08, 1.28, and 1.25 times ↑ risk, respectively)
   5. PANDAS
      i. *Pediatric Autoimmune Neuropsychiatric Disorders Associated with Streptococcal Infection*
      ii. Still a theory of etiology
      iii. Etiology may be antibodies to the streptococcal bacteria cross-reacting with the basal ganglia
      iv. Structural similarities between the streptococcal cell surface and proteins of the basal ganglia
      v. http://www.pandasnetwork.org

## III. DSM-5 DIAGNOSTIC CRITERIA[245]
A. Obsessions, compulsions, **or both**
B. Obsessions as defined by:
   1. Recurrent & persistent thoughts, urges, or images that are experienced, at some time during the disturbance, as intrusive and unwanted, & that in most individuals cause marked anxiety or distress.
   2. The individual attempts to ignore or suppress such thoughts, urges, or images, or to neutralize them with some other thought or action (i.e., by performing a compulsion).
C. Compulsions are defined by:
   1. Repetitive behaviors (e.g., hand washing, ordering, checking) or mental acts (e.g., praying, counting, repeating words silently) that the individual feels driven to perform in response to an obsession or according to rules that must be applied rigidly.
   2. Behaviors or mental acts are aimed at preventing or reducing anxiety or distress, or preventing some dreaded event or situation; however, these behaviors or mental acts are not connected in a realistic way with what they are designed to neutralize or prevent, or are clearly excessive.
D. Symptoms cause marked distress, are time consuming (>1 hr/d), or significantly interfere with the person's normal routine
E. With good, poor, or absent insight (Insight means that at some point, person recognizes that their thoughts and behavior are excessive or unreasonable)

## IV. PATHOPHYSIOLOGY -- Unknown
A. Serotonin mediated
   1. A 5HT agonist, m-CPP (*meta-chlorophenylpiperazine [trazodone's metabolite]*) worsens symptoms
   2. 5HT antagonists worsened symptoms after successful clomipramine treatment
B. May involve some dysfunction in the orbitofrontal cortex, anterior cingulate cortex, and striatum
   1. PET studies suggest a hyperfunctioning "loop" in the brain

## V. TREATMENT
   ✪*Patients generally respond best to the highest tolerable doses (sometimes above max), and response takes much longer than treating depression (6-12 weeks or more), and is rarely 100% complete*✪

A. Duration of treatment should be weighed against side effects in the individual
  1. Relapse rates high if treatment is discontinued (odds ratio 2.43 times) compared to placebo[304]
B. **Clomipramine** (Anafranil®)[821]
  1. TCA approved for OCD in 1989, including children 10-17-years-old
  2. 97% protein bound
  3. T½ = 31 - 37 hrs
  4. Drug interactions similar to other TCAs (e.g. QT-prolonging drugs, anticholinergics)
  5. Clomipramine is superior to SSRIs, which are superior to other antidepressants
  6. Dosage is 25-250 mg/d -- max. dose N.T.E. 250 mg/d (exponential ↑ in seizures)
    i. Available in 25, 50, and 75 mg capsules
  7. Side Effects: dry mouth (80%), dizziness and tremor (>50%) , fatigue (38%), sexual dysfx. (up to 70%), seizures (0.5 - 2.2%) -- dose related
C. **SSRIs** - ALL are FDA-approved, except citalopram & escitalopram
  1. *See Chapter on Antidepressants for more information*
  2. **Fluoxetine** (Prozac®) – also approved for pediatric patients aged 7-17 years
  3. **Sertraline** (Zoloft®) – also approved for pediatric patients aged 6-17 years
  4. **Paroxetine** (Paxil®) - NOT approved in children
  5. **Fluvoxamine** (Luvox®) – its only FDA-approved indication (also, pediatric patients aged 7-17 years)
D. Repetitive Transcranial Magnetic Stimulation (rTMS)
  1. FDA approved on 8/17/2018
    i. https://www.accessdata.fda.gov/cdrh_docs/reviews/DEN170078.pdf
    ii. Brainsway Deep Transcranial Magnetic Stimulation System (dTMS)

# VI. POTENTIAL FUTURE TREATMENTS FOR OCD IN STUDY
A. Agomelatine
B. **Antibiotic** treatment trial for the PANDAS/PANS Phenotype (minocycline, penicillin, azithromycin)
C. BHV-4157 in adults in Phase II and III
D. Bitopertin (RO4917838) in Combination with SSRIs
E. **Cannabinoids** (marijuana and dronabinol for Trichotillomania and OCD)
F. D-cycloserine[357] in Phase III (from clinicaltrials.gov)
  1. Glycine-gated NMDA agonist
  2. Studied as augmentation of Cognitive Behavioral Therapy (CBT) for Pediatric OCD[822]
G. Ketamine – for adults
H. N-Acetylcysteine (NAC) 2000 mg **+** fluvoxamine a day shows great promise[823]
  1. Also being studied for Grooming Disorders (trichotillomania/hair pulling, onychophagia/nail biting, excoriation/pathological skin picking)[824,825]
I. Nitrous Oxide
J. **Oxytocin** administration in body dysmorphic disorder (BDD) and OCD
K. Rapastinel (Formerly GLYX-13)
L. **Sarcosine** (N-Methylglycine) - a dietary supplement in Phase II
M. SLC7A11 – a protein stimulant
N. **Tolcapone** in Phase II/III by the University of Chicago (Clinical trials ID# NCT03348930)
O. **Troriluzole** (**BHV4157**) by Biohaven Pharmaceutical and Yale University
  1. Glutamate modulator in Phase II/III for Obsessive-compulsive disorders
  2. Orphan Drug Approved for Spinocerebellar degeneration
  3. Also in Phase III for Anxiety disorders and Phase II/III for Alzheimer's disease
P. **Drugs in study for similar disorders**
  1. **Vortioxetine** for the Treatment of Hoarding Disorder in Phase III
  2. **Subthalamic Stimulation** in Phase II for Tourette's Syndrome
  3. **N-Acetyl Cysteine** in Phase II for Pathologic Skin Picking
  4. **SXC-2023** by Promentis Pharmaceuticals in Phase II for Impulse Control Disorders

# VII. AUGMENTATION STRATEGIES FOR TREATMENT-RESISTANT OCD PATIENTS
A. Lithium (300-1800 mg/d) **+** clomipramine (25-250 mg/d)
B. Buspirone (20-60 mg/d) **+** fluoxetine (20-80 mg/d)
C. Fenfluramine (30-60 mg/d) **+** fluoxetine / fluvoxamine (50-300 mg/d) / clomipramine
D. Haloperidol (1-20 mg/d) or pimozide (1-2 mg/d) **+** SSRI **+** lithium
E. ADD carbamazepine (400-1200 mg/d), clonazepam (2-4 mg/d), desipramine (10-300 mg/d), valproic acid (500-3000 mg/d), or verapamil (240-480 mg/d)
F. Caffeine 300 mg/day, dextroamphetamine 30 mg/day, and morphine 30 mg once a week have shown positive efficacy in small studies as augmentation strategies[826]
G. MAOIs
H. Antiandrogens
I. Behavioral therapy or Computer-based Cognitive Behavioral Therapy (CBT)[827]
J. Psychosurgery (capsulotomy or cingulotomy)
K. Successful in case studies
  1. Ondansetron/granisetron, topiramate, lamotrigine, pindolol, riluzole, memantine, glycine
  2. Risperidone and aripiprazole have best evidence of efficacy[828]
L. Treatments that have not worked in studies for OCD augmentation
  1. Thyroid, clonazepam, desipramine, inositol, naltrexone, oxytocin

I. Personality disorders are dysfunctional characteristics of a person's personality. These disorders are incongruent with societal "norms". It is believed that infants begin forming their personality in the first 2 years of life. Personality disorders have a large environmental component but may also have a genetic component. People with personality disorders are often unaware of their condition and may feel persecuted by society due to the way they are treated by others. They are divided into Clusters and Types (*see DSM-5*[244] for detailed information). Varying combinations of dysfunction in affectivity, cognition, interpersonal function, and impulse control are observed, based on the type of personality disorder and the cluster into which the disorder is categorized. In the DSM-IV-TR, personality disorders are diagnosed under **Axis II**, along with intellectual disabilities.

A. **Cluster A**: The *odd and eccentric cluster* includes the paranoid, schizoid, schizotypal personality d/o.

B. **Cluster B**: The *dramatic, emotional, erratic cluster* includes the histrionic, narcissistic, antisocial, and borderline personality d/o.

C. **Cluster C**: The *anxious or fearful cluster* includes avoidant, dependent, and obsessive-compulsive personality d/o.

II. **Cluster A**

A. **Paranoid personality** generally manifests within the early adulthood years and is primarily associated with an intense distrust due to assuming that the motives of others are malicious. Because of the preoccupation with unjustified doubts, a paranoid person may perceive even innocuous interactions as an attack upon his or her character. The result of such an extreme suspicion is that interpersonal relationships are strained and the ability to interact becomes stunted.

B. **Schizoid personality** types have a blunted affect that is associated with feelings of detachment. Those with a schizoid personality type may not desire close relationships but rather choose to be solitary. Because they are prone to not show much emotion, others perceive them as having an emotionally cold disposition.

C. Those with a **schizotypal personality** type display a dysfunction in the ability to interact interpersonally due to discomfort. The discomfort does not arise from a negative self-image however, but rather the actual act of having to interact. Schizotypal personality types may also demonstrate cognitive distortions, odd speaking patterns and experience strange perceptual occurrences that influence their behavior.

III. **Cluster B**

A. **Histrionic personality** is characterized by a pattern of excessive emotionality and attention seeking. Histrionic types tend to not be happy unless they are the center of attention. In order to gain attention, they may be easily swayed by fads, become overly trusting, and may even interact with others in an inappropriately sexual manner. Displays of emotion are overly dramatic and theatrical, yet are actually superficial and may change immediately.

B. **Narcissistic personality** types are prone to grandiose fantasies with the need for admiration. Generally lacking empathy, narcissists are arrogant and feel a sense of entitlement. They expect others to acknowledge their supposed superiority and will feel overly jealous if others receive praise.

C. Those with an **antisocial personality** demonstrate a pervasive pattern of disregard for and violation of the rights of others. They are extremely impulsive and will show disregard for the safety of others and themselves. Because of this, and that they fail to conform to social norms, they tend to participate in unlawful activities and lack remorse for those whom they have wronged.

D. **Borderline personality** is associated with instability in self-image and interpersonal relationships. Impulsivity that may lead to self-harm, such as substance abuse and promiscuous sex, is typically demonstrated. In many cases, relationships are polarized such that a pattern of extreme idealization and devaluation are expressed. This may lead to feelings of emptiness and frantic efforts to avoid imagined abandonment.

IV. **Cluster C**

A. **Avoidant personality** types tend to show dysfunction in the ability to interact interpersonally due to discomfort. Unlike the schizotypal personality, however, the discomfort in this case is due to feelings of self-inadequacy. Because of the fear of shame, ridicule, or rejection, those with avoidant personalities may choose to not interact at all. The feeling of inferiority is so pervasive that new activities are rarely attempted, and relationships are seldom formed.

B. Those with a **dependent personality** tend to be extremely clingy and display an excessive need to be taken care of. They are prone to experience separation anxiety and will attempt to find another relationship quickly if one ends. It tends to be difficult for them to make everyday decisions and they go out of their way to have others take responsibility for major decisions.

C. An **obsessive-compulsive personality** is characterized by an inflexible and rigid strive for perfection. It may be rigid to the point that projects and tasks cannot be completed because they are not perfect enough. The preoccupation with details, rules, lists, and organization can be extremely invasive to the point that it affects interpersonal function.

## V. PHARMACOTHERAPY

A. ★★*NO MEDICATIONS ARE INDICATED TO TREAT A PERSONALITY DISORDER*★★

B. Borderline Personality Disorder
  1. Evidence-based medicine lacks support for pharmacotherapy[829-831]
  2. However, polypharmacy is common[832]
    i. Over 50% of patients are on more than 2 psychotropics
    ii. Over 11% of patients take more than 5 psychotropics simultaneously
  3. Some medications may be indicated to ↓ symptoms, such as depression, paranoia, & impulsivity
    i. Quetiapine 150-300 mg/d has shown significant improvement in the Zanarini Rating Scale for Borderline Personality Disorder (82% response vs. 48% placebo)[833]
    ii. American Psychiatric Association 2001 guidelines recommend pharmacotherapy as adjunctive treatment of symptoms such as affective instability, impulsivity, psychotic-like symptoms, and self-destructive behavior[834]
    iii. Pharmacotherapy is not cost effective and not a substitute for behavioral psychotherapy[835]
      a. If used, time-limited monotherapy preferred over polypharmacy
    iv. 2009 (to 2016) National Institute for Health & Clinical Excellence (NICE) guidelines discourage pharmacotherapy[836]
  4. Currently, Brexpiprazole (Rexulti®) by Lundbeck is in Phase II study for Borderline Personality Disorder

I. PTSD affects 7.7 million adults, or 3.5% of the U.S. population[296]
  A. Occurs when an individual is exposed to a traumatic event in which both were present:
    (1) Person (experienced, witnessed, or confronted) with an event that involved actual or threatened death, serious injury, or physical integrity to self or others.
    (2) The individual's response involved intense fear, helplessness or horror.
  B. Women are more likely to be affected than men.
  C. Rape is the most likely trigger of PTSD
    1. 65% of men and 45.9% of women who are raped will develop the disorder.
  D. Combat is the most common trauma for men
  E. Childhood sexual abuse is a strong predictor of lifetime likelihood for developing PTSD.
II. Acute Stress Disorder – occurs 3 days to <u>1 month</u> after traumatic event
  A. Prevalence estimated at 5 to 20%
  B. Person can be involved or just witness a traumatic event
  C. 1 in 4 youth experience maltreatment in their lifetime (1 in 7 in the last year)[254]
    1. "Trauma survivors" more likely to be easily distracted and have attention, mood, & conduct problems
    2. On the Pediatric Symptoms Checklist (PSC), young trauma survivors screened 94% positive for PTSD, 68% positive for severe depression, and 63% positive for Bipolar.
    3. 96% are at risk for future psychosis

---

**III. DSM-5 DIAGNOSIS**
**Re-experiencing (One or more)**
- Intrusive Memories (IMs)
- Nightmares (NMs)
- Feel as if traumatic event recurring
- Intense psychological distress at exposure to internal or external cues symbolizing/resembling traumatic event
- Physiologic reactivity on exposure to internal/external cues symbolizing/resembling traumatic event.
- Avoidance (Three or more)
**Thoughts/feelings/conversations associated with trauma**
- Activities, places, people that arouse recollections of the trauma
- Feeling of detachment/estrangement from others
- Inability to recall an important aspect of trauma
- Markedly diminished interest in activities
- Restricted range of affect
- Sense of foreshortened future
**Hyperarousal (Two or more)**
- Difficulties concentrating
- Exaggerated startle response
- Hypervigilance
- Irritability/Angry outbursts
- Difficulties sleeping

---

**IV. PHARMACOLOGIC RECEPTOR TARGETS**[837-839]
  A. $5HT_{2A}$ receptor antagonists
    1. Increase in restorative slow wave sleep (SWS) and decrease in waking after sleep onset
  B. *Alpha₁* receptor antagonists - reduce trauma-related nightmares and sleep disturbances
  C. Histamine₁ ($H_1$) receptor antagonists - ↓ wakefulness and ↑ restorative slow wave sleep
**V. PHARMACOLOGIC TREATMENT**[348,840]
  A. Duration of treatment should be weighed against side effects in the individual
    1. Relapse rates are high if treatment is discontinued (odds ratio 2.45 times) vs. placebo[304]
  B. First-line therapy: All SSRIs or SNRIs
    1. Only paroxetine & sertraline are FDA-approved medications
  C. Second-line therapy: mirtazapine, nefazodone, tricyclic antidepressants (TCAs), and phenelzine
    1. Propranolol (Inderal®) and other *beta*-blockers
      i. 2015 meta-analysis concluded it was ineffective in *preventing* PTSD post-trauma[841]
      ii. It is believed to impair the memory consolidation process
      iii. In a series of placebo-controlled trials, 40 mg administered prior to or just after memory reactivation effectively neutralized a conditioned fear response (i.e., defensive startle response)[842]
      iv. Propranolol indirectly targets the protein synthesis required for reconsolidation by inhibiting norepinephrine-stimulated CREB phosphorylation of fear memory while sparing declarative memory of memory formation (PTSD was not prevented, but symptoms were reduced)
      v. Trauma memory reactivation statistically ↓ (vs. placebo) when studied for reconsolidation therapy[843]
    2. *Alpha*-2 agonists - Guanfacine (although shown to reduce nightmares in children)
    3. Yohimbine (*alpha₂* antagonist) - readily crosses BBB and can produce CNS effects (intrusive memories, flashbacks, nightmares, agitation, etc.)

D. **Not** recommended as monotherapy
  1. Guanfacine, anticonvulsants (tiagabine, topiramate, or valproate) as monotherapy
  2. Bupropion, buspirone, trazodone, anticonvulsants (lamotrigine or gabapentin) or atypical antipsychotics as monotherapy
  3. Benzodiazepine monotherapy (although given to 30-74% of patients)
    i. Benzodiazepines <u>can worsen</u> the severity of PTSD[844]
    ii. Causes worse psychotherapy outcomes, ↑ aggression and depression, and substance use
    iii. They do <u>not</u> prevent PTSD from occurring
    iv. As post-trauma prophylaxis, they can actually <u>increase</u> the risk of developing PTSD
E. Avoid caffeine, stimulants, and alcohol (40-50% comorbidity with substance use disorders)
F. Pharmacotherapy in children not recommended due to negative studies (unless comorbidities exist)[845]
G. Adjunctive treatments
  1. Atypical antipsychotics (e.g., risperidone, olanzapine, quetiapine) if psychotic symptoms present
  2. Prazosin - Alpha$_1$ blocker - for sleep/nightmares[808] – crosses the BBB
    i. Very high doses (e.g., up to 50 mg QHS or divided TID) may be required to be effective[846]
    ii. Average dose for men is usually higher than for women
    iii. A large multicenter VAMC trial in 2018 did not show superiority over placebo at 26 weeks[847]
    iv. 2016 Meta-analysis showed *significant symptom improvement* over placebo on nightmares, overall PTSD symptoms, clinical global improvement, sleep quality, hyperarousal symptoms, dream content, and total sleep time[848]
  3. Trazodone, buspirone, gabapentin (for insomnia), valproic acid
H. Other therapies studied
  1. To prevent PTSD development after a traumatic event
    i. Propranolol (up to 160 mg/d), sertraline, and IV hydrocortisone[348]
  2. IV ketamine (0.5 mg/kg) shown effective in studies[849-851]
  3. Blueberries were found to be effective in a rat-model of PTSD, because they ↑ serotonin[852]
  4. Eye Movement and Desensitization and Reprocessing Therapy (EMDR)

# VI. POTENTIAL FUTURE TREATMENTS FOR PTSD IN STUDY
A. BNC-210 (IW-2143) by Bionomics and Ironwood Pharmaceuticals
  1. "GABA modulator" – a negative allosteric modulator (antagonist) of the α7 nicotinic Ach receptor
  2. Doses of 150 mg, 300 mg and 600 mg BID for 12 weeks studied
  3. Also in Phase II trials for agitation in dementia, PTSD and Generalized Anxiety Disorder
B. Brexpiprazole (Lu AF41156, OPC-34712; Rexulti) by Otsuka/Lundbeck
  1. Phase III for Post-traumatic stress disorders
C. NBTX-001 (the noble gas xenon) by Nobilis Therapeutics[430]
  1. Antagonist of NMDA, AMPA, nicotinic ACh (α4β2), 5HT$_3$, & plasma membrane Ca$^{2+}$ ATPase
  2. Currently in Phase III trials using the Zephyrus™ inhalational Device
  3. Also in Phase II for Irritable Bowel Syndrome (IBS), Alzheimer's Disease, & Parkinson's Disease
D. NYX-783 by Aptinyx in Phase II trials for PTSD (FDA Fast Track status)
E. Oxytocin (Syntocinon) nasal spray
  1. In two Phase IV trials at Massachusetts General Hospital (ClinicalTrials.gov Identifier: NCT01631682) and Yale University (ClinicalTrials.gov Identifier: NCT02546570)
F. Ropivacaine 0.5% (7 to 10 mL) into the right-side stellate ganglion (collection of nerves at the base of the neck at the level of the C6 anterior tubercle) administered twice, 2-weeks apart
  1. Stellate ganglion block used for pain since the 1940's
  2. Blocks sympathetic nerve impulses to the body and may "reboot" the system to its pre-trauma state by providing negative feedback to the amygdala
  3. In 108 military service men, showed significant ↓ in PTSD symptoms at 8 weeks vs. placebo
  4. Side effects were mild, but the potential for serious effects exists (e.g., seizures or Horner syndrome - characterized by right-sided droopy red eye and constricted pupil)
G. SRX246 by Azevan Pharmaceuticals in Phase II clinical trials (expected completion in June 2020)
  1. ClinicalTrials.gov Identifier: NCT02733614
  2. MOA: Vasopressin 1$_a$ receptor antagonist
  3. Phase II trials have already completed for childhood Intermittent Explosive & Disorder
  4. Vasopressin 1$_a$ receptor antagonists are intended to reduce stress, fear, aggression, depression, and anxiety, as shown in preclinical tests
H. Tianeptine oxalate (TNX-601) by Servier and Vela Pharmaceuticals
  1. Atypical μ-opioid receptor agonist and AMPA receptor modulator
  2. Already marketed in Europe for Alcoholism, Anxiety disorders, and Major Depressive Disorder in Europe under the brand names "Coaxil", "Stablon" and "Tatinol"
  3. Not currently in study in the U.S. – Phase I for PTSD planned for 2020
I. Tonmya® (TNX-102 SL) by Tonix Pharmaceuticals[853]
  1. Sublingual cyclobenzaprine HCl
    i. 5HT$_{2A}$, alpha$_1$, and H$_1$ antagonist
  2. One Phase III study showed significant efficacy at 5.6 mg (2 x 2.8 mg tablets) QHS
    i. https://clinicaltrials.gov/ct2/show/NCT03062540
  3. 37% of research patients experienced oral hypoesthesia (tongue/mouth numbness)
J. Verucerfont (GSK-561679, NBI-77860) by Neurocrine Biosciences
  1. CRF1 receptor antagonist in Phase II for Post-Traumatic Stress Disorders and Alcoholism

I. Recommendations from the American Heart Association (AHA), The American College of Cardiology Foundation (ACCF), and Heart Rhythm Society (HRS)

II. NORMAL QTC SHOULD BE < 420-440 ms *(NOTE: QTc is not the same as QT)*
  A. QTc is a corrected value that adjusts for factors such as heart rate (RR)
    1. Bazett's formula for $QTc = QT \div \sqrt{RR}$
    2. Fridericia's formula for $QTc = QT \div \sqrt[3]{RR}$
    3. Hodges formula for $QTc = QT + 1.75 \times (RR-60)$
  B. Recommended high QTc in males is **> 450 ms** and in females **> 460 ms**
    1. A short QTc in men and women is < 390 ms
  C. For high risk drugs with known QT-prolonging effects, 12-lead EKGs should be performed before therapy begins and after the optimal dose is reached
    1. For IV medications, continuous telemetry or remote telemetry monitoring is recommended
    2. Caution is advised with concomitant use of 2 low, medium, or high risk medications
    3. Arizona Center for Education and Research on Therapeutics (AZCERT)
      i. Responsible for the CredibleMeds® website & database (www.crediblemeds.org)
  D. FDA suggests discontinuing a medication if QTc > 500 ms or an ↑ of 60 ms from baseline occurs
    1. FDA benchmarks require drug trials to report an ↑ of **10 to 20 ms** or more in trials[864]
  E. QT interval **>500 ms** ↑s' risk for ventricular tachyarrhythmia, *torsades de pointes*, & sudden death
    1. For each **10 ms** ↑ above 500 ms, the risk of *torsades de pointes* (TdP) ↑ **by 5-7%**
  F. From APA resource document: "*there is no absolute QTc interval at which a psychotropic should not be used*"[865] – if benefits outweigh risks

III. CONGENITAL LONG QT SYNDROME (LQTS)
  A. A genetically inherited (or acquired) condition in which the QT-interval is longer than normal
    1. Prevalence is 1 per 2,000-10,000 people, but **may not be** evident unless an EKG is performed
      i. 10% of patients have normal QTc
  B. TdP may present as symptoms of palpitations, lightheadedness, syncope, seizures, sudden death in family members < 55 y.o., or congenital deafness of family members
    1. Peak risk of sudden cardiac death - children and young adults (≈ 8,000 deaths a year)
    2. 5-10% of patients who develop drug-induced TdP are carriers of gene mutations related to LQTS
  C. When **QTc >500 ms**, there is a 2-3 x ↑ risk of TdP
  D. Treat with IV magnesium, *beta*-blockers, implantable cardiac defibrillators, or pacemakers
  E. Conditions that can ↑ risk of death
    1. Low $Mg^{2+}$, low $K^+$, low $Ca^{2+}$, bradycardia, dehydration, sleeping, 2nd and 3rd degree AV block, other medical conditions
      i. e.g., anorexia, renal or hepatic dysfunction, hypothyroidism, diabetes, exercise (swimming, outdoor sports), heart failure, male sex, and QT-prolonging medications (dose-related)
    2. Drug interactions on CYP450 that increase a QT-prolonging drugs' concentration
    3. Combination of an antipsychotic + antidepressant can result in QTc ↑ of 24 ± 21 ms[866]
    4. In situations where there are ≥ 2 QT-prolonging medications, approx. 15% have QT-prolongation, and 10% will have QTc > 500 ms (avg. increase of 31 ms)[867]

IV. DRUGS THAT PROLONG QTC (PARTIAL LIST)
  A. Class I and III anti-arrhythmics
  B. Macrolide & quinolone antibiotics, pentamidine, & SMX/TMP (Bactrim)
  C. Azole antifungal agents
  D. Anti-malarial drugs
  E. Anti-emetics (e.g., dolasetron, ondansetron, droperidol)
  F. Anti-retrovirals (e.g., atazanavir, saquinavir)
  G. Methadone, amphetamines, and cocaine
  H. Propofol, sotalol, arsenic trioxide, albuterol
  I. Fosphenytoin, tacrolimus
  J. Tyrosine kinase inhibitors (used for cancer or inflammation)

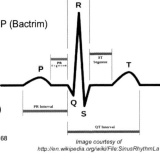

Image courtesy of
http://en.wikipedia.org/wiki/File:SinusRhythmLa

V. PSYCHIATRIC MEDICATIONS THAT PROLONG QTC
  A. Tricyclic antidepressants - Amitriptyline (8.5 ms ↑ QTc), maprotiline (13.9 ms ↑ QTc), nortriptyline (35.3 ms ↑ QTc)[868]
  B. SSRIs (e.g., citalopram, escitalopram)[869,870]
    1. Citalopram 10-20, 40, and 60 mg/d can ↑ QTc by 7.8-8.5, 12.6-16.5 and 18.5 ms respectively
    2. Escitalopram can ↑ QTc by 4.5-6.4 ms at up to 20 mg/d (10.7 ms at 30 mg/d - above max dose)
  C. Bupropion can cause QT-reduction (average 19.2 ms in one study)[871]
  D. Antipsychotics
    1. Chlorpromazine, thioridazine (↑ up to 30 ms), haloperidol (esp. given IV), fluphenazine, clozapine, ziprasidone (avg. 15.9 ms), iloperidone, quetiapine (avg. 5.7 ms), risperidone (avg. 3.6 ms), pimozide
    2. Perphenazine can cause QT-reduction
    3. There is a 3 x increased risk of sudden cardiac death in antipsychotic users[872]
  E. Lithium (18.6 ms avg. QTc ↑)
  F. Dementia medications (e.g., donepezil, galantamine), amantadine
  G. VMAT2 inhibitors (for tardive dyskinesia)

I. ETIOLOGY AND PATHOPHYSIOLOGY OF SCHIZOPHRENIA[877]
  A. In Greek, it is derived from *skhizein* (to split) and *phren* (mind)
    1. Swiss psychiatrist, *Eugene Bleuler*, separated symptoms into positive & negative > 100 yrs ago
    2. Previously called "Dementia Praecox" by *Emil Kraepelin* – meaning *premature madness*
      i. That term used from late 1800s to mid-1900s
  B. A chronic mental disorder characterized by psychosis and an inability to function in society based on a loss of reality testing
    1. Most patients experience a prodromal phase prior to their first psychotic episode, characterized by negative symptoms, cognitive deficits, and social awkwardness
    2. Affects 0.27 to 0.83% of the population[878]
    3. Among the top 10 leading causes of health disability
    4. Usually manifests in early adulthood, with premorbid IQ below ½ to 2 standard deviations[879]
      i. Males have earlier onset, but lifetime risk is equal for males and females
    5. Life expectancy reduced by 10-20 years[880]
    6. May be detectable from deficits in auditory sensory processing and tone-matching[881-883]
      i. ↓ ability to match tones or to detect the 'musicality' of speech (prosody)
      ii. Auditory cortex-level dysfunction
      iii. A computerized automated speech analysis algorithm has been developed to listen to natural speech patterns of youths at high-risk for psychosis[884]
        a. Their speech patterns predicted later psychosis with 100% accuracy
    7. Retinal imaging may one day help identify people with Schizophrenia
      i. Eye-movement abnormalities were observed with a 98.3% accuracy of identifying schizophrenia[885]
      ii. Wider retinal venules also observed
  C. Abnormal endocannabinoid system (ECS) signaling "tone"[886]
    1. Patients with schizophrenia have a significantly higher expression of cannabinoid-1 (CB1) receptors on their peripheral immune cells
    2. Significantly higher anandamide (endogenous cannabinoid) levels in CNS fluid and blood
      i. When in remission, anandamide levels return to normal
      ii. Cannabidiol increases anandamide levels, but reduces positive symptoms
    3. Marijuana use can increase the risk of developing schizophrenia by over 3-fold[887,888]
      i. High potency (high THC content) marijuana can increase the risk over 5-fold
  D. Putatively, schizophrenia is believed to be the result of *too much* DA activity in the mesolimbic area and *too little* DA activity in the mesocortical area
    1. Excess $D_2$ receptors in the brain / mesolimbic area
    2. Down-regulated $5HT_{2A}$ receptors in the frontal cortex
      i. $5HT_{2A}$ blockade ↑ DA in the mesocortical area (frontal cortex) and nigrostriatal pathway
  E. Cognitive therapy can significantly ↓ symptoms in patients who choose not to take medication[889]
  F. Genetic inheritance[880,890,891,892]
    1. 10% incidence if a 1st degree relative or parent has schizophrenia
    2. 40% incidence if both parents have schizophrenia
    3. 3% incidence if a 2nd degree relative has schizophrenia
    4. 40 to 81% concordance for identical twins (9-11% for fraternal twins)
    5. MicroRNA (miRNA-137) variations are associated with schizophrenia[893]
    6. At least 108 genetic loci associated with schizophrenia[894]
    7. May have to do with mitochondrial dysfunction
  G. Environment, inflammation, and infections
    1. Higher concentrations of *Lactobacillus* phage phi-adh (a bacteriophage that invades *Lactobacillus gasseri*) found in the mouths of schizophrenia patients[895]
    2. Environmental factors, such as *Toxoplasma Gondii* (found in 1/5 of schizophrenia pts)[896]
    3. Inflammation is suspected - from evidence that minocycline, aspirin, estrogen, and N-acetylcysteine help reduce psychotic symptoms[897,898]
      i. Increased antibody levels have been found to some Epstein-Barr (EBV) viral proteins[899]
    4. Glutamate dysfunction is also implicated[449,900,901]
      i. Autoimmunity to $D_2$ & NMDA receptors found in 19% of pediatric new psychosis vs. 0% controls
    5. 19 study meta-analysis found Vit D deficient people were 2.16x more likely to have schizophrenia
      i. 65% of schizophrenia patients were deficient in Vitamin D[902]
    6. Other theories include oxidative stress, ↓ nitric oxide biosynthesis, impaired anti-apoptotic signaling, reduced neurotropics (nerve growth factors) and dysfunction of GABA[903]
  H. Anti-N-methyl-D-aspartate (NMDA) receptor encephalitis[904]
    1. Relatively new diagnosis (since 2007) of encephalitis caused by antibodies to NMDA receptors
    2. Mostly occurs in younger females
      i. Teratomas (primarily in the ovaries) are found in half of female patients
    3. Presents as abrupt onset psychosis, seizures, memory problems, dyskinesias, and instability of autonomic functions of the body (e.g., blood pressure, incontinence, drooling)
      i. Patients are often misdiagnosed as having Schizophrenia
    4. Diagnoses with a spinal tap (CSF) revealing antibodies to the NMDA receptor

5. Treatment involves removing the teratoma (if present), corticosteroids, IV immunoglobulins, plasmapheresis, cyclophosphamide, rituximab, azathioprine, mycophenolate, methotrexate
6. Most patients recover, but some have severe functional impairments or die
I. Psychotic episodes cause progressive loss of cortical and subcortical gray matter[905-908]
  1. Mostly frontal and temporal cortices, hippocampus, amygdala, and thalamus
  2. A decline in growth factors causes shrinkage of the neuropil
    i. Reduces synaptic connections, dendrite length, & the number and size of dendritic extensions
    ii. May be from chronic inflammatory state
    iii. Childhood-onset schizophrenia - Loss estimated at 1-3% per year for the first 5 years [909]
    iv. Only SGAs prevent and reverse neurotoxicity[910,911] → FGAs worsen it
J. Early intervention in the "prodromal" (i.e., pre-psychotic) stage may prevent schizophrenia[912]
  1. Prodromal symptoms can present 2-5 years before a psychotic break
    i. Prodrome: Loss of cognitive & psychosocial functioning, atypical interests & beliefs, mild disorganized thinking or speech, minor hallucinations or delusions, and *negative* symptoms
    ii. Positive symptoms develop late in the prodromal phase (perceptual abnormalities, ideas of reference, and paranoia)
  2. >20% of these individuals will progress to psychosis in 1 year / >50% in 4 years
    i. Psychotherapy, antipsychotics, or both can reduce the risk of progression to schizophrenia

## II. DEFINITIONS OF CORE PSYCHOTIC SYMPTOMS
A. Delusions - fixed false beliefs not open to change even when evidence contradicts them; termed bizarre if implausible and not derived from ordinary experience
B. Hallucinations - involuntary sensory experiences not related to external stimuli. Usually are auditory with Schizophrenia. Visual and tactile hallucinations may be related to illicit substances.
C. Disorganized thinking or speech - person cannot keep their thoughts coherent. They may have loose associations of widely varied topics.
  1. Includes catatonia or abnormal motor behavior (unrelated to drugs)

## III. ADDITIONAL PSYCHOTIC SYMPTOMS
A. Grossly disorganized or catatonic behavior - unpredictable or silly behavior, or a great decrease in the response to external stimuli
  1. Catatonia is best treated with *high doses* of benzodiazepines or psychostimulants
B. Negative symptoms - (*see next page*)

## IV. DIAGNOSES OF PSYCHOTIC DISORDERS[245]
A. Brief Psychotic Disorder – ≥ 1 core symptom of psychosis with or without ancillary symptoms
  1. Lasts at least 1 day and remits in < 30 days
B. Schizophreniform Disorder – At least 1 core symptom of psychosis + 1 other symptom
  1. Psychosis that lasts 1 to 6 months
C. Schizophrenia – At least 1 core symptom of psychosis + 1 other symptom
  1. Psychosis must persist > 6 months
D. Schizoaffective Disorder – Meets full diagnosis of Schizophrenia + a mood episode exists
  1. Bipolar type or Depressive type
    i. Some believe it is actually misdiagnosed Bipolar Disorder[913]

## V. PATHOPHYSIOLOGY OF 4 DOPAMINERGIC PATHWAYS INVOLVED WITH ANTIPSYCHOTIC USE
A. These 2 involve antipsychotic's mechanism of action:
  1. Mesolimbic pathway: "the reward, pleasure pathway" associated with addiction, schizophrenia, & depression
    i. Over-activation → Positive symptoms
  2. Mesocortical pathway: involves cognitive control, motivation, and emotional response
    i. Under-activation → Negative symptoms
    ii. *Note*....First generation antipsychotics (FGAs) can induce negative symptoms and cognitive impairment, because they block dopamine here too[914]
B. These 2 involve antipsychotic's unintended side effects:
  1. Nigrostriatal pathway: involved with movement / relaxation of muscles
    i. Dopamine blockade from antipsychotics → movement disorders and extrapyramidal symptoms
  2. Tuberoinfundibular pathway: regulates the secretion of prolactin from pituitary gland
    i. Dopamine blockade from antipsychotics → increases prolactin secretion

## VI. UNDERLYING TRIGGERS OF DELIRIUM AND PSYCHOSIS
A. Schizophrenia is somewhat a diagnosis of exclusion
B. Must eliminate potential causes before a diagnosis is concluded

| C. Medical Illnesses | |
|---|---|
| o Syphilis | o Lewy body dementia |
| o Parkinson's disease | o Alzheimer's disease |
| o Huntington's disease | o CVA / stroke |
| o Lupus | o Frontotemporal lobar degeneration |
| o Infections (e.g., UTIs, URIs) | o Traumatic brain injury |
| o Anti-NMDA receptor encephalitis | o Myxedema[607] (severe hypothyroidism - 5-15%) |
| o Dehydration | o Advanced HIV or other viral infections (e.g., Creutzfeldt-Jakob disease) |
| o Pituitary tumor | |

D. Medications / Drugs
- Antibiotics
- Antimalarial agents
- Marijuana
- Cocaine / amphetamines
- LSD / PCP / psilocybin / other hallucinogens (5HT$_{2A}$ agonists)
- Bath salts / Spice / K2 / Flakka
- Parkinson's medications
- Corticosteroids
- Clonidine
- Opiates
- Varenicline (Chantix®)
- Other various "street drugs"
- Benzodiazepines
- Z-drugs (e.g., zolpidem, eszopiclone, zaleplon)
- Leukotriene Inhibitors (e.g. Singulair® (montelukast), Accolate® (zafirlukast), Zyflo® (zileuton) and Zyflo CR®)[915]

## VII. SPECIFIC TARGET SYMPTOMS OF SCHIZOPHRENIA: POSITIVE, NEGATIVE, & COGNITIVE

A. **POSITIVE SYMPTOMS**: things that happen that should not happen
- Delusions
- Conceptual disorganization
- Excitement
- Suspiciousness / persecution
- Grandiosity
- Hostility
- Hallucinations

Typical & Atypical Antipsychotics treat these symptoms

B. **NEGATIVE SYMPTOMS**: things that should happen and do not happen
1. *The 5 A's:*
- Affect (generally flat or incongruent)
- Alogia (relative absence of speech)
- Avolition / apathy (lack of emotion, enthusiasm, and initiative)
- Attention (poor or lack of)
- Anhedonia (absence of pleasure)
2. Also:
- Difficulty in abstract thinking
- Lack of spontaneity
- Flow of conversation
- Stereotyped thinking
- Blunted mood
- Emotional withdrawal
- Poor rapport

*ONLY* Atypical **Antipsychotics** treat these symptoms

C. **COGNITIVE SYMPTOMS**
1. Executive function - i.e., learning from one's mistakes
2. Anosognosia – The inability to believe that one has schizophrenia
   i. A difficult symptom of schizophrenia
   ii. Greatly contributes to non-adherence

## VIII. ANTIPSYCHOTIC CLASSES AND RECEPTORS
A. Typical antipsychotics (1st Generation / FGAs)
   1. Primary mechanism of action is to block D$_2$ receptors
B. Atypical antipsychotics (2nd Generation / SGAs)
   1. Primary mechanism of action is to block D$_2$ receptors and 5HT$_{2A}$ receptors
C. No antipsychotic is perfect, so they may also block histamine (H$_1$), acetylcholine (Ach), *alpha* (α$_1$), and other receptors, which can add to side effects
   1. Binding to other receptors may contribute to cardiometabolic side effects, specifically 5HT$_{2C}$, Muscarinic (M$_3$) and H$_1$ receptors
   2. Metabolic effects occur when the ratio of binding affinities (Ki) of 5HT$_{1A}$:H$_1$ or 5HT$_{2C}$:H$_1$ is > 1
      i. Based on Dr. Rappa's own calculations using established binding affinities[916-918]
         a. Binding affinities are greatest at the lowest numbers
         b. Ratios above equate to much more antihistamine effect than 5HT$_{1A}$ or 5HT$_{2C}$ antagonism
      ii. The higher the ratio, the more cardiometabolic effects are seen
      iii. Another analysis showed weight gain with H$_1$, α$_{1A}$, 5HT$_{2C}$, and 5HT$_6$ receptor affinities[919]
D. **Black Box Warning** for all antipsychotics about potential ↑ risk of death in patients with dementia
   1. ↑ risk of stroke may be associated with high doses, high anticholinergic effects, and α$_2$ binding[920]
E. Atypicals may ↑ risk of aspiration, urinary retention, acute kidney injury, & hypotension in the elderly[921]
F. New *Warning and Precaution* added to all antipsychotic medications
   1. May cause somnolence, postural hypotension, or motor and sensory instability, which may lead to falls and, consequently, fractures or other injuries
   2. In > 65 yrs old - there is a 52% ↑ risk of falls and 50% ↑ risk of non-vertebral fractures[922]
G. Chlorpromazine dose equivalents for SGAs are impossible to determine due to the variety of mechanisms of action, although some have tried[923]

## IX. EFFECTS OF NICOTINE
A. An estimated 60-90% of schizophrenia patients smoke cigarettes for anxiolytic effects, enhanced attention, and pro-cognitive effects[924]
B. Smoking induces CYP1A2 enzymes and lowers clozapine, olanzapine, and others' levels
C. Smoking cessation with bupropion SR (with or without nicotine replacement) should be routinely offered to patients
D. α7 nicotinic partial agonists are being studied for helping cognition in schizophrenia patients[925,926]

## X. ANTIPSYCHOTIC EFFECTIVENESS[927]

A. First-episode patients respond much better than in repeated episodes based on Positive and Negative Syndrome Scale (**PANSS**) & Brief Psychiatric Rating Scale (**BPRS**) scores[928]
   1. Minimal response (>20% reduction): 81% versus 51%
   2. Good response (>50% reduction): 52% versus 23%
   3. Approximately 2/3 of patients will respond to each antipsychotic[929]
   4. 20% may see significant improvement, and in some cases, may have full recovery[930]
   5. Clozapine is the most effective to date[931]
   6. Olanzapine, risperidone, and amisulpride (non-US drug) are more effective than haloperidol[932]
   7. Meta-analysis showed that haloperidol was inferior to SGAs in 1st episode patients[933]
   8. Predictors of antipsychotic response[928]
      i. Higher total baseline symptom severity
      ii. Treatment-naïve patients
      iii. Shorter illness duration
B. OPTiMiSE study found that it is best to keep a 1st episode patient on the 1st antipsychotic tried for at least 10 weeks to see a response[934,935]
   1. If no response, start clozapine
   2. Current recommendations are to fail at least 2 antipsychotics before starting clozapine.
C. Based on 3 meta-analyses, if no symptom improvement after 2 weeks of starting an antipsychotic, it's 90% likely not to work, and patients may benefit from a treatment change[928,936]
   1. Must assess medication adherence before declaring medication non-effective[937]
   2. If partial improvement in first 2 weeks, then optimize dose and reassess at 4 weeks
   3. If still partial response at 4 weeks, continue up to 8 weeks before switching medications
   4. If no response at 4 weeks, guidelines suggest a switch to another antipsychotic
D. A drug must block between 65 and 78% of $D_2$ receptors in the striatum to reduce psychosis
   1. 2 mg to 5 mg/d of haloperidol achieves maximal blockade in this range[938-944]
E. Some atypical antipsychotics never exceed 78% due to transient (i.e., loose) $D_2$ binding
   1. Result is little or no EPS (e.g., quetiapine, clozapine)
F. Chronic receptor blockade causes DA receptors to upregulate[945]
   1. Sudden discontinuation of blockade (i.e., med non-adherence) causes overstimulation of receptor
   2. "Supersensitivity psychosis" can result
G. Initial high doses of antipsychotics do **not** equate to faster or better response[946-948]
   1. Antipsychotics can take up to 6-8 weeks (or longer) for response
   2. Refer to *page 16* for "TIME FRAME FOR MEDICATIONS TO SHOW EFFICACY"
   3. Sedation does not equal response
   4. Neurotoxicity can occur with high dose antipsychotics[949]
   5. Neurolepsis is likely to be misconstrued as a good drug effect (*see page 86*)
H. Medication adherence is defined as patients taking $\geq$ 80% of their prescribed medications[950]
   1. Various studies use from 67-95% ranges to define adherence
I. With full medication adherence, relapse rate in Schizophrenia is about 3% per year[951]
   1. With 1st episode - guidelines suggest continuing medication up to 2 years
   2. With recurrent episodes – treat with medications from 5 years to indefinitely
   3. Non-adherence with medications estimated at 50% over 1 year
      i. Without medication, relapse rate is 77% in 1 year and 90% in 2 years
      ii. 5-year follow-up study of 1st episode treatment responsive patients showed an 82% cumulative risk of a 1st relapse and a 5x greater risk of a 1st or 2nd relapse if not taking medication[952]
   4. Atypical antipsychotic long-acting injectables (LAIs) should be considered for non-adherent patients and as first-line maintenance therapy[953,954]
      i. Controversy exists as to whether or not LAIs actually prevent relapse[955,956]
J. Up to 30% of patients may be "treatment refractory" to antipsychotics
   1. May consider clozapine or slow titration above maximum recommended doses
   2. Polypharmacy should ONLY be considered when clozapine has failed or during a cross-titration in switching from one antipsychotic to another
K. Up to an estimated 40% of patients with first-episode psychosis are NOT being treated correctly[957]
   1. e.g., too high of dose, polypharmacy, addition of antidepressants or stimulants (without need), or received no antipsychotic at all
L. Antipsychotic polypharmacy does not increase therapy's initial effectiveness
   1. **Antipsychotic polypharmacy can increase the risk for re-hospitalization, diabetes, EPS, sedation, seizures, metabolic effects, mortality, and sudden cardiac death**[947,958-962]
   2. 2019 study in Finland found a 7-13% lower risk of psychiatric rehospitalization from non-specific antipsychotic polypharmacy compared with any monotherapy[963]
      i. Combination of clozapine & aripiprazole associated with 14-23% lower risk of rehospitalization
M. **2017 meta-analysis-based antipsychotic augmentation strategies of 42 possible cotreatments**[964]
   1. Only the following add-on therapies to an antipsychotic significantly improved symptoms:
   2. For *overall* symptoms: add any antidepressant, lamotrigine, estrogen, lithium, N-acetylcysteine, minocycline, topiramate, adenosine modulators, buspirone, NSAID, or modafinil/armodafinil
   3. For *positive* symptoms: add lamotrigine, estrogen, adenosine modulator, topiramate, or NSAID
   4. For *negative* symptoms: add any antidepressant, 5HT₃ antagonist, lamotrigine, minocycline, acetylcholinesterase inhibitor, testosterone/estrogen, topiramate, or modafinil
   5. No augmentation strategy was superior for clozapine

# XI. EXPERT CONSENSUS GUIDELINES

A. All treatments are in addition to psychosocial therapies & support
B. All guidelines recommend weighing the side effects of the medication against the benefits to each individual patient

| | PORT 2009[965] | WFSBP 2012[948] | NICE 2014[966] | EPA 2015[967] | Canadian Guidelines 2017[937] | APA 2004 / 2009 / 2019 draft[968,969] |
|---|---|---|---|---|---|---|
| 1st choice for 1st episode | FGA or SGA (except OLZ or CLZ) | Low dose FGA < SGA Preferably OLZ, RIS, QUE or HAL | SGA or FGA at optimum dosage for 4-6 weeks | Low dose SGA | Low dose FGA, SGA or LAIA for 2-8 weeks. If effective, treat > 18 months | FGA or SGA |
| Primary negative or cognitive symptoms | – | SGA ± adjunctive mirtazapine | Art therapy | – | – | CLZ, other SGA, or adjunct antidepressant |
| For repeat episodes (2nd choice) | FGA or SGA | Moderate dose for > 2-8 weeks | SGA or FGA, (try an SGA before considering CLZ) | – | Low to moderate dose FGA or SGA, or LAIA for non-adherence or pt. preference. Treat > 2-5 years | SGA |
| Treatment-resistant | CLZ | CLZ | CLZ | – | CLZ for > 8-12 weeks at a dose of >400 mg/d with therapeutic levels | CLZ |
| 4th choice | – | Switch to another SGA (preferably OLZ or RIS), LAIA or CLZ augmentation (with RIS or LMT), or ECT | CLZ serum levels & augmentation for > 8-10 weeks | – | Insufficient evidence for a specific recommendation | SGA (OLZ), CLZ augmentation, ECT |
| Other | Low-freq. (1 Hz) rTMS | Topiramate for weight control / valproate for aggression and hostility | Smoking cessation therapies / LAIA if patient prefers | – | CLZ is a preferred treatment for psychosis associated with aggression | CLZ is a preferred tx for psychosis assoc. with chronic suicidal thoughts /aggression. Consider an LAIA for chronically non-adherent pts. |

< - preferred less than > - more than ± - with or without
PORT - Patient Outcomes Research Team         EPA - European Psychiatric Association
NICE - National Institute for Health and Clinical Excellence
APA - American Psychiatric Association
WFSBP - World Federation of Societies of Biological Psychiatry
CLZ = clozapine        HAL = haloperidol
LMT = lamotrigine     OLZ = olanzapine        QUE = quetiapine        RIS = risperidone
*(For other abbreviations used, see pages 7-8)*

# XII. RISK OF SUICIDE & VIOLENCE[970-974]

A. 2/3 of healthcare providers see people with schizophrenia as "dangerous"
B. 20-40% of people with schizophrenia attempt suicide
   1. 2 X more likely than violent behaviors
   2. Medication adherence = protective factor for suicide and violent behavior in dozens of studies
   3. LAIAs reduce rate of violent acts by 40%

# XIII. NON-PSYCHIATRIC USES OF ANTIPSYCHOTIC MEDICATIONS

A. Anti-emetic - because of dopamine blockade in the CTZ (chemoreceptor triggered zone)
   1. e.g., trimethobenzamide (Tigan®) and prochlorperazine (Compazine®)
B. Anti-pruritic - because of $H_1$ blockade
C. Pre-anesthesia with opiates - e.g., droperidol
D. Gastrointestinal "prokinetic" agent - e.g., metoclopramide (Reglan®)
E. Tourette's syndrome (Note: aripiprazole is approved)

## XV. WARNINGS AND PRECAUTIONS FOR ALL ANTIPSYCHOTICS

A. ALL antipsychotics can cause weight gain, hyperglycemia, hyperlipidemia, orthostatic hypotension, falls, leukopenia, neutropenia, agranulocytosis, seizures/convulsions, potential for cognitive and motor impairment, body temperature regulation, suicide and dysphagia

1. Suicide in children & young adults (up to age 24) if also FDA-approved for depression (any kind)

## XVI. SIDE EFFECTS OF TYPICAL ANTIPSYCHOTICS (ALSO CALLED 1$^{ST}$ GENERATION / FGAs)

A. Related to the potency of the drug on $D_2$ blockade (*see RELATIVE POTENCIES on page 90*)

B. **Low potency** drugs are highest in anticholinergic, antihistaminic, *alpha*$_1$ blockade (i.e., orthostatic hypotension), but are low in EPS

C. **High potency** drugs are high in EPS, but low in anticholinergic and other side effects

D. Neuroleptic – from Greek "*neuro*" and "*lēptikos*" means to "seize the nerve"

1. Refers to EPS as a side effect -- A "zombie"-like state of indifference and detachment

2. "Neurolepsis" or "Ataraxy" - an altered state of consciousness, indicated by quiescence, reduced anxiety, diminished motor activity, calmness, and apathy to the surroundings

3. Somnolence may occur, but generally the person can be roused & can respond to commands[976]

E. *Secondary negative symptoms - because of $D_2$ blockade in the pre-frontal cortex*[914]

F. Extrapyramidal Side Effects (EPS)

1. EPS is from an imbalance between dopamine and acetylcholine (Ach) in the brain

2. 5HT$_2$ blockage can increase DA in the striatum and frontal cortex, which reduces EPS and helps with Negative Symptoms

3. DA normally inhibits Ach release

i. *If you block DA, then you have to artificially block Ach to* ↓ *EPS*

DA↓ / Ach↑

## XVII. FOUR TYPES OF EPS AND THEIR TREATMENTS

A. Acute Dystonia

1. Sudden onset of muscle contraction

2. An *emergency* situation

3. Examples: torticollis, blepharospasm, oculogyric crisis, trismus, retrocollis, laryngospasm

4. Treat with an I.M. medication because of more rapid onset vs. oral medication

i. Benztropine mesylate (Cogentin®) injection[105]

a. FDA-approved for treating EPS reactions

b. Usual dose is 1 to 4 mg IM prn, either QD or BID

c. Supplied as 2 mL ampules - 1 mg/mL

d. Anticholinergic effects: tachycardia, dry mouth, urinary retention, constipation, hyperthermia

ii. Diphenhydramine HCL (Benadryl®) injection[977]

a. Has both anticholinergic and antihistaminic effects

b. Pregnancy Category B

c. Usual dose is 10 to 50 mg IV (rate NTE 25 mg/min) or deep IM up to 100 mg if required prn

1. Maximum daily dosage is 400 mg

d. Available in 50 mg/mL single-dose 1 mL vials or 50 mg/mL in a 1 mL single-use syringe

iii. Lorazepam (Ativan®) injection (C-IV)[978]

a. Usual dose is 2 mg prn, up to 4 mg a day

b. If used *intravenously*, it must be *diluted* 1:1 with a compatible solution

c. Keep in a *refrigerator* at 2° to 8°C until use

1. Stable for 30 days at room temperature (discard if longer)

d. Peak concentrations in 3 hours

e. >90% bound to plasma proteins

f. Conjugated, not metabolized, so doses may need to be ↓ in renal failure pts.

g. Pregnancy Category D

h. Drug interactions: probenecid or valproate – give ½ usual dose

1. Oral contraceptives - It may be necessary to increase the dose of lorazepam

i. Available in 1 mL Carpuject™ single-dose cartridges of 2 mg/mL & 4 mg/mL

B. Pseudoparkinsonism

1. Resembles Parkinson's Disease (e.g., masked face, shuffled gait, bradykinesia)

2. 15 - 60% of patients

3. Test for this with an AIMS test (Abnormal Involuntary Movement Scale)

4. Do **not** treat with DA agonists -- Treat with **p.o.** anticholinergics or amantadine

5. Anticholinergics

i. Note: ALL anticholinergic drugs are contraindicated in patients with narrow angle glaucoma

ii. Benztropine mesylate (Cogentin®)[106,107]
  a. Usual dose is 0.5 mg up to a maximum of 6 mg/d (divided BID)
  b. Has both anticholinergic and antihistaminic effects / side effects
  c. Available in 1 mg tablets & 0.4 mg/mL oral solution
iii. Trihexyphenidyl / benzhexol (Artane®)
  a. FDA-approved for treating EPS
  b. Usual dose is 2 to 15 mg/d (divided TID)
  c. Best tolerability if given with meals
  d. Time to peak: 1.3 hours
  e. Half-life: 33 hours
  f. Available in: 2 mg & 5 mg tablets and 2 mg/5 mL elixir
iv. Diphenhydramine (Benadryl®)[53,979]
  a. Not FDA approved for EPS
  b. Usual dose is 50-300 mg/d
  c. Protein binding: 98.5%
  d. Metabolism: CYP2D6 (major) / CYP1A2, CYP2C9 and CYP2C19 (all minor)
  e. Half-life: varies from 4 to 18 hours depending on age of patient (average adult = 9 hours)
  f. Availability: 12.5, 25, & 50 mg tablets & capsules / 12.5 mg/ml, 12.5 mg/5 ml & other liquids
6. Biperiden (Akineton) – Discontinued and no longer in production
7. Amantadine
i. MOA is not well understood
ii. A weak, non-competitive NMDA receptor antagonist[980]
iii. Pre-synaptically enhancing the release of dopamine and inhibiting its reuptake
iv. Post-synaptically, acts directly on the DA receptor, and upregulates D2 receptors *in vivo*
v. Common side effects: nausea, dizziness (lightheadedness), and insomnia
  a. Since it works on DA receptors, it may cause hallucinations, psychosis, impulsive behaviors, depressed mood, and somnolence
vi. Major drug Interactions:
  a. Anticholinergic drugs (enhances anticholinergic side effects)
  b. Hydrochlorothiazide & triamterene reduce the clearance of amantadine
vii. Overdose deaths have been reported, with the lowest acute lethal dose of 1 gram
viii. Renally eliminated, so adjust doses for renal impairment
ix. Available in 100 mg tablets and 50 mg/5 mL suspension
x. Symmetrel[109] (Endo Pharmaceuticals Inc.)
  a. FDA approved for the treatment of drug-induced extrapyramidal reactions
  b. Usual dose is 100 to 400 mg daily in divided doses (BID)
  c. Half-life has averaged 16 ± 6 hours
  d. Onset of action usually within 48 hours
  e. Available in 100 mg capsules & 50 mg per 5 mL fruit punch flavored syrup
xi. Osmolex ER™[75] (amantadine ER) by Vertical Pharmaceuticals, LLC
  a. Indicated for the treatment of drug-induced EPS and Parkinson's Disease in adults
  b. Initial dosage is 129 mg orally once daily in the *morning*
    1. Dose can be increased weekly to a maximum daily dose of 322 mg QAM
  c. 85% is excreted unchanged in urine
  d. Available in: 129 mg, 193 mg, and 258 mg extended-release tablets
xii. Gocovri™[76] (Adamas Pharma LLC)
  a. Not FDA approved for EPS, but is approved for treating dyskinesia in Parkinson's disease
  b. Contraindicated in patients with end-stage renal disease
  c. Initial dosage is 137 mg QHS
    1. After 1 week, should increase to the recommended daily dosage of 274 mg QHS
    2. Capsules can be opened, and contents sprinkled on soft food
  d. Available in 68.5 mg and 137 mg extended-release capsules
C. Akathisia -- internal and external restlessness, fidgetiness
1. Occurs in 10-36% of patients
2. Most common type of EPS with SGAs & high potency FGA agents
3. Not to be confused with anxiety or "agitation"
4. Associated with an increased risk of *suicidal ideation*[981]
5. Test for this with the BARS (Barnes Akathisia Rating Scale)
6. Treat with *beta* blockers or benzodiazepines
i. Propranolol (Inderal®) is the drug of choice
  a. Usual dose is 20 to 120 mg/d divided BID or TID (titrate slowly!!!)
  b. Propranolol is highly lipophilic and easily crosses the blood-brain barrier
  c. 90% bound to plasma proteins
  d. Half-life: 3 to 6 hours
  e. Propranolol is a substrate, as well as a weak inhibitor of CYP2D6
  f. Drug interactions
    1. Increased blood levels with inhibitors of CYP2D6, CYP1A2, and CYP2C19
    2. Decreased blood levels with EIAEDs (many anticonvulsants) and smoking
    3. Propranolol increases the blood levels of diazepam, warfarin, & triptans (migraine drugs)
  g. Available in 10, 20, 40, 60, and 80 mg tablets
ii. Metoprolol and other *beta* blockers have also been used successfully

D. Tardive Dyskinesia (TD)[914,982,983]
1. Involuntary movements of the face, mouth, arms, legs
2. From DA receptor up-regulation
3. People who get early EPS side effects may be more likely to develop TD
4. FGAs: Incidence of 5% per year (prevalence 20-30% for long-term users)
5. SGAs: Incidence of 0.8% (5.3% in those >65 y.o.) per year
6. 60-70% of cases are mild, but approx. 3% are severe[984]
7. May be irreversible and can be extremely disabling
8. Treatments shown to improve TD include clonazepam and ginkgo biloba[985]
9. Newly approved class of drugs: Vesicular Monoamine Transporter 2 (VMAT2) inhibitors
   i. MOA: Decreases uptake of monoamines into synaptic vesicles
      a. Also depletes monoamines from nerve terminal stores
   ii. All VMAT2 inhibitors are contraindicated in those on MAOIs or reserpine
   iii. All have warnings (not black box) about somnolence, QT-prolongation, and NMS
   iv. All can increase risk of akathisia and parkinsonism
   v. All bind to melanin-containing tissues in the eyes, skin, & hair
      a. No monitoring required, but be aware of possibility of long-term ophthalmologic effects
   vi. Safety data in pregnancy and lactation is lacking
   vii. Valbenazine (Ingrezza®)[111] (Neurocrine Biosciences, Inc.)
      a. Indicated for Tardive Dyskinesia
         1. Granted Orphan Drug status by the FDA for pediatric *Tourette Syndrome*
      b. Dosage: 40 mg QD with or without food
         1. Stay at 40 mg for those with moderate or severe hepatic impairment, are receiving strong CYP3A4 or CYP2D6 inhibitors, or who are poor CYP2D6 metabolizers
         2. Do not give with strong CYP3A4 inducers
         3. Not recommended in those with severe renal impairment (CrCl <30 mL/min)
         4. After one week, increase to 80 mg QD
      c. Common side effects: somnolence (11%), akathisia, arthralgia, and vomiting
      d. Long-term monitoring for prolactin elevations and cholestasis (↑ alkaline phosphatase and bilirubin) recommended
      e. Highly protein bound (>99%)
      f. Half-life (t½): 15-22 hours
      g. Metabolized by CYP3A4/5 and CYP2D6
      h. Inhibits p-glycoprotein
      i. Available in a dose-titration kit, and 40 mg & 80 mg capsules (very expensive)
   viii. Deutetrabenazine (Austedo®)[110] (Teva Pharmaceuticals)
      a. Indicated for Chorea associated with Huntington's Disease and Tardive Dyskinesia
      b. BBW: Depression and suicidality in patients with Huntington's Disease
         1. Contraindicated in patients who are actively suicidal or have untreated depression
      c. Usual dose 6 mg po BID with FOOD
         1. Doses can be increased weekly to a maximum of 48 mg/day (divided BID)
         2. Adjust doses in those on strong CYP2D6 inhibitors or are poor CYP2D6 metabolizers
            i. Max dose is 36 mg/d (divided)
      d. Up to 85% protein bound
      e. Half-life (t½): 9-10 hours
      f. Common side effects: Somnolence, diarrhea, dry mouth, and fatigue
      g. Metabolized mainly by carbonyl reductase
         1. Secondary major metabolism by CYP2D6 / Minor metabolism by CYP1A2 and CYP3A4/5
      h. Available in 6, 9, & 12 mg tablets (very expensive)
      i. Currently being studied for Tourette Syndrome & Dyskinetic Cerebral Palsy (tevapharm.com)
   ix. Tetrabenazine (Xenazine®)[112] (Lundbeck)
      a. Not FDA approved for TD, but recommended as an option by the APA[968]
         1. Indicated for Chorea associated with Huntington's Disease
      b. BBW: Depression and suicidality in patients with Huntington's Disease
         1. Contraindicated in patients who are actively suicidal or with hepatic impairment
      c. Usual starting dose is 12.5 mg a day
         1. Increase to 12.5 mg BID after each week
         2. Max single dose should not exceed 25mg
         3. Patients requiring doses above 50 mg/day should be genotyped for CYP2D6
            i. If a poor metabolizer, max daily dose NTE 50 mg (25 mg BID)
            ii. If an extensive/intermediate metabolizer, max daily dose of 100 mg divided BID-TID
         4. Reduce dose if given with strong CYP2D6 inhibitors
      d. Protein binding averages 70% (includes parent drug + 2 active metabolites)
      e. Half-live averages 8 hours (includes parent drug + 2 active metabolites)
      f. Metabolized mainly by CYP2D6, with some contribution of CYP1A2
      g. Available in 12.5 & 25 mg tablets
10. Other treatments with inconclusive or insufficient data
    i. Acetazolamide, bromocriptine, thiamine, baclofen, Vitamins E and B6, selegiline, melatonin, nifedipine, levetiracetam, buspirone, *yi-gan san*, botulinum toxin type A, ECT, α-methyldopa, reserpine, other antipsychotics, and deep brain stimulation in the pallidum

# XVIII. OTHER POTENTIAL SIDE EFFECTS WITH TYPICAL ANTIPSYCHOTICS (FGAS)

A. Anticholinergic (e.g., dry mouth, blurred vision, constipation)
B. Pigmentary retinopathy
C. Seizures
D. Photophobia / Photosensitivity
E. Hyperprolactinemia[986]
  1. Bone demineralization, amenorrhea, gynecomastia
  2. Sexual dysfunction in 25-60% of patients
F. Dermatological rash and blue-gray skin discoloration
G. Thermoregulation difficulties ("poikilothermia")
H. Hepatologic issues (Up to 50% have transiently ↑ed LFTs)
I. Hematologic (blood dyscrasias including agranulocytosis)
J. Cardiovascular
  1. Arrhythmias (may be responsible for sudden death)
  2. Tachycardia from vagal inhibition, reflex tachycardia, and quinidine-like effects
K. Rabbit syndrome - a long-term side effect of peri-oral tremors occurring at a frequency of 5 Hz
L. Neuroleptic Malignant Syndrome (NMS)[987-990]
  1. A rare, potentially life-threatening, idiopathic, yet iatrogenic, reaction to neuroleptic agents
    i. Can also occur from Parkinson's medications and phenothiazine anti-emetics
    ii. Mortality, once reported at 20 to 30% is now estimated at 5.6 to 12%
      a. Mortality is from respiratory failure (pulmonary emboli), CV collapse, myoglobinuric renal failure, arrhythmias, or diffuse intravascular coagulation (DIC)
      b. Older patients have greater mortality risk
  2. Occurs in 0.02% to 1.4% of patients receiving antipsychotics
    i. Those with a genetic polymorphism of the $D_2$ receptor (taqI A, A1 allele ) may be at 10 x ↑ risk
    ii. In 2018, 862 cases were reported to the FDA[991]
      a. Aripiprazole was the most common drug reported to the FDA as the suspected agent
    iii. More common in younger male patients (2:1 vs. females)
  3. Usually occurs in first 2 weeks of drug initiation, dose change, or drug therapy change
    i. Sudden withdrawal of a dopamine agonist (i.e., for Parkinson's disease) can cause NMS
    ii. Inhaled surgical anesthetics have been reported to cause NMS
  4. Incidence ↑ with low serum iron (normal: 60 to 170 mcg/dL), dehydration, agitation, & exhaustion
  5. Highest occurrence with chlorpromazine and high-potency neuroleptics (i.e., haloperidol)
  6. Lowest occurrence with the long-acting depot formulations and atypical antipsychotics
  7. Symptoms develop over 24 to 72 hours
    i. "Lead pipe" muscle rigidity (may be so intense that it leads to rhabdomyolysis and necrolysis)
    ii. Diffuse tremors, dystonic reactions in upper extremities (i.e., trismus), agitation, catatonia, akinesia, sialorrhea, dysarthria, altered consciousness/stupor, tachypnea, and urinary retention
    iii. Malignant hyperthermia ($\geq$104°F/40°C), diaphoresis, tachycardia, fluctuations in BP
  8. Mental Status changes may result from hyperthermia, anticholinergic effects, or hypoactivity of the dopaminergic system in the mesocortical area
  9. LABS
    i. Elevated WBC/ CBC with or without left shift
    ii. Elevated CPK (creatinine phosphokinase) from muscle rigidity – in the thousands
      a. Increases in CPK and potassium indicates skeletal muscle necrosis (rhabdomyolysis)
      b. Myoglobinuria leads to acute renal failure – hemodialysis may be needed
      c. Increased liver enzymes (ALT and AST)
  10. NMS TREATMENT
    i. Discontinue neuroleptic immediately & decrease hyperthermia (e.g., cooling blankets)
    ii. Maintain renal function and correct electrolyte abnormalities
    iii. IV benzodiazepines for muscle relaxation
    iv. Dantrolene (Dantrium®) to relax skeletal muscles
      a. Dose: 1 mg/kg IV initially; repeat dose prn until symptoms subside, up to max of 10 mg/kg
      b. Oral dose is 100-200 mg/d
      c. May reverse muscle rigidity / rhabdomyolysis and may decrease temperature
    v. Bromocriptine 2.5-5 mg two to six times a day
    vi. Amantadine may also be used (100 mg po BID)
    vii. ECT used if other treatments fail
  11. Recurrence rate is between 13% and 37% if rechallenged with an antipsychotic
    i. Recommended to delay rechallenge for at least 2 weeks to reduce recurrence
  12. Neuroleptic Malignant Syndrome Information Service: www.nmsis.org
  13. Malignant Hyperthermia Association of the United States: https://www.mhaus.org/nmsis/

# XIX. RAPID TRANQUILIZATION FOR VIOLENT BEHAVIORS

★ **Combining Benzodiazepines + Antipsychotics work the fastest in decreasing psychotic aggression and acute manic symptoms**
  ▪ **For prn use only**

▶ A combination of Haldol® + Ativan® + Cogentin® or Benadryl® is nicknamed a "cocktail"
▶ Also sometimes referred to as a "B52" (50 mg Benadryl® + 5 mg Haldol® + 2 mg Ativan®)

## XX. TYPICAL ANTIPSYCHOTICS (1ST GENERATION ANTIPSYCHOTICS) IN ORDER OF INCREASING POTENCIES:

A. **Chlorpromazine (Thorazine®)**[196]
1. 1st antipsychotic discovered by accident on 12/11/1950 by 2 Rhone-Poulenc chemists in France
   i. They were looking for better anesthetics for surgery
   ii. Called it a "pharmacologic lobotomy" and "artificial hibernation"
   iii. Found that this class of drugs are good antiemetics
2. Later discovered tricyclic antidepressants (TCAs)
3. Dosing is from 25 mg po TID up to 1000 mg a day (divided) – sometimes more is needed
4. Available in 10, 25, 50, 100, and 200 mg tablets
5. 92-97% protein binding
6. Side effects can be serious and significant (as on previous pages)
   i. Rare cholestatic jaundice (0.5%) & hepatic granulomas
   ii. Hyperglycemia, photosensitivity (3%)
7. Moderate CYP2D6 inhibitor
8. IM injection can be painful & not compatible with lorazepam or benztropine in the same syringe[992]
   i. Dose is 25-50 mg IM TID as necessary for aggression
   ii. If used IV, must be diluted with saline to a final concentration of 1 mg/mL
9. Also used for intractable hiccups, acute intermittent porphyria, "presurgical apprehension", tetanus, and as an antiemetic
10. Approved for Bipolar Disorder and for the treatment of severe behavioral problems in children ages 6 months to 12-years-old

B. **Thioridazine (Mellaril®)**[205]
1. Highest of all neuroleptics in anticholinergic effects
2. Lowest of all neuroleptics in EPS
3. BBW about QTc prolongation (as per latest P.I.)
4. Max dose **800 mg/d** due to pigmentary retinopathy
5. Up to 60% incidence of retrograde ejaculation and other types of sexual dysfunction

C. **Molindone (Moban®)**[203]
1. Moderate EPS, low sedation and anticholinergic effects
2. May cause more akathisia than other FGAs[993]
3. Only agent reported not to cause wt. gain
4. Less effect on lowering seizure threshold
5. Contraindications: severe CV disorders

D. **Loxapine (Loxitane®)**[201]
1. Inhaled loxapine powder (Adasuve®)[202]
   i. FDA-approved 12/2012 through a restricted ADASUVE REMS (www.adasuverems.com) program (Risk Evaluation and Mitigation Strategy) because of *risk of bronchospasm* (BBW)
   ii. Made by Alexza Pharmaceuticals and indicated for the acute treatment of agitation associated with schizophrenia or bipolar I disorder in adults
   iii. Caution in respiratory patients
   iv. Half-life is ≈ 8 hours
   v. Dose is 10 mg (thermal aerosolizer)
      a. Peaks in 2 min., similar to an injection
2. Oral dose is 10-100 mg/d (÷ BID to QID)
3. Active metabolite is amoxapine (Asendin®)
   i. Metabolized by CYP1A2, 3A4 and 2D6
4. Blocks $D_2$ and serotonin $5HT_{2A}$ receptors
   i. Like an atypical, but is not one
5. Moderate EPS/anticholinergic effects
   i. Low weight gain
6. Inhibits P-glycoprotein

E. **Perphenazine (Trilafon®)**[204]
1. Mid-potency
2. Also to treat intractable hiccups and n/v
3. Metabolized by CYP2D6

F. **Trifluoperazine (Stelazine®)**[207]
1. Also has anxiolytic indication
2. Dosing is 2-50 mg divided BID-QID

G. **Thiothixene (Navane®)**[206]
1. Hi potency, hi EPS
2. Moderate anticholinergic effects
3. Approved for children > 12-years-old
4. Dosage: 10-60 mg/d divided BID-TID

**RELATIVE POTENCIES:**
*(lowest to highest)*
**100 mg Chlorpromazine (Thorazine®) =**
100 mg Thioridazine (Mellaril®)
10 mg Molindone (Moban®)
10 mg Loxapine (Loxitane®)
8-10 mg Perphenazine (Trilafon®)
5 mg Trifluoperazine (Stelazine®)
4-5 mg Thiothixene (Navane®)
2 mg Haloperidol (Haldol®)
2 mg Fluphenazine (Prolixin®)

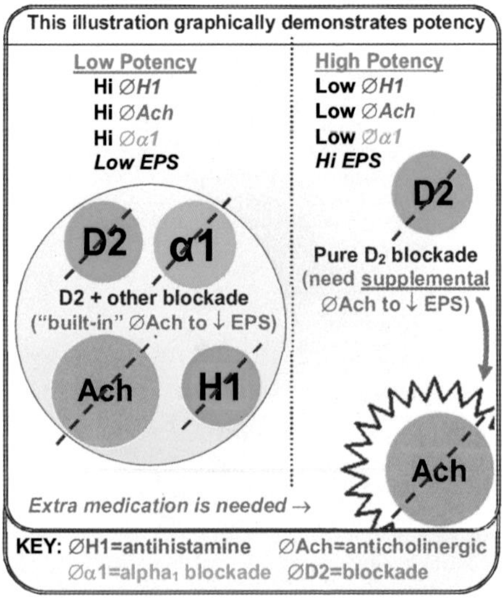
This illustration graphically demonstrates potency
Low Potency
Hi ∅H1
Hi ∅Ach
Hi ∅α1
Low EPS
High Potency
Low ∅H1
Low ∅Ach
Low ∅α1
Hi EPS
D2
α1
Ach
H1
D2 + other blockade
("built-in" ∅Ach to ↓ EPS)
D2
Pure D2 blockade
(need supplemental ∅Ach to ↓ EPS)
Ach
Extra medication is needed →
KEY: ∅H1=antihistamine ∅Ach=anticholinergic
∅α1=alpha1 blockade ∅D2=blockade

H. Haloperidol (Haldol®)[199]
1. Very little anticholinergic side effects, high EPS, less sedation, little CV effects
   i. High doses can prolong QT-interval
2. Approved for Tourette's syndrome & for psychosis/behavioral problems in children > 3-years-old
3. Recommended dose is 2-5 mg/d (range: 1-30 mg/d, with a max oral dosage of 100 mg/day)[994,995]
   i. Package insert recommends 0.5-2 mg PO 2-3 times/day for adults with moderate symptoms
      a. For patients severe, chronic, or treatment-resistant symptoms, 3-5 mg PO 2-3 times/day
      ii. The Patient Outcome Research Team (PORT) consensus guidelines recommend a dosage for
         acute therapy of 6-20 mg/day (maintenance therapy recommended is 6-12 mg/day)
   iii. Available as a tablet, liquid, short-acting and long-acting injectable
   iv. IV administration is not FDA-approved, and may result in QT-prolongation[861]
4. Combined IM benztropine, diphenhydramine, or hydroxyzine in the same syringe is *supposedly*
   incompatible[996], but testing shows that it is compatible for 4 hrs after being mixed[992]
5. Metabolized by CYP3A4, CYP2D6, p-glycoprotein, & CYP1A2 (minor)
   i. Clearance is significantly increased by smoking and inducers
   ii. Ultra-rapid metabolizers of CYP2D6 will also require a much higher dose
   iii. Oral half-life is 14-37 hours
6. Also available as haloperidol decanoate in sesame oil[200]
   i. Caution in those with sesame allergy
      a. Incidence: 0.09% (of elderly) to 0.33% (of young people)[997]
      b. Oil is never absorbed into the body, although immune system may encapsulate it
         1. Pulmonary micro-emboli can accumulate from lymphatic absorption[998]
   ii. Administered Q 4 weeks dosing via *Z-track injection method*
   iii. Dosed at 10-20 times the total daily oral dose
   iv. Give no more than 100 mg on first dose (Z-track method), then give the rest in 3-7 days
   v. Maximum volume per injection site – 3 mL / Maximum dose – 450 mg / month
   vi. Plasma levels peak 6 days after injection
   vii. NEVER give haloperidol decanoate I.V.
7. High amounts found in breast milk
   i. Infants can experience EPS
8. Conc. in the CNS is 20 times that of blood
9. Caution in patients with QTc-prolongation
10. Protect oral dosage forms from light
11. Combinations with lithium can ↑ risk of
    neurotoxicity and encephalopathy
12. **NOTE:** 28 published study reveal that
    haloperidol (and other FGAs) are highly
    neurotoxic and should no longer be utilized in practice[903]
   i. Cause apoptotic cell death, reduce neurotropins/BDNF, and ↓ hippocampal neuroplasticity[910]

Z-Track injection method — skin — subcutaneous tissue — muscle — Use side of hand to pull tissue to one side — depot medication

I. Fluphenazine (Prolixin®)[197]
1. High EPS
2. Available as a decanoate/IM depot in sesame oil[198]
   i. Injected Q 2-3 weeks at 1.25 times the total daily oral dose (max 100 mg/dose)
   ii. Given via Z-track injection method or subcutaneous administration possible
   iii. 1.2% benzyl alcohol preservative
3. Contraindications: sub-cortical brain damage, comatose, or severely depressed states
4. Monitoring: routine CBC w/diff due to incidence of blood dyscrasias
5. Plasma levels observed can vary up to 40-fold in patients receiving the same dose
6. Smoking (CYP1A2 inducer) significantly reduces plasma fluphenazine levels

XX. ATYPICAL ANTIPSYCHOTICS – Work on multiple symptoms of schizophrenia
A. An atypical (SGA) is an antipsychotic that has a lower risk of EPS and prolactin elevations, and
   affects positive, negative, and cognitive symptoms of schizophrenia
   1. Atypicals are associated with possible akathisia and metabolic effects
B. Atypicals increase neurogenesis through neurotrophic growth factors into the hippocampus,
   whereas typicals are associated with neuronal apoptosis and necrosis[903]
C. Aripiprazole (Abilify®)[208] - Otsuka Pharmaceutical
1. Also approved for:
   i. Adjunctive treatment of Major Depressive Disorder (has a BBW about suicide)
   ii. Acute Treatment of Manic and Mixed Episodes associated with Bipolar I
   iii. Tourette's disorder (ages 6 to 18 years)
   iv. Irritability Associated with Autistic Disorder (ages 6 to 17 years)
   v. Approved for bipolar (ages 10-17) and schizophrenia (ages 13-17) in adolescents
2. Structurally similar to trazodone and buspirone[633]
3. As an arylpiperazine, it possesses antidepressant activity
4. MOA: DA partial agonist, $5HT_{1A}$ partial agonist; $5HT_{2A}$ antagonist; $5HT_7$ antagonist; $5HT_{2C}$ partial
   agonist; moderate *alpha$_1$* & $H_1$ blockade
5. > 99% protein bound
6. VERY LONG half-life: 75 hours + 96 hours for its active metabolite
7. Metabolized by CYP2D6 and CYP3A4
   i. Adjust doses for poor metabolizers or with CYP450 inducers/inhibitors
   ii. Aripiprazole and dihydroaripiprazole are efflux transporter (P-gp) substrates

8. Side effects: headache, anxiety, insomnia, N/V, lightheadedness, akathisia, constipation
    i. WARNING: Pathological Gambling and Other Compulsive Behaviors may increase
9. Excreted in human breast milk
    i. May cause EPS and/or withdrawal effects in neonates exposed during the 3rd trimester
10. Dosing: 10-15 mg/d (up to a max of 30 mg/d) usually given in the AM due to possible insomnia
11. Immediate-acting IM injection is 9.75 mg in 1.3 mL sterile water (max of 3 injections a day)
    i. *Not available currently in the US due to poor sales*
12. Tablets available in 2, 5, 10, 15, 20, and 30 mg strengths
    i. Liquid available in 1 mg/mL orange-flavored solution
    ii. DiscMelt® (ODT) tablets available in vanilla-flavored 10 and 15mg
13. Abilify Maintena™[209] - Aripiprazole monohydrate LAI injection - Otsuka Pharmaceutical
    i. Also approved for Maintenance monotherapy treatment of Bipolar I disorder in adults
    ii. Prefilled dual-chamber syringe
    iii. Dose: 400 mg in the gluteal or deltoid muscle monthly (can be reduced to 300mg)
    iv. Adjust doses with CYP2D6 and CYP3A4 inhibitors and poor metabolizers
    v. **Avoid** with patients on CYP3A4 inducers
    vi. 2 weeks of Abilify oral overlap therapy is recommended
    vii. Peak plasma levels in 4 days (deltoid) and ~ 5-7 days (gluteal)
    viii. Cmax is 31% higher for deltoid vs. gluteal site
    ix. Half-life is ≈ 30-46 days once steady state is reached
    x. Shown to improve Quality of Life compared to Invega Sustenna®[999]
14. Abilify Mycite (aripiprazole tablets with sensor) - Otsuka Pharmaceutical
    i. A drug-device combination product comprised of aripiprazole tablets embedded with an Ingestible Event Marker (IEM) sensor intended to track drug ingestion (cost ≈ $1650)[1000]
15. Aristada™[210] (aripiprazole lauroxil) – Alkermes, Inc.
    i. 4 to 8-week long-acting IM injection[1001]
    ii. Uses the LinkeRx™ microcrystal (micron-sized particle) technology platform from Alkermes
        a. A proprietary linker lipid ester of aripiprazole with a chemical tail
    iii. A prodrug of N-hydroxy-methyl aripiprazole, which is a prodrug of aripiprazole
    iv. Doses studied: 441 mg, 662 mg, 882 mg or 1064 mg administered Q 4, 6, or 8 weeks
    v. Dosing
        a. 441 mg (deltoid or gluteal), 662 mg (gluteal) or 882 mg monthly (gluteal)
            1. Lowest dose = deltoid or gluteal / larger doses = gluteal only
        b. 441 mg Q 4 weeks = 10 mg/d oral
        c. 662 mg Q 4 weeks = 882 mg Q 6 weeks = 1064 mg Q 8 weeks all ≈ 15 mg/d oral
        d. Dose of 882 mg Q 4 weeks modeled to be ≈ equivalent to 20 mg/d oral
        e. Essentially, dose ≈ 44 x daily oral aripiprazole dose
        f. Efficacy and side effects similar between doses[1002]
        g. Adjust doses if given with inducers or inhibitors of CYP2D6 or CYP3A4
        h. Monitor for pathological gambling and other compulsive behaviors
    vi. Once injected, drug is systemically released over 46 days
    vii. Plasma levels peak in ≈ 1 month
    viii. 3 weeks of oral overlap is recommended
    ix. Primary side effect: akathisia
        a. Weight gain was not as significant as with the monohydrate (Abilify Maintena)
    x. Half-life is < 2 months
    xi. Available in 441, 662, 882 & 1064 mg pre-filled syringes
    xii. Special information
        a. Tap syringe 10 times, then shake vigorously for a minimum of 30 seconds before use
        b. If syringe is not used within 15 minutes, shake again for 30 seconds
        c. Aristada™ is a "shear thinning" liquid (the opposite of a non-Newtonian fluid)
            1. Viscosity is reduced when shaken and pushed fast through the syringe
16. Aristada Initio™[211] (aripiprazole lauroxil) – Alkermes, Inc.
    i. Utilizes a nano-crystalline milled dispersion of aripiprazole lauroxil to ↑ the rate of dissolution
    ii. Administered as a one-time injection given into gluteal or deltoid muscle
    iii. Dose = 675 mg (volume = 2.4 ml) injection
    iv. Must be given with 30 mg of oral aripiprazole (replaces 3 weeks of oral overlap)
        a. When combined with 30 mg oral aripiprazole, therapeutic levels are reached within 4 days
    v. Given a regularly scheduled Aristada™ injection on same day or up to 10 days after Initio™
    vi. Reaches systemic circulation on the 1st day (peak in 16-35 days)
    vii. Avoid use in known CYP2D6 poor metabolizers or co-administration with strong CYP2D6 or CYP3A4 inhibitors or inducers
D. Asenapine (Saphris®)[212] – also approved for Bipolar + *Pediatric Bipolar* – Allergan Inc.
    1. Available in 2.5 mg, 5 mg, and 10 mg sublingual tablets (black cherry flavored)
        i. For Schizophrenia: 5 mg SL BID / For Bipolar Disorder: 10 mg SL BID
        ii. Administration: Food and water should be avoided for 10 minutes after dissolving the tablet under the tongue. Do not swallow the tablet.
    2. Elimination of asenapine is primarily through direct glucuronidation by UGT1A4 and oxidative metabolism by cytochrome P450 isoenzymes (predominantly CYP1A2)
        i. Weak inhibitor of CYP2D6
        ii. May increase paroxetine levels 2-fold (reduce paroxetine dose as needed)

iii. Reduce dose with concomitant strong CYP1A2 inhibitors (e.g., fluvoxamine) as needed
iv. Antihypertensive drugs may be more effective due to asenapine's $\alpha_1$ blockade
3. Half-life: 24 hours
 i. In elderly, concentrations are 40% higher compared to younger patients[1003]
4. 95% protein bound
5. Caution if given with QT-prolonging medications or in cardiac-risk patients
6. Common side effects: akathisia, somnolence, dizziness, ↑ appetite & weight (esp. with children)
 i. Oral site reactions:
  a. Ulcers, blisters, peeling/sloughing, and inflammation[1003]
  b. Hypoesthesia and/or oral paresthesia (usually resolves within an hour)
 ii. Serious allergic reactions and angioedema have been reported to the FDA
7. Asenapine *transdermal* system (Secuado®)[213] by Noven Therapeutics – Approved 10/2019
 i. Daily patch delivery system applied to the hip, abdomen, upper arm, or upper back area
 ii. Available in 3.8 mg/24 hr, 5.7 mg/24 hr, and 7.5 mg/24 hr patches
 iii. Peak concentrations in 12-24 hours
 iv. Half-life is approx. 30 hours
 v. Adverse skin site reactions (erythema & pruritis) are common (≈14.5% vs. 4% with placebo)
  a. More common in black/African American patients
 vi. Avoid external heat sources to patch (↑ rate and extent of absorption)
 vii. Contraindicated in severe hepatic impairment (Child Pugh C)
E. Brexpiprazole (Rexulti®)[214] - Otsuka Pharmaceutical Co.
1. Also approved as adjunctive therapy to antidepressants for major depressive disorder
2. Available in 0.25 mg, 0.5 mg, 1 mg, 2 mg, 3 mg, and 4 mg tablets
 i. For Schizophrenia: 2-4 mg QD / For MDD adjunct: 1-3 mg QD
 ii. Adjust doses in poor metabolizers or with strong CYP2D6 or CYP3A4 inducers/inhibitors
 iii. Reduce dose in moderate to severe hepatic or renal impairment (CrCl<60 ml/min)
3. MOA: partial $5HT_{1A}$ agonist, partial $D_2$ agonist, and $5HT_{2A}$ antagonist
 i. Also antagonizes $H_1$, $M_1$, $5HT_{2B}$, $5HT_7$, $\alpha_{1A}$, $\alpha_{1B}$, $\alpha_{1D}$, and $\alpha_{2C}$ receptors
4. >99% protein bound
5. Metabolized by CYP3A4 and CYP2D6 to DM-3411 (*inactive* metabolite)
 i. Patients on strong CYP2D6 or CYP3A4 inhibitors – Give half of usual dose
 ii. Patients on strong/moderate CYP2D6 with strong/moderate CYP3A4 inhibitors – Give ¼ dose
 iii. In known CYP2D6 poor metabolizers taking strong/moderate CYP3A4 inhibitors – Give ¼ dose
 iv. Patients on strong CYP3A4 inducers - double the usual dose
6. Half-life is 91 hours (DM-3411's half-life is 86 hours - *not therapeutically significant*)
7. Side effects
 i. High fasting glucose (9-10%)
 ii. ≥ 7% increase in body weight (20-30%)
 iii. ↑ cholesterol (6-9%), ↑ LDL cholesterol (2%), ↓ HDL cholesterol (15%), ↑ triglycerides (13-17%)
 iv. Dyspepsia, diarrhea, akathisia, tremor, sedation, ↑ CPK
 v. No QTc prolongation seen, even at 4 x maximum dose
8. Pregnancy and lactation
 i. Animal data shows it is not teratogenic at high doses, but ↑ deaths did occur with lactation
 ii. No human data available on pregnancy and lactation
  a. Use in 3rd trimester can result in EPS/neonatal withdrawal symptoms
F. Cariprazine (Vraylar®)[215] - Forest Labs[215,544,1004]
1. Also approved for acute treatment of manic or mixed episodes of Bipolar I and for bipolar depression
2. MOA: $D_2$, $D_3$, & $5HT_{1A}$ partial agonist, and $5HT_{2B}$ & $5HT_{2A}$ antagonist (weak $H_1$ & $\alpha_{1A}$ blockade)
 i. More $D_3$ than $D_2$ selective ($D_3$ receptor stimulation has been shown to promote neurogenesis[1005])
3. 91-99% protein bound
4. Metabolized by CYP3A4 to 2 active metabolites
 i. Didesmethylcariprazine (DDCAR) and desmethylcariprazine (DCAR)
 ii. Reduce dose by 50% with strong CYP3A4 inhibitors
  a. Not recommended with strong CYP3A4 inducers or in severe renal impairment
 iii. Half-life: 2-5 days (2-3 weeks for active metabolite, DDCAR)[1006]
5. Available in 1.5 mg, 3 mg, 4.5 mg, and 6 mg capsules
 i. For schizophrenia: 1.5 mg to 6 mg/day / Bipolar: 3 mg to 6 mg/day
6. Side effects: EPS (19-26%), akathisia (13-20%), dyspepsia, vomiting, somnolence, restlessness
 i. Low risk of weight gain and metabolic side effects
7. Better than risperidone on Positive and Negative Syndrome Scale (PANSS) for negative symptoms[1007]
8. In Phase III trials for the relapse prevention of Schizophrenia
G. Clozapine (Clozaril®, Fazaclo® orally disintegrating tablet, Versacloz™ liquid)[216-218]
1. Discovered in 1952, but withdrawn in 1975 due to agranulocytosis, but remarketed in 1988 with blood monitoring requirements - Novartis Pharmaceuticals and others
2. Clozapine is underutilized for fear of side effects and required monitoring[1008,1009]
3. Indicated for *Treatment-Resistant Schizophrenia* and to *reduce the risk of suicidal behavior* in schizophrenia/schizoaffective disorder
 i. "*Treatment-Resistant*" means that a patient must fail trials of at least 2 antipsychotics at adequate doses for at least 6 weeks duration

ii. Guidelines suggest using clozapine if patient is chronically suicidal or overly aggressive
   a. To reduce suicide risk, patients must be continued for > 2 years of therapy
iii. Approx. 30-60% considered treatment-resistant will respond to clozapine[928,937,1010]
iv. Real-world studies in Sweden and Finland found clozapine to be superior to both FGAs & SGAs
    with less all-cause discontinuations, in lowering mortality rates, better outcomes regarding
    overall symptoms, and preventing re-hospitalizations & treatment failures[1011-1012,1013]
4. Structural analogue of loxapine, asenapine, olanzapine, and quetiapine
5. See **Black Box Warnings** on *page 9*
6. $D_1$ > $D_2$, $D_4$, $5HT_2$, $5HT_3$, $5HT_6$, and $5HT_7$ antagonist
7. Also blocks *alpha2*, cholinergic, histaminic receptors
8. Half-life: 8-12 hours
9. Dosing: 25-900 mg/d (slow titration)
   i. Tablets available: 25 & 100 mg / Versacloz™: 50 & 100 mg/mL suspension - Tasman Pharma
   ii. Fazaclo® mint-flavored ODT: 12.5, 25, 100, 150, & 200mg - Jazz Pharmaceuticals, Inc.
10. Metabolism mainly via CYP3A4, CYP1A2, and CYP2D6
   i. Patients concomitantly using strong CYP1A2 inhibitors – give 1/3 usual dose
    a. E.g., fluvoxamine, ciprofloxacin, enoxacin
   ii. Concomitant use of strong CYP3A4 inducers is not recommended
   iii. If discontinuing a CYP1A2 or CYP3A4 Inducer, may need to reduce dose
    a. E.g., CYP1A2 inducer (e.g., tobacco smoke)
    b. E.g., CYP3A4 inducer (e.g., carbamazepine)
11. Cigarette smoking (CYP1A2 inducer) will ↑ metabolism, so larger doses may be needed
12. Pregnancy Category B
13. QT-prolongation warning added to prescribing information
14. Side effects: drowsiness, dizziness, reflex tachycardia, orthostatic hypotension, N/V, fever,
    visual disturbances, constipation, weight gain, hyperglycemia, colitis, angioedema, skin
    pigmentations, rhabdomyolysis, and more (***very little EPS***)
   i. Cardiomyopathy and myocarditis (incidence of 0.015% to 8.5%)
    a. Estimated 0.28% mortality
    b. May be immune-mediated, with symptoms of shortness of breath, tachycardia, fever, fatigue,
      chest pain, palpitations, and peripheral edema
    c. If suspected, get Cardiologist consult, EKG, C-reactive protein, and troponin (I & T subtypes)
   ii. Dose-related seizures (1 to 4.4% - Avg. 2.8%) – especially from a rapid titration[968,1014]
   iii. Salivation (sialorrhea) / drooling - in up to 40% of patients
    a. Treat with anticholinergics given sublingually (tropicamide[1015] ($M_4$ antagonist), atropine eye
      drops or chewing gum, ipratropium) or antihypertensives (propranolol, clonidine, terazosin)
    b. Glycopyrrolate (Robinul®) - available as an oral soln. (Cuvposa®)[1016] for drooling in children
      & as an inhalation soln. (Lonhala® Magnair®) & powder (Seebri® Neohaler®) for COPD
   iv. RARE: agranulocytosis (0.38-0.73%)
    a. Requires weekly monitoring of ANC (Absolute Neutrophil Count) (not WBCs as before) for
      the first 6 months, then Q 2 weeks for the next 6 months, then Q 4 weeks thereafter[1017,1018]
    b. New ANC requirement is 1000 cells/microliter or more
    c. *Clozapine REMS program* coordinates ALL requirements for registering, monitoring,
      prescribing, dispensing, and receiving clozapine
    d. All prescribing physicians MUST be certified through the program to prescribe clozapine
      1. Go to www.clozapinerems.com for details
    e. For patients of African descent with BEN (Benign Ethnic Neutropenia)[1019-1023]
      1. Hemoglobin, mean corpuscular volume (MCV) serum transferrin saturation (TS), ↑ serum
        ferritin, WBC and ANC of those of African descent can be lower than in Europeans[1024]
      2. For patients with BEN, ANC must be 500 cells/microliter or more
      3. Previously ineligible patients for clozapine can potentially now be considered for it
      4. Draw blood late in the day - Neutrophils peak between 7 and 8 PM[1025]
      5. Lithium 300-600 mg/d been tried successfully to ↑ ANC for prophylaxis[1026-1030]
      6. Have patient avoid strenuous exercise, which can ↓ ANC
15. Clozapine levels >350-400μg/L for optimal response (*clozapine:norclozapine ratio >2:1*)[1031-1037]
   i. The therapeutic response begins to appear at 100μg/L
   ii. Toxic range: Greater than 1000μg/L
H. Iloperidone (Fanapt®)[219] - Vanda Pharmaceuticals
   1. Starting dose: 1 mg po BID
   i. Titrate up slowly to avoid orthostatic hypotension (due to *alpha1* blockade)
   ii. Target dosage is 12-24 mg per day divided BID (titrate slowly to reduce orthostatic hypotension)
   2. Half-life: 18-37 hours
   3. Metabolized by CYP2D6 and CYP3A4
   i. Give ½ usual dose in poor CYP2D6 metabolizers or on a strong CYP2D6 or CYP3A4 inhibitor
   4. Acts as a weak P-glycoprotein inhibitor
   5. Side effects: dizziness, dry mouth, fatigue, nasal congestion, orthostatic hypotension,
    somnolence, tachycardia, and weight gain
   i. Rare: priapism (from *alpha1* blockade)
   6. Not a first-line agent due to QT-prolongation (**not a BBW**)
   i. Contraindicated to be given with other QT-prolonging drugs
   7. Not recommended in severe hepatic impairment

8. A long-acting injectable using microsphere technology is being studied[1038]
   i. Available in 1 mg, 2 mg, 4 mg, 6 mg, 8 mg, 10 mg and 12 mg tablets
I. Lurasidone (Latuda®)[220] – Sunovion Pharmaceuticals
   1. Also approved for Bipolar Depression (with or without valproate or lithium)
   2. Antagonist of $D_2$, $5HT_{2A}$, $5HT_7$ receptors, & partial agonist at $5HT_{1A}$ receptor (possibly anxiolytic)
   3. Pregnancy Category B
   4. Half-life: 18 hours
   5. Metabolized via CYP3A4 to 2 active and 2 inactive metabolites
   i. Use ½ usual dose with moderate CYP3A4 inhibitors
   ii. CONTRAINDICATED with strong CYP3A4 inhibitors
      a. E.g., clarithromycin, darunavir, elvitegravir, grapefruit & grapefruit juice, indinavir, tipranavir, ketoconazole, lopinavir, mibefradil, nelfinavir, ritonavir, saquinavir, and voriconazole
   iii. CONTRAINDICATED with strong CYP3A4 inducers
      a. E.g., avasimibe, carbamazepine, phenytoin, rifampin, St. John's Wort
   6. Schizophrenia dose: 40 mg to 80 mg (up to 160mg) QD with FOOD (> 350 calories)
   7. Bipolar dose: 20 mg to 60 mg QD with FOOD (> 350 calories)
   i. Food increases absorption by 2-3 times
   8. Available in 20 mg, 40 mg, 80 mg and 120 mg tablets
   9. Dose should not exceed 40 mg/d in those with severe hepatic/renal impairment (CrCl < 50 mL/min) or those taking Diltiazem
   10. Common side effects: dose-related akathisia, nausea, somnolence, pseudoparkinsonism
   11. Recent data reveals that lurasidone can reduce metabolic effects (e.g., weight), daytime sedation, and prolactin levels from other atypicals[1039]
   12. Data shows efficacy in MDD with subsyndromal hypomania[1040]
J. Olanzapine (Zyprexa®/Zydis®)[221] – Eli Lilly and Company
   1. Approved for acute Bipolar treatment and maintenance (incl. child/adolescents) and *TRD*
   2. Structural analogue of clozapine
   3. 93% protein bound
   4. Half-life: 21-54 hours
   5. Metabolism mainly via CYP1A2 & CYP2D6, and glucuronidation
   6. Dosing: 2.5-20 mg daily *(higher doses well tolerated)*
   7. Available in non-scored 2.5, 5, 7.5, 10, 15, & 20 mg tabs
   i. Non-flavored, sweetened 5, 10, 15, & 20 mg ODT (non-scored)
   8. Side effects: drowsiness, dizziness, akathisia, weight gain
   i. Not recommended in the elderly due to anticholinergic effects (see Beers List)
   9. Cigarette smoking (CYP1A2 inducer) & valproic acid[1041] will ↑ metabolism, so need larger doses
   10. Rapidly-acting olanzapine IM injection (10 mg vial)
   i. Must be reconstituted with 2.1 mL of sterile water (makes 5 mg/mL concentration)
   ii. Dose is 10 mg which can be repeated in 2-4 hours – Max. of 3 injections (30mg)
   iii. Do not give within 1 hour of a *benzodiazepine* or CNS depressants – leads to bradycardia, hypotension, & other cardiovascular complications
   iv. Not approved for subcutaneous or IV administration, but Emergency Dept. studies have been done with successful outcomes[1042,1043]
   11. Zyprexa Relprevv®[222] - long-acting IM depot - Eli Lilly and Company
   i. BBW  Risk of severe sedation (including coma) and/or delirium after each injection
      a. 0.07% risk for each injection = ~1 per 1400 injections
      b. Patient must be observed for at least 3 hours in a registered facility with ready access to emergency response services
      c. Called "Post-injection Delirium/Sedation Syndrome" (PDSS)
      d. Proper injection technique is crucial to reduce incidence
      e. Occurs in under an hour in 80% of patients
      f. Can resemble alcohol intoxication
      g. All patients should mostly recover within 72 hours
      h. No specific remedy is suggested. Just supportive care
      i. Only available through a restricted distribution program (required REMS program)
      j. Deaths have been reported to the FDA from very high olanzapine blood levels[1044]
   ii. Insoluble salt complex with pamoic acid
      a. Once injected into gluteal muscle, the salt complex slowly dissolves
         1. In blood vessels or plasma, it dissociates into olanzapine and pamoic acid
         2. Pamoic acid is non-pharmacologically active and excreted unchanged
      b. Dose ≈ 30 x oral dose divided over the 2-4 week interval
         1. In a DBPCT, doses of 210 mg Q 2 weeks, 300 mg Q 2 weeks and 405 mg Q 4 weeks were equally effective and well tolerated[1045]
      c. Doses: 150, 210 or 300 mg Q 2 weeks OR 300 or 405 mg Q 4 weeks
         1. Maintenance dose is generally 30 x oral dose divided by Q 2 or 4 weeks
            i. 10 or 15 mg a day = 300 mg or 405 mg every 4 weeks
            ii. 10, 15, or 20 mg a day oral = 150 mg, 210 mg, or 300 mg (max dose) every 2 weeks
         2. Loading doses
            i. Those on 10 mg/d oral, load with 210 mg every 2 weeks or 405 mg every 4 weeks
            ii. Those on 15–20 mg/d of oral should be loaded with 300 mg every 2 weeks
      d. Plasma levels peak in 2-7 days

      1. Given Q 2 weeks, trough levels are 50% of peak
      2. Given Q 4 weeks, trough levels are 25% of peak
   e. Half-life is ≈ 1 month
   f. Availability: Powder for suspension for IM use only: 210 mg/vial, 300 mg/vial, & 405 mg/vial
      1. Must be reconstituted with provided diluent
      2. Needle-Pro® syringes with needle protective device should be used
      3. Drug is stable for 24 hours and must be used in that time frame
      4. Vigorous shaking is required to suspend the mixture
12. Adding melatonin to olanzapine showed it lessened weight gain, abdominal obesity, and triglycerides, and had a positive impact on psychotic symptoms vs. olanzapine alone[1046]
13. A single dose of olanzapine 10 mg shown to ↓ glucose effectiveness, ↑ fasting glucose for over 4 hours, ↓ serum cortisol, and lower fasting free fatty acid levels in healthy volunteers[1047]

K. **Paliperidone (Invega®)**[223] – 9-hydroxy-risperidone (active metabolite of risperidone)
  1. Extended-release once daily dosing (OROS system) - Janssen Pharmaceutica
   i. Tablets should not be chewed or crushed; may see tablet shell in stool
  2. Less EPS than risperidone
  3. Approved for adolescent Schizophrenia (ages 12-17) and adult Schizoaffective Disorder
  4. Available as 1.5 mg, 3 mg, 6 mg, & 9 mg extended-release tablets
  5. Recommended dose: 6 mg/d -- Max dose: 12 mg/d
  6. 59% renal elimination with some metabolism by CYP2D6 and CYP3A4
  7. ↑ dose when giving with a strong inducer of <u>both</u> CYP3A4 and P-gp (e.g., carbamazepine)
  8. Weak inhibitor of P-gp at high doses
  9. **Invega Sustenna®**[224] (paliperidone palmitate) extended-release injectable suspension
   i. Made with NanoCrystal® technology - Janssen Pharmaceutica
     a. Increased surface area of nanocrystals leads to initial rapid release
     b. Does not require an oral overlap
     c. Hydrolysis of paliperidone palmitate results in free paliperidone + palmitic acid
   ii. Also approved for Schizoaffective Disorder
   iii. Initial dose of <u>234 mg</u> on day 1 and then <u>156 mg</u> one week later (± 4 days) in *deltoid only*
   iv. After 1st injection, plasma levels of active paliperidone are detectable on 1st day
     a. Plasma levels peak in < 2 weeks / Half-life is 25-49 days
   v. Recommended monthly maintenance dose is <u>117 mg</u> (range 39-234mg)
     a. Administered in the deltoid or gluteal muscle (gluteal absorption is 28% lower than deltoid)
   vi. Not recommended if CrCl < 50 ml/min
   vii. Reduce dose if CrCl > 50, but < 80 ml/min
   viii. *Avoid using with a strong inducer of CYP3A4 and/or P-gp*
   ix. Monitor for extremely rare anaphylaxis (even if oral meds well tolerated)
   x. Available in 39 mg, 78 mg, 117 mg, 156 mg, and 234 mg prefilled syringes
   xi. Does NOT need refrigeration or reconstitution
   xii. Must shake vigorously for 10 seconds before administration
     a. Inject within 5 minutes or re-shake
  10. **Invega Trinza™**[225] (paliperidone palmitate) extended-release injectable suspension
   i. 3-month formulation (half-life is > 3 to 4 months) - Janssen Pharmaceutica
   ii. Patients should be stabilized on Invega Sustenna® for > 4 months before using
   iii. NanoCrystal® technology
     a. Uses larger particle size resulting in slower dissolution and a longer dosing interval
   iv. Time to schizophrenia symptom relapse is significantly delayed vs. placebo[1048]
   v. Not recommended if CrCl < 50 ml/min
   vi. Deltoid injections result in a 11-12% higher Cmax compared to gluteal
   vii. Available in prefilled syringes: 273 mg, 410 mg, 546 mg, and 819 mg
   viii. Shake syringe vigorously for at least 15 seconds prior to injection
   ix. Inject within 5 minutes of shaking vigorously

| *Converting from Sustenna to Trinza* | | | | |
|---|---|---|---|---|
| Most recent dose of Sustenna | 78mg | 117mg | 156mg | 234mg |
| Start Trinza at this dose* | 273mg | 410mg | 546mg | 819mg |
| *Trinza dose is 3.5 x Sustenna dose | | | | |

L. **Pimavanserin tartrate (Nuplazid™)**[226] - ACADIA Pharmaceuticals Inc.
  1. Approved for treating hallucinations and delusions associated with Parkinson's disease psychosis
  2. MOA: inverse agonist & antagonist at $5HT_{2A}$ receptors (and to a lesser extent at $5HT_{2C}$ receptors)
  3. Usual dose: 34 mg QD with or without food
   i. Reduce dose to 10 mg QD with concomitant strong CYP3A4 inhibitors
   ii. Avoid use with concomitant strong or moderate CYP3A4 inducers
  4. Has a warning (**non-BBW**) about QT-prolongation
   i. Do not give in combination with other drugs known to prolong QT interval
  5. Common side effects: peripheral edema, confusion, and nausea
  6. Use with caution in patients with severe renal impairment and end stage renal disease
  7. ≈ 95% protein bound
  8. Half-life of pimavanserin & active N-desmethylated metabolite ≈ 57 and 200 hours, respectively
  9. Metabolized by CYP3A4 (major), CYP3A5 (major), CYP2J2 (minor), and CYP2D6 (minor)

i. Reduce dose if given with a strong CYP3A4 inhibitor
ii. Avoid use if patient is receiving a moderate or strong CYP3A4 inducer
10. Available in 34 mg capsules & 10 mg tablets
11. Currently in Phase II trials for the treatment of Negative Symptoms of Schizophrenia
M. Quetiapine (Seroquel®/Seroquel XR®)[227] - AstraZeneca
 1. Approved for Bipolar depression (Seroquel XR® only), pediatric patients, and add-on for MDD
 2. Structural analogue of clozapine
 3. Dosing: Initiate at 50-100 mg BID; average: 600-800 mg/d *(higher doses well tolerated)*
  i. Bipolar depression: Average dose approx. 300 mg/d
  ii. Seroquel XR is dosed QD in the evening <u>without</u> food or <u>with</u> a light snack (<300 cal)
  iii. Availability: 50 mg, 150 mg, 200 mg, 300 mg, 400 mg tablets
 4. Half-life: 6-7 hours
 5. 83% protein bound and 100% bioavailable
 6. Partially metabolized by CYP3A4
  i. Norquetiapine – major active metabolite with high $5HT_2$ and $M_1$ (muscarinic) blockade
 a. Also NE reuptake inhibitor
 7. Drug interactions
  i. If patient is taking a strong CYP3A4 inhibitor – reduce dose to 1/6th usual dose
  ii. If patient is taking a strong CYP3A4 inducer – increase dose up to 5 times usual dose
  a. E.g., Phenytoin ↑s quetiapine clearance by 500%
  iii. Avoid use in any patient with concomitant QT-prolonging medications
 8. Side effects: dizziness, postural hypotension, drowsiness, dry mouth, ↑ lipids, wt. gain
  i. New warnings (11/2018) added about rare leukopenia, neutropenia and agranulocytosis, and
   anticholinergic effects
 9. Little to no EPS or prolactin elevations seen across dose range
 10. Drug of choice in Parkinson's dementia/psychosis and Lewy Body Dementia patients
 11. Has abuse/misuse potential due to its sedative/anxiolytic effects
 12. Do <u>NOT</u> use for insomnia (as a hypnotic agent)
N. Risperidone (Risperdal®/ Risperdal® M-Tab/Risperdal Consta®/Perseris™)[228]
 1. $D_2$ antagonist (affects positive symptoms) and $5HT_{2A}$ antagonist (affects negative symptoms)
 2. *Alpha₁* and *alpha₂* blockade (see info for Remeron (mirtazapine) on page 54)
 3. Approved for Bipolar (ages 10-17) and Schizophrenia (ages 13-17) in adolescents, and irritability
  in autistic children & adolescents (ages 5 to 17)
 4. Average dose is 4-5 mg/d (National average)
 5. Available as 0.25 mg, 0.5 mg, 1 mg, 2 mg, 3 mg, & 4 mg tablets
  i. Risperdal M-Tabs: 0.5, 1, 2, 3, & 4 mg peppermint-flavored ODT *(contains phenylalanine)*
  ii. Unflavored oral solution (1 mg/ml)
 6. Metabolized by CYP3A4 and CYP2D6
  i. Patients on CYP3A or Pgp inducers – increase dose up to double usual dose
  ii. Patients on CYP2D6 inhibitors – Do not exceed 8 mg a day
 7. Half-life is approx. 20 hours (shorter in CYP2D6 extensive-metabolizers)
 8. Side effects: Sedation, orthostatic hypotension, dose-related EPS (No anticholinergic effects)
  i. In autism study - headache (6%), epistaxis (6%) and pyrexia (6%)
  ii. Prolactin elevations are higher than with haloperidol
 9. Risperdal® Consta®[229] kit – IM Depot formulation- Janssen Pharmaceutica
  i. Approved as monotherapy for Bipolar I Disorder with or without Li⁺ / valproate
  ii. Risperidone encapsulated into polymeric microspheres
   a. Drug release occurs by erosion of the PLGA polymer
   b. Approx. 1% of risperidone (on surface of the microspheres) is released within 24 h
   c. Polymer erodes over 4–6 weeks
   d. Lag period of ≈ 3 weeks after injection
  iii. Plasma levels peak in 3-4 weeks / Half-life is 3-6 days
  iv. 3 weeks of oral Risperdal overlap therapy is needed when starting Consta
  v. Relative risk reduction of relapse of 84.7% in 1 year vs. oral risperidone[1049]
  vi. EPS occurs in 10 & 24% receiving 25 & 50 mg Q 2 weeks, respectively
  vii. Dose: 12.5 to 25 mg IM injection (deltoid or gluteal) given Q 2 weeks (Max is 50mg)
  viii. Store in refrigerator (or out for up to 7 days), protected from light / needs reconstitution
   a. Reconstituted injection must be used within 6 hours
  ix. Monitor for extremely rare anaphylaxis (even if oral meds well tolerated)
  x. Available in vial kits of 12.5 mg, 25 mg, 37.5 mg, and 50 mg
 10. Perseris™[230] - *Subcutaneous* long-acting risperidone – Indivior PLC
  i. Administered Q 4 weeks subcutaneously in the abdomen only with patient supine
  ii. Dosing depends on stabilized oral daily dosage
   a. 90 or 120 mg (equivalent to 3 to 4 mg a day of oral, respectively)
   b. Not recommended for patients stable on less than 3 mg/day or higher than 4 mg/day
  iii. Interactions with strong CYP2D6 inhibitors / CYP3A4 inducers & inhibitors
  iv. No oral overlap needed
  v. Plasma levels peak in 4-6 hours and again in 10-14 days
  vi. Half-life is 9-11 days
  vii. Available in 90 mg (0.6 ml) & 120 mg (0.8 ml) dual-syringe vial kits for reconstitution
  viii. One syringe with risperidone powder & other with a prefilled liquid delivery system (Atrigel)

a. Syringes require 60 cycles to mix (1 cycle = pushing contents back & forth in each syringe)

b. Store in refrigerator, but warm to room temperature (up to 7 days) before administering

O. Ziprasidone (Geodon®)[231] – Pfizer Pharmaceuticals

1. $5HT_{2A}$, $5HT_{2C}$, $5HT_{1D}$ antagonist/$5HT_{1A}$ agonist > $D_2$, $D_3$ antagonist; moderate *alpha₁*, histamine₁ blockade and 5HT, NE reuptake inhibition

2. Dosing: Initiate at 20 mg BID with food; average dose: 160 mg/d divided BID with food

3. Up to two-fold absorption ↑ with food (Dose it at MEAL TIMES)

4. Immediate-acting IM injection is available in 20 mg/mL vial

   i. Can give 10 mg every 2 hours or 20 mg every 4 hours (max of 40 mg a day)

5. Half-life: 7 hours (2-5 hours for IM injection)

6. > 99% protein bound

7. Side effects: ↑ QT interval, akathisia, anorexia, depression, diarrhea, hallucinations, headache, hostility, insomnia, N/V, rash

8. Drug interactions: drugs that prolong QT interval (quinidine, sotalol, thioridazine, etc.); carbamazepine ↓ levels 36%; ketoconazole ↑ levels 33%

9. Metabolized by CYP3A4; weak inhibitor of CYP2D6 (high dose)

10. QT-prolongation is dose-related

    i. EKG recommended in patients at risk for cardiac complications

11. May be associated with rare skin reaction (DRESS - Drug Reaction with Eosinophilia and Systemic Symptoms)[1050]

## XXI. POTENTIAL FUTURE TREATMENTS FOR SCHIZOPHRENIA IN STUDY[1051,1052]

A. Various *transdermal delivery systems* are under investigation (creams, films, gels, nano-systems, patches, solutions, & sprays)[1053]

1. Asenapine (nano-system, spray, gel, ointment, lotion, foam, aerosol, film)

2. Aripiprazole (liquid, gel)

3. Blonanserin (patch in Phase III trials)

4. Chlorpromazine (gel)

5. Haloperidol (nano-system)

6. Olanzapine (nano-system, patch)

7. Prochlorperazine (microneedles)

8. Quetiapine (cream)

9. Risperidone (nano-system, patch)

B. ADX-1149 - Addex Therapeutics with Janssen Pharmaceuticals[1054]

1. A first-in-class, potent, small molecule positive allosteric modulator (PAM) of metabotropic glutamate receptor 2 (mGluR2), a Family C class of G Protein Coupled Receptors (GPCR)

C. ALKS 3831 - Alkermes plc developed combination product of olanzapine + samidorphan to mitigate the metabolic effects of olanzapine[581]

1. 12-week study - 37% less weight gain with ALKS 3831 than olanzapine

2. 24-week study of 561 patients (ENLIGHTEN-2) of ALKS 3831 vs. olanzapine[1055]

   i. Weight gain was less with ALKS 3831 vs. olanzapine (p=0.003)

   ii. Overall, 36% of ALKS 3831 and 25% of olanzapine patients gained weight

   iii. A new drug application (NDA) to the FDA to be submitted in the fall of 2019

   iv. *https://clinicaltrials.gov/ct2/show/NCT02694328*

3. Also applying for manic or mixed episodes associated with bipolar I disorder as a monotherapy or adjunct to lithium or valproate and for maintenance treatment of bipolar I disorder

4. Fixed dosage strengths for ALKS 3831 include 10 mg of samidorphan co-formulated with 5 mg, 10 mg, 15 mg or 20 mg of olanzapine

D. APN-1125 by Alpharmagen; CoMentis in Phase I/II

1. α7 nicotinic acetylcholine receptor partial agonist

E. Aripiprazole transdermal patch (AQS-1301) by Aequus Pharmaceuticals in Phase I

F. Aripiprazole oral soluble oral film by CMG Pharmaceutical in Phase I

G. Aripiprazole monohydrate by Otsuka Pharmaceutical 2 month injectable (Phase I completed)

H. ASP-4345 by Astellas Pharma US (Phase II) - D1 receptor modulator

I. AUT-00206 by Autifony Therapeutics; University of Manchester; Univ. of Newcastle upon Tyne

1. Shaw potassium channel modulator currently in Phase I trials

2. Granted Orphan Drug Status for Fragile X syndrome

J. Avisetron (AVN-211) - Avineuro Pharmaceuticals

1. A strong $5HT_6$ receptor antagonist and weak $5HT_{2B}$ antagonist

2. Phase III trials underway and Phase II trials in progress for cognitive dysfunction

K. AVP-786/AVP-923 (deuterium-modified dextromethorphan + quinidine) – Otsuka/Avanir Pharma

1. Sigma-1 (σ1) receptor agonist, SNRI, and NMDA receptor antagonist

2. Phase II/III for Negative symptoms of schizophrenia

L. AXS-05 (bupropion + dextromethorphan fixed-dose combination) - Axsome Therapeutics

1. A fixed-dose combination of bupropion and dextromethorphan (DXM)

2. Currently in Phase II/III trials for agitation

M. Basmisanil (RG-1662, RO-5186582) by Chugai Pharmaceutical/Roche

1. Phase II for the treatment of CIAS Cognitive Impairment Associated with Schizophrenia

2. GABA receptor α subunit-containing negative allosteric modulator

N. BI 425809 by Boehringer Ingelheim

1. In Phase II schizophrenia (combination with Computerized Cognitive Training)

O. BI-409306 (SUB-166499) by Boehringer Ingelheim
  1. A phosphodiesterase 9A inhibitor in Phase II (also for Alzheimer's)
P. BIIB-104 (PF-04958242) by Biogen & Pfizer in Phase II Fast Track
  1. Positive allosteric modulator (PAM) of AMPA receptor (AMPAR), ionotropic glutamate receptor
  2. For the treatment of CIAS Cognitive Impairment Associated With Schizophrenia
Q. Bitopertin (Hoffmann-La Roche)
  1. A glycine reuptake inhibitor for negative symptoms
  2. 10, 30, or 60 mg/d were significantly superior to placebo in an 8-week trial[1056]
R. Blonanserin[1057] (Lonasen®) - Sumitomo Pharmaceutical (Suzhou) Co., Ltd.
  1. Currently only available in China and Japan
  2. Study compared with risperidone
  3. Higher risk of akathisia than risperidone
S. Brexpiprazole (OPC-34712) SQ or IM (single dose) by Otsuka Pharmaceutical (Phase I)
T. Brilaroxazine (RP5063, RP-5000, oxaripiprazole) - Reviva Pharmaceuticals
  1. Currently in Phase II/III (https://adisinsight.springer.com/drugs/800035778)
  2. Also being studied for a variety of other psychiatric conditions (e.g., schizoaffective disorder)
  3. MOA: A dopamine-serotonin system stabilizer on D2, D3, and D4 receptors and $5HT_{1A}$ & $5HT_{2A}$ receptors as a partial agonist. May also affect $5HT_7$, H1, D1, D5, $5HT_6$, $5HT_3$, *Alpha*-1B receptor sites, and serotonin transporter (SERT)
U. Cannabidiol (CBD; GW-42003, GWP-42003, GWP-42003-P, ECP-012A; Arvisol, Epidiolex)
  1. Cannabinoid receptor modulator, antioxidant, other actions
  2. Many studies in Phase II are underway by GW Pharmaceuticals, Yale University, University of Alabama, University of Utah, University of Maryland, and others
V. Coumadin - linked to a decrease or long-term remission of psychotic symptoms in schizophrenia
  1. Normalization of tissue-plasminogen activator (tPA) is the postulated mechanism of action[1058]
  2. No further studies have been conducted
W. CTP-692[1059] - Concert Pharmaceuticals, Inc.
  1. A deuterium-modified analog of D-serine (endogenous NMDA receptor co-agonist)
  2. The Company intends to advance the program into a Phase II trial in the fourth quarter of 2019
X. D-Cycloserine[357] 50 mg a day in Phase III and IV trials
Y. DORIA®; Risperidone ISM® extended-release by Rovi – completed Phase II trials
  1. ISM = *In situ* microparticles implant (https://www.rovi.es/en/ism)
  2. Intramuscular injection (gluteus or deltoid) reaches therapeutic levels in plasma within the first few hours after the drug is administered with no supplemental oral risperidone required
  3. 4 week duration of effect
Z. Erteberel (LY-500307, SERBA-1) by Eli Lilly & Company
  1. Estrogen Receptor *Beta*-agonist (ERβ agonist ) in Phase II
AA. Evenamide (NW-3509) - Newron Pharmaceuticals [Phase III supposed to start at end of 2019]
  1. MOA: Selective voltage-gated sodium channel blocker
  2. For add-on therapy for the treatment of schizophrenia (Phase IIb)
  i. Also being studied as adjunctive therapy of clozapine treatment-resistant Schizophrenia (TRS)
AB. F-17464 by Pierre Fabre Medicament (Phase II completed)
  1. A $D_3$ receptor antagonist, $5HT_{1A}$ receptor partial agonist, and weak D receptor partial agonist
AC. FKF02SC (TGOF-02N) by Fabre-Kramer Pharmaceuticals (Phase II)
  1. $5HT_2/D_2$ antagonist atypical antipsychotic, with highest receptor binding for $D_2$, $D_3$, $5HT_{2C}$, $5HT_{2A}$, $\alpha_1$ and $H_1$ receptors, and moderate affinity for $D_1$, $D_4$ and $5HT_{1A}$ receptors
  2. T½ from 3.24 to 3.84 hours
AD. Huperzine A is currently in Phase II & III trials for Alzheimer's and Schizophrenia
  1. https://clinicaltrials.gov/ct2/results?term=Huperzine
AE. Iloperidone LAI by Vanda Pharmaceuticals in Phase I and II – preparing for Phase III trials
  1. Monthly depot (crystalline and microparticle formulations)
AF. KarXT (trospium chloride/xanomeline) by Karuna Pharmaceuticals (Phase II)
  1. Combined $M_1$ and $M_4$ muscarinic acetylcholine receptor agonist and peripherally-selective muscarinic acetylcholine receptor antagonist
AG. Lu AF11167 by Lundbeck
  1. For the negative symptoms of schizophrenia
  2. Possible MOA: a potent and selective inhibitor of the PDE2A & PDE10A enzyme
  3. Doses currently being studied in Phase II trial: 1-2 mg/day or 3-4 mg/day
AH. Lu AF35700 by Lundbeck (Phase III completed 12/2019)
  1. $D_1$, $5HT_{2A}$, and $5HT_6$ receptor antagonist
  2. 10 and 20 mg doses being tested
AI. Lumateperone (ITI-007)[586] - Intra-cellular Therapies
  1. On FDA's Fast Track for approval for acute or residual symptoms of Schizophrenia
  2. A new drug application was submitted to the FDA in the fall of 2018
  3. FDA postponed for Schizophrenia by end of 2019
  4. Other possible future indications: bipolar depression (Phase III), depression, autism, and sleep
  i. Phase III trial for behavioral disturbances in dementia was terminated, because of inefficacy
  5. MOA: $5HT_{2A}$ receptor antagonist (60 x more affinity than to dopamine)
  i. A dopamine receptor phosphoprotein modulation (DPPM)
    a. Partial agonist of presynaptic D2 receptors and an antagonist of postsynaptic D2 receptors
  ii. A 5HT transporter blocker, with some D1 receptor affinity & indirect glutamatergic modulation

AJ. MK-8189 by Merck is in Phase II trials for schizophrenia as of the summer of 2019
  1. MOA is unknown
  2. As of 9/25/19, a Phase I continuation trial is also underway
AK. N-acetylcysteine (NAC) as adjunctive therapy for negative symptoms[1060]
  1. Doses of 1000 to 2700 mg divided BID used in most trials
AL. NaBen® - Sodium benzoate[1061] (SND-11, SND-12, SND-13, SND-14; Clozaben) by SyneuRx
  1. In Phase II/III trials for adolescent schizophrenia
  2. MOA: D-amino acid oxidase inhibitor
  3. Granted orphan drug status for refractory schizophrenia in combination with clozapine (12/2011)
AM. Neboglamine (CR-2249, XY-2401; nebostinel) by Rottapharm in Phase II
  1. NMDA receptor glycine-site positive allosteric modulator
AN. OMS-824 (OMS-643762) by Omeros Corporation (trials are currently suspended)
  1. A phosphodiesterase 10A inhibitor
AO. Oxytocin (Syntocinon) - 24 IU Intranasally one time only
  1. Phase IV for Oxytocin on Satiety Signaling in People with Schizophrenia to determine if oxytocin is effective for the prevention/treatment of weight gain and overeating in people with schizophrenia
  2. By the Maryland Psychiatric Research Center
    i. ClinicalTrials.gov Identifier: NCT01614093
  3. Also in Phase IV trials for its effects on Social Cognition Skills Training in Schizophrenia
    i. By the University of California, Los Angeles
    ii. ClinicalTrials.gov Identifier: NCT03245437
AP. Paliperidone palmitate (R092670) 6-month formulation (700 & 1000 mg equivalent [mg eq])[1062]
  1. Recruiting for participants in Phase III trials as of fall 2019 (Janssen Research & Development)
AQ. Pimavanserin (ACP-103, BVF-048; Nuplazid) – $5HT_{2A}$ receptor inverse agonist
  1. In Phase II for adjunctive therapy of Negative Symptoms in Schizophrenia
  2. https://www.acadia-pharm.com/pipeline/
AR. Pomaglumetad methionil (DB-103, LY-2140023, LY-2812223) by Denovo Biopharma & Eli Lilly
  1. MOA: acts on glutamic acid mGlu2/3 receptors
  2. Phase I trials completed, and showed significant efficacy in Phase II clinical trials (p-value < 0.05) but failed to achieve the desired effect in the Phase III pivotal trials
  3. New Phase II trial was set to begin in 2019
AS. Pyridoxamine (BST-4001, K-163, K-163SZ; Pyridorin) by NephroGenex/Kowa in Phase II
  1. Vitamin B, advanced glycosylation end-product inhibitor, oxygen radical scavenger
AT. RG7906 (RO6889450) by Roche in Phase II trials for the negative symptoms associated with Schizophrenia
AU. Risperidone (BB0817, EN 3342) by Braeburn Pharmaceuticals
  1. A 6-month *Implant* in Phase 3 study
  2. Non-biodegradable drug-eluting stent
AV. Roluperidone (CYR-101, MIN-101, MT-210) - Minerva Neurosciences
  1. For monotherapy of negative symptoms in schizophrenia (Phase III)
  2. MOA: $5HT_{2A}$ and sigma$_2$ antagonist
  3. Doses studied: 32 mg or 64 mg
AW. Rykindo® (LY03004) Luye Pharma – Risperidone microspheres - FDA application submitted
AX. Sarcosine[1063] (N-Methylglycine)
  1. A dietary supplement that has pharmacological activity to boost functioning of the glutamatergic N-methyl-d-aspartate receptor (NMDAR)
  2. Being studied for the prevention and treatment of schizophrenia (Phase II)
AY. SEP-363856[1064] - Sunovion Pharmaceuticals Inc. and PsychoGenics Inc.
  1. Granted breakthrough therapy designation by FDA after positive Phase II (SEP361-201) trial[1065]
  2. MOA: believed to activate TAAR1 (trace amine-associated receptor 1) and $5HT_{1A}$ receptors
  3. Phase III DBPC trial of once-daily doses of 50 or 75 mg (n=245) - planned start Oct. 2019
    i. Statistically superior on Positive and Negative Syndrome Scale (PANSS), Clinical Global Impressions-Severity (CGI-S), PANSS sub-scale scores, & the Brief Negative Symptom Scale (BNSS) total score
  4. Side effects (only slightly more than placebo): somnolence, agitation, nausea, and dyspepsia
AZ. Sulforaphane (derived from broccoli sprouts)[1066] in Phase II/III studies
  1. Affects production of glutamate from glutathione to increase levels in the brain
BA. SUVN-D4010 by Suven Life Sciences
  1. $5HT_4$ receptor agonist - Phase I for Schizophrenia & Alzheimer's
  2. Suven has another compound (SUVN-I6107) that is a muscarinic receptor-1 positive allosteric modulators (M1-PAM), and M1/M4 agonist compound for depression, cognition and psychosis
  3. They appear to be devoid of cholinergic side effects
  4. http://www.suven.com/drugdiscoveryresearch.aspx#clinical-pipeline-section
BB. TAK-041 by Takeda
  1. G Protein-Coupled Receptor 139 (GPR139) protein agonist
  2. Completed a Phase I study for Cognitive Impairment Associated with Schizophrenia (CIAS) with negative symptoms in September 2019.
  3. Currently in Phase II study in the United Kingdom
BC. TAK-831 by Takeda in Phase II
  1. D-amino acid oxidase inhibitor
  2. For Cognitive Impairment Associated with Schizophrenia (CIAS)

BD. **TS-134** (TS-1341) by Taisho Pharmaceutical in Phase I study for Schizophrenia
BE. **Other potential future drug mechanisms:**
  1. PDE (phosphodiesterase) receptors inhibitors of: PDE10 (10A specifically) and PDE1
  2. D1 receptor antagonists
  3. Glutamate/NMDA receptor antagonists
   i. Found to cause *Olney lesions* in rodents
    a. Vacuoles that may precede permanent cell death in the brain
  4. Group I and group II metabotropic glutamate receptor allosteric modulators
  5. Adjunctive estradiol in women of childbearing age[1067]

## XXII. COMPLEMENTARY AND ALTERNATIVE THERAPIES
A. Repetitive Transcranial Magnetic Stimulation (rTMS) at 1Hz over the left temporoparietal cortex can help with acute treatment of persistent auditory hallucinations[965,1068]
  1. Treatment over the dorsolateral prefrontal cortex helps negative symptoms
B. Electroconvulsive Therapy (ECT) with antipsychotic therapy

## XXIII. RECOMMENDED METABOLIC MONITORING[1069,1070]

| (may be conducted more frequently as indicated) | Baseline | 4 weeks | 8 weeks | 12 weeks and then quarterly | Every 6 months | Annually |
|---|---|---|---|---|---|---|
| Personal / Family History | A / P | | | A | | A / P |
| Height / weight (BMI) | A / P | A / P* | A / P* | A / P* | | A |
| Waist Circumference | A | | | A | | A |
| Blood Pressure | A / P | | | A/P | P | A |
| Fasting Plasma Glucose | A / P | | | A/P | P | A |
| Fasting Lipid Profile | A / P | | | A/P | P | A then ≤ 5 yrs |

A = Adults   P = Pediatrics   * = At every visit (+ assess diet, exercise, sexual dysfx, & smoking)
Pediatric patients should also have a thyroid panel and prolactin level checked regularly

## XXIV. USEFUL INFORMATION[960,961,1071-1073]

♦ **ALL** Atypicals are effective for Bipolar mania but only some for Bipolar Depression
♦ **Dementia** – **Black Box Warning with ALL antipsychotics** - ↑ **risk of death by 1.6-1.7X**
♦ **ALL atypicals have the potential to cause weight gain and diabetes**

## XXV. ORAL ANTIPSYCHOTICS

| Typical | Atypical (2nd Generation) | | |
|---|---|---|---|
| *Low to High potency:* | *-azoles:* | *-apines:* | *-idones:* |
| Chlorpromazine (Thorazine) Thioridazine (Mellaril) Molindone (Moban) Loxapine (Loxitane) Perphenazine (Trilafon) Trifluoperazine (Stelazine) Thiothixene (Navane) Haloperidol (Haldol) Fluphenazine (Prolixin) | Aripiprazole (Abilify) Brexpiprazole (Rexulti) | Loxapine (low dose) Clozapine (Clozaril) Olanzapine (Zyprexa) Quetiapine (Seroquel) Asenapine (Saphris) | Risperidone (Risperdal) Ziprasidone (Geodon) Paliperidone (Invega) Iloperidone (Fanapt) Lurasidone (Latuda) |
| | *Unique:* Cariprazine (Vraylar) / Pimavanserin (Nuplazid) | | |

## XXVI. ANTIPSYCHOTIC RELATIVE DIFFERENCES

### SGA CARDIOMETABOLIC SIDE EFFECTS
*Risk of diabetes in psychiatric patients is 2-4x that of the non-psychiatric population (approx. 13%).
Antipsychotic medications can double that risk.
Even higher risk if antipsychotics combined with antidepressants (especially in children).*
Abilify = Geodon = Cariprazine = Latuda ≤ Fanapt ≤ asenapine < Invega = Risperdal = Seroquel ≤ Rexulti ≤ Thorazine ≤ CloZaril ≤ Zyprexa
*(almost alphabetical by Brand name)*
→ Consensus guidelines from 2004 say that if patients develop diabetes or weight gain, they should be switched to Geodon or Abilify.[1069] Update should now include Latuda and Vraylar.

# XXVII. ANTIPSYCHOTICS AND THEIR OTHER FDA-APPROVED INDICATIONS (AS OF 1/2020)

| Indication:  /  Antipsychotic: | Acute mania | Bipolar depression | Bipolar mixed episodes | Bipolar maintenance | Pediatric bipolar | Pediatric schizophrenia | Irritability in autism | TRD/ MDD add-on |
|---|---|---|---|---|---|---|---|---|
| Aripiprazole | ✓ | | ✓ | | age≥10 ± | age≥13 | age≥6 | ✓ |
| Aripiprazole LAIA | | | | ✓ | | | | |
| Aripiprazole lauroxil LAIA | | | | | | | | |
| Asenapine | ✓ ± | | age≥10 | ✓ | age≥10 ± | | | |
| Brexpiprazole | | | | | | | | ✓ |
| Cariprazine | ✓ | ✓ | ✓ | | | | | |
| Iloperidone | | | | | | | | |
| Lurasidone | | age≥10 ± | | | | age≥13 | | |
| Olanzapine | ✓ ± | | ✓ | age≥13 | age≥13 | age≥13 | | |
| Olanzapine LAIA | | | | | | | | |
| Paliperidone | S.A.D. ± | | | | | age≥12 | | |
| Paliperidone LAIA | S.A.D. ± | | | S.A.D. ± | | | | |
| Paliperidone 3-mo. LAIA | | | | | | | | |
| Quetiapine | ✓ ± | ✓ | | ✓ ± | age≥10 ± | age≥13 | | |
| Quetiapine XR | ✓ ± | ✓ | ✓ | ✓ ± | | | | ✓ |
| Risperidone | ✓ ± | | ✓ | | age≥10 ± | age≥13 | age≥5 | |
| Risperidone LAIA | | | | ✓ ± | | | | |
| Risperidone SQ LAIA | | | | | | | | |
| Ziprasidone | ✓ | | ✓ | ✓+ | | | | |

✓ = yes  
LAIA = Long-acting injectable antipsychotic  
S.A.D. = Schizoaffective disorder  
± = with or without adjunctive lithium or valproic acid  
+ = with adjunctive lithium or valproic acid  
TRD = Treatment-resistant depression (adjunct therapy)

# XXVIII. ANTIPSYCHOTIC PLASMA LEVELS[968,1075-1081]

A. An expert consensus workgroup from Germany, Switzerland, Austria, and Italy recommend routine therapeutic drug monitoring of olanzapine, haloperidol, perphenazine, and fluphenazine, based on expert opinions and drug therapy trials.[1082,1083]

| Drug | Therapeutic Range ( ng/ml) | Toxic Levels ( ng/ml) | Time to peak (hours) | Protein binding (%) |
|---|---|---|---|---|
| **FIRST GENERATION ANTIPSYCHOTICS / TYPICALS** | | | | |
| Chlorpromazine (Thorazine®) | 30-100 / 30-300 | > 350 / 600 | < 3 | 90-99 |
| Fluphenazine (Prolixin®) | 0.2-2 / 1-10 | 50-100 / 15 | < 2 | 99 |
| Haloperidol (Haldol®) | 5-20 / 1-10 | > 50 / 15 | 2-6 | 89-93 |
| Loxapine (Loxitane®) | 10-30 / 5-10 | >1000 / 20 | 1.5-3 | 97 |
| Molindone (Moban®) | ~500 | None yet established | 1.5 | 76 |
| Perphenazine (Trilafon®) | 0.8-2.4 / 0.6-2.4 | >50 / 5 | 1-3 | 91-99 |
| Thioridazine (Mellaril®) | 100-2000 / 100-200 | 2500-5000 / 400 | 1-4 | 96-99 |
| Thiothixene (Navane®) | 2-15 | 100 | 1-2 | 90 |
| Trifluoperazine (Stelazine®) | 1-10 | 100-200 | 1.5-6 | 90-99 |
| **SECOND GENERATION ANTIPSYCHOTICS / ATYPICALS** | | | | |
| Aripiprazole (Abilify®) | 109–585 / 100-500 | > 210+ / 1000 | 3-5 | >99 |
| Asenapine (Saphris®) | 4-62+ / 1-5 | > 62+ / 10 | 0.50 | |
| Brexpiprazole (Rexulti®) | 4-40 | 280 | 4 | 99 |
| Cariprazine (Vraylar®) | 10-20 | 40 | 3-6 | 91-97 |
| Clozapine (Clozaril®) | 350-500 / 350-600 | > 700 / 1000 | 1-6 | 97 |
| Iloperidone (Fanapt®) | 5-10 | 20 | 2-4 | 92-97 |
| Lurasidone (Latuda®) | 60-135+ / 15-40 | > 135+ / 120 | 1-3 | 99 |
| Olanzapine (Zyprexa®) | 20-30 / 20-80 | > 200 / 100 | 6 | 93 |
| Paliperidone (Invega®) | 20-60+ / 20-60 | > 60+ / 120 | 24 | 74 |
| Quetiapine (Seroquel®) | 100-1000 / 100-500 | > 1800 / 1000 | 1.5 | 83 |
| Risperidone (Risperdal®) – includes 9-OH-risperidone | 20-60 / 20-60 | 1800 (fatal) / 120 | 1 | 90 |
| Ziprasidone (Geodon®) | 20-60 / 50-200 | > 220 / 400 | 6-8 | >99 |

⊕ From unconfirmed sources

*Values in RED are from reference source # 1082*

## XXIX. DOSE ADJUSTMENTS WITH INHIBITORS/INDUCERS OR POOR METABOLIZERS

| NAME | CYP1A2 | CYP2C9/19 | CYP2D6 | CYP3A4 | P-gp |
|------|--------|-----------|--------|--------|------|
| **Typical 1st Generation Antipsychotics (common ones only)** | | | | | |
| Chlorpromazine (Thorazine®) | | | X | | |
| Fluphenazine (Prolixin®) | | | | | |
| Haloperidol (Haldol®) | X | | X | X | |
| Loxapine (Loxitane®/Adasuve®) | | | | | X |
| Molindone (Moban®) | | | | | |
| Perphenazine (Trilafon®) | | | PX | | |
| Thiothixene (Navane®) | X | | | | |
| Trifluoperazine (Stelazine®) | X | | | | |
| **Atypical 2nd Generation Antipsychotics** | | | | | |
| Aripiprazole (Abilify®) | | | PX | X! | |
| Asenapine (Saphris®) | | | | | |
| Brexpiprazole (Rexulti®) | | | PX | X | |
| Cariprazine (Vraylar®) | | | | X! | |
| Clozapine (Clozaril®, Versacloz®) | X | | PX | X! | |
| Iloperidone (Fanapt®) | | | PX | X | |
| Lurasidone (Latuda®) | | | | X! | |
| Olanzapine (Zyprexa®/Relprevv) | X | | | | |
| Paliperidone (Invega®/Sustenna) | | | | X | X |
| Pimavanserin (Nuplazid™) | | | | X! | |
| Quetiapine (Seroquel/XR®) | | | | X | |
| Risperidone (Risperdal®/Consta) | | | X | X | |
| Ziprasidone (Geodon) | | | | | |
| X = Dose modification of antipsychotic needed     ! = Avoid with strong inhibitors or inducers | | | | | |
| P = Dose adjustments needed in Poor Metabolizers | | | | | |

## XXX. ADJUSTMENTS FOR RENAL AND HEPATIC IMPAIRMENTS

| NAME | RENAL | HEPATIC |
|------|-------|---------|
| **Typical 1st Generation Antipsychotics** | | |
| Chlorpromazine (Thorazine®) | Use with caution | Use with caution |
| Fluphenazine (Prolixin®) | Use with caution | Contraindicated |
| Haloperidol (Haldol®) | ----- | ----- |
| Loxapine (Loxitane®/Adasuve®) | ----- | ----- |
| Molindone (Moban®) | | Use with caution |
| Perphenazine (Trilafon®) | Contraindicated | Use with caution |
| Thioridazine (Mellaril®) | ----- | Reduce dose |
| Thiothixene (Navane®) | ----- | Reduce dose |
| Trifluoperazine (Stelazine®) | ----- | Contraindicated |
| **Atypical 2nd Generation Antipsychotics** | | |
| Aripiprazole (Abilify®) | ----- | ----- |
| Asenapine (Saphris® SL) | ----- | Contraindicated |
| Brexpiprazole (Rexulti®) | Reduce dose | Reduce dose |
| Cariprazine (Vraylar®) | Not recommended if severe | Not recommended if severe |
| Clozapine (Clozaril®, Versacloz®) | Dose adjustment may be needed | Dose adjustment may be needed |
| Iloperidone (Fanapt®) | ----- | Not recommended if severe |
| Lurasidone (Latuda®) | Reduce dose | Reduce dose |
| Olanzapine (Zyprexa®/Relprevv) | ----- | Use with caution |
| Paliperidone (Invega®/Sustenna) | ↓ dose if CrCl is 50-80 ml/min<br>Not recommended if < 50 ml/min | ----- |
| Pimavanserin (Nuplazid™) | Use with caution if severe | ----- |
| Quetiapine (Seroquel/XR®) | ----- | Reduce dose |
| Risperidone (Risperdal®/Consta) | Reduce dose and monitor | Reduce dose and monitor |
| Ziprasidone (Geodon) | ----- | Use with caution |

## XXXI. INJECTABLE ANTIPSYCHOTICS

| IMMEDIATE-ACTING | |
|------|------|
| **Typical:** | **Atypical:** |
| Haldol® (haloperidol)<br>Thorazine® (chlorpromazine)<br>Numerous others | Geodon® (ziprasidone)    Abilify® (aripiprazole)<br>Zyprexa® (olanzapine) (no BZDs w/in 2 hrs) |
| **LONG-ACTING (LAIAs)** | |
| **Typical:** | **Atypical:** |
| Prolixin Decanoate®<br>(fluphenazine)<br>Haldol Decanoate®<br>(haloperidol) | Abilify Maintena™ (aripiprazole) / Aristada™ (aripiprazole lauroxil)<br>Risperdal Consta® / Perseris™ (risperidone)<br>Invega Sustenna® / Invega Trinza™ (paliperidone palmitate)<br>Zyprexa Relprevv® (olanzapine) (Q 2-4 weeks) |

| FIRST GENERATION ANTIPSYCHOTICS / TYPICALS | | | |
|---|---|---|---|
| Drug | Metabolism enzymes / transporters | Half-life (hours) | Affected by smoking? |
| Chlorpromazine (Thorazine®) | CYP2D6 (major), CYP1A2 (minor), CYP3A4 (minor) substrate | 23-37 | Yes |
| Fluphenazine (Prolixin®) | CYP2D6 (major) substrate | 4.4-16.4 | Yes – ↓ ~50% |
| Haloperidol (Haldol®) | CYP2D6 (major), CYP3A4 (major), CYP1A2 (minor) substrate; 50-60% glucuronidation | 14-37 | Yes |
| Loxapine (Loxitane®) | CYP1A2 (minor), CYP2D6 (minor), CYP3A4 (minor) substrate; P-gp inhibitor | 7.61 ± 1.87 | No |
| Molindone (Moban®) | CYP2D6 | 1.5 | Yes |
| Perphenazine (Trilafon®) | CYP2D6 (major) substrate, CYP1A2 (minor), CYP2C19 (minor), CYP2C9 (minor), CYP3A4 (minor) substrate | 9-12 | No |
| Thioridazine (Mellaril®) | CYP2D6 (major) substrate and moderate inhibitor, CYP2C19 (minor) substrate | 5-27 | No |
| Thiothixene (Navane®) | CYP1A2 (major) substrate | 34 | Yes |
| Trifluoperazine (Stelazine®) | CYP1A2 (major) substrate | 3-12 | Yes |
| SECOND GENERATION ANTIPSYCHOTICS / ATYPICALS | | | |
| Aripiprazole (Abilify®) | CYP2D6 (major), CYP3A4 (major) substrate | aripiprazole: 75 dehydro-aripiprazole: 94 | No |
| Asenapine (Saphris®) | CYP1A2 (major), CYP2D6 (minor), CYP3A4 (minor) substrate; glucuronidation by UGT1A4; CYP2D6 weak inhibitor | ~24 | No |
| Brexpiprazole (Rexulti®) | CYP3A4 (major), CYP2D6 (major) substrate | 91 | No |
| Cariprazine (Vraylar®) | CYP3A4 (major), CYP2D6 (minor) substrate | 48-96 | No |
| Clozapine (Clozaril®) | CYP1A2 (major), CYP2A6 (minor), CYP2C19 (minor), CYP2C9 (minor), CYP2D6 (minor), CYP3A4 (minor) substrate | 12 | Yes – ↓ by 23% |
| Iloperidone (Fanapt®) | CYP2D6 (major), CYP3A4 (minor) substrate, CYP3A4 weak inhibitor | ~ 24 | No |
| Lurasidone (Latuda®) | CYP3A4 (major) substrate, CYP3A4 weak inhibitor | 18-40 | No |
| Olanzapine (Zyprexa®) | CYP1A2 (major), CYP2D6 (minor) substrate; metabolized via direct glucuronidation | Oral and short-acting IM: Children: (10 to 18 years): 37.2 ± 5.1; Adults: 30 | Yes – ↓ by 40% |
| Paliperidone (Invega®) | P-gp/ABCB1, CYP2D6(minor), CYP3A4 (minor) substrate | 23; Renal impairment (CrCl <80 mL/min): 24-51 | No |
| Pimavanserin (Nuplazid™) | CYP3A4 | 57 & 200 for active metabolite | No |
| Quetiapine (Seroquel®) | CYP3A4 (major), CYP2D6 (minor) substrate | Adults: ~6; XR: ~7 Children (12-17 years): 5.3 | No |
| Risperidone (Risperdal®) | CYP2D6 (major), CYP3A4 (minor), P- gp/ABCB1 substrate, N-dealkylation (minor), CYP2D6 weak inhibitor | Avg: ~ 20 Extensive metabolizers: Risp.: 3 / 9-OH-Risp.: 21 Poor metabolizers: Risp.: 20 / 9-OH-Risp.: 30 | No |
| Ziprasidone (Geodon®) | CYP1A2 & CYP3A4 (minor) substrates, glutathione aldehyde oxidase | Adults: 7 Children: 3.3-4.1 | No |

XXXIII. ANTIPSYCHOTIC RECEPTOR BINDING AFFINITIES (LEAST TO MOST) [861,862,931,968,986,1084-1088]

**RELATIVE 5HT₁ₐ ACTIVITY (helps with negative symptoms and reduced EPS side effects)**
chlorpromazine = haloperidol = loxapine = molindone = perphenazine = olanzapine < fluphenazine = thioridazine = thiothixene = trifluoperazine = paliperidone = risperidone < asenapine < clozapine = lurasidone = quetiapine < iloperidone < aripiprazole = cariprazine = ziprasidone < brexpiprazole

## RELATIVE D2 BLOCKADE BINDING AFFINITIES (FGAs AND SGAs)

aripiprazole = brexpiprazole = cariprazine < clozapine = quetiapine < loxapine = molindone = thioridazine = iloperidone = olanzapine < chlorpromazine = haloperidol = trifluoperazine = asenapine = lurasidone = paliperidone = risperidone = ziprasidone < fluphenazine = perphenazine = thiothixene

## RELATIVE *ALPHA*-2 BINDING AFFINITIES (increases sympathetic outflow from the CNS)

fluphenazine = haloperidol = loxapine = thiothixene = trifluoperazine = quetiapine < chlorpromazine = molindone = perphenazine = thioridazine = aripiprazole = clozapine = olanzapine = ziprasidone < lurasidone = paliperidone < asenapine = iloperidone = risperidone < brexpiprazole

## XXXIV. ANTIPSYCHOTIC RELATIVE RISKS (LEAST TO MOST)[859,861,862,927,931,961,968,986,1089,1090]

### HYPERGLYCEMIA

fluphenazine = loxapine = molindone = perphenazine = thioridazine = thiothixene = trifluoperazine = aripiprazole = lurasidone = asenapine = paliperidone = ziprasidone < chlorpromazine = brexpiprazole = haloperidol = cariprazine = iloperidone = quetiapine = risperidone = olanzapine < clozapine

### HYPERLIPIDEMIA

ziprasidone = cariprazine = iloperidone = lurasidone < loxapine = molindone = thiothixene = aripiprazole = brexpiprazole = paliperidone = risperidone = haloperidol < chlorpromazine = fluphenazine = perphenazine = thioridazine = trifluoperazine = asenapine < clozapine = olanzapine = quetiapine

### WEIGHT GAIN

ziprasidone = haloperidol < fluphenazine = loxapine = molindone = perphenazine = thioridazine = thiothixene = trifluoperazine = aripiprazole = lurasidone = cariprazine = chlorpromazine < asenapine = brexpiprazole = paliperidone = risperidone = quetiapine = iloperidone < clozapine = olanzapine

### QT$_C$ PROLONGATION (DOSE-RELATED)

fluphenazine = loxapine = molindone = perphenazine = thiothixene = trifluoperazine = brexpiprazole = cariprazine = lurasidone = aripiprazole = asenapine = clozapine = iloperidone = olanzapine = paliperidone = risperidone < chlorpromazine = quetiapine = ziprasidone = haloperidol (especially IV) = thioridazine

### PROLACTIN ELEVATION

aripiprazole < cariprazine = clozapine < quetiapine < brexpiprazole = asenapine = olanzapine = iloperidone = ziprasidone ≤ lurasidone < haloperidol << paliperidone = risperidone

### ANY TYPE OF EPS (akathisia, pseudoparkinsonism, acute dystonia, & tardive dyskinesia)

thioridazine = clozapine = iloperidone = quetiapine < aripiprazole = brexpiprazole = cariprazine = ziprasidone < chlorpromazine = olanzapine < asenapine = paliperidone < loxapine = molindone = perphenazine = trifluoperazine = lurasidone = risperidone < fluphenazine = haloperidol = thiothixene

### AKATHISIA (SPECIFICALLY)

iloperidone < quetiapine < brexpiprazole < ziprasidone < paliperidone < aripiprazole < asenapine < olanzapine < risperidone < cariprazine < lurasidone

### ORTHOSTATIC HYPOTENSION & *ALPHA*-1 BINDING AFFINITIES

molindone < cariprazine < fluphenazine = haloperidol = loxapine = perphenazine = thiothixene = trifluoperazine = aripiprazole = lurasidone = brexpiprazole < asenapine = paliperidone = risperidone = ziprasidone = olanzapine = quetiapine < chlorpromazine = thioridazine = clozapine = iloperidone

### SEDATION (H1 BINDING AFFINITIES)

haloperidol = molindone = lurasidone < iloperidone < fluphenazine = thioridazine = trifluoperazine = aripiprazole = brexpiprazole = cariprazine = risperidone = ziprasidone < chlorpromazine = loxapine = perphenazine = thiothixene = asenapine = clozapine = olanzapine = paliperidone = quetiapine

### SEIZURE RISK

fluphenazine = haloperidol = loxapine = molindone = perphenazine = trifluoperazine = aripiprazole = asenapine = brexpiprazole = cariprazine = iloperidone = lurasidone = paliperidone = risperidone = ziprasidone < chlorpromazine = thioridazine = olanzapine = quetiapine < thiothixene = clozapine

### ANTICHOLINERGIC EFFECTS (M1 BINDING AFFINITIES)

fluphenazine = haloperidol = molindone = perphenazine = thiothixene = aripiprazole = asenapine = brexpiprazole = cariprazine = iloperidone = lurasidone = paliperidone = risperidone = ziprasidone < clozapine < loxapine = trifluoperazine = quetiapine < chlorpromazine < thioridazine = olanzapine

## A. SUSTAINING MECHANISMS OF LONG-ACTING INJECTABLE ANTIPSYCHOTICS (LAIAs)

| LAIA NAME | VEHICLE |
|---|---|
| Aripiprazole | Water (lyophilized powder of poorly soluble aripiprazole monohydrate crystals) |
| Aripiprazole lauroxil & Olanzapine pamoate | Water (suspension of nanocrystals of poorly soluble salts) |
| Haloperidol decanoate & Fluphenazine enanthate/decanoate | Sesame oil solution of lipophilic prodrug (esterification of a hydroxyl handle in blood) |
| Paliperidone palmitate | Water (suspension of nanocrystals of ester made with palmitic acid) |
| Risperidone (Consta®) | Water (suspension of biodegradable polymeric microspheres) |
| Risperidone (Perseris™) | Water (suspension of biodegradable polymers) |

## B. NEEDLE SIZES FOR LONG-ACTING INJECTABLE ANTIPSYCHOTICS

| LAI | DELTOID | GLUTEAL |
|---|---|---|
| Abilify Maintena® | 1-inch 23G in non-obese or 1½-inch 22G in obese patients | 1½-inch 22G for non-obese patients / 2-inch 21G for obese patients |
| Aristada® | 441 mg only: 1-inch 21G or 1½-inch 20G | 441, 662, 882, or 1064mg: 1½-inch 20G or 2-inch 20G |
| Aristada Initio® | 1-inch 21G or 1½-inch 20G | 1½-inch 20G or 2-inch 20G |
| Prolixin Decanoate® | N/A | 1 to 2-inch, 21G or larger |
| Haldol Decanoate® | N/A | 1 to 2-inch, 21G or larger |
| Zyprexa Relprevv® | N/A | 1½-inch 19G needle |
| Invega Sustenna® | 1-inch 23G (wt. <90 kg) or 1½-inch 22G (wt. >90 kg) | 1½-inch 22G |
| Invega Trinza® | 1 to 1½-inch 22G TW needle | 1½-inch 22G TW needle |
| Risperdal Consta® | 1-inch 21G ultra TW needle | 2-inch 20G TW needle |
| Perseris™ | SubQ in Abdomen only: 5/8-inch 18G safety needle | |

## C. LAIA ADMINISTRATION

| LAIA | Use as a loading dose? | Pre-mixed? | How supplied? | Pre-injection instructions? | Injection site(s)? |
|---|---|---|---|---|---|
| Abilify Maintena® | NO | NO | 400 mg dual chamber PFS / 300 mg vial of lyophilized powder | Follow instructions in kit for reconstitution. Shake up to 60 sec to maintain suspension. | D or G |
| Aristada® | NO | YES | 441, 662, 882 & 1064 mg PFS | Tap syringe 10 times, shake vigorously for > 30 sec. (Use within 15 min. or re-shake) | G (D - 441 mg) |
| Aristada Initio® | YES | YES | 675 mg PFS | Tap 10 X & shake vigorously for > 30 sec. (Use within 15 min. or re-shake) | D or G |
| Prolixin® Decanoate | YES | YES | 25 mg/mL sesame oil susp. in 5 mL vials & ampules | Withdraw & Inject medication with a 21G (or larger bore) needle | SQ or G (max.100 mg Q 2 weeks) |
| Haldol® Decanoate | YES | YES | 50 & 100 mg/mL sesame oil susp. in ampules, single & multidose vials | Withdraw & inject medication with a 21G (or larger bore) needle | G (max. 450 mg/mo) |
| Zyprexa Relprevv® | YES | NO | 210, 300, & 405 mg vial kits | Tap vial & inject included diluent. Tap vial before removing suspension with syringe & shake prior to use | G |
| Invega Sustenna® | YES | YES | 39, 78, 117, 156, & 234 mg PFS | Shake vigorously for 10 sec. (Use within 5 min. or re-shake) | D or G |
| Invega Trinza® | N/A | YES | 273, 410, 546, & 819 mg PFS | Shake vigorously for 15 sec. (Use within 5 min. or re-shake) | D or G |
| Risperdal Consta® | NO | NO | 12.5, 25, 37.5, & 50 mg vial kits | Sit at room temp for 30 min., then shake 10 sec. just prior to use | D or G |
| Perseris™ | NO | NO | 90 & 120 mg dual-syringe vial kits | Room temp for 15 min., connect 2 syringes and push liquid back & forth into each syringe for 5 cycles, then more rapidly for another 55 cycles | SQ |

PFS = Pre-filled Syringe   D=Deltoid   G=Gluteal   SQ=Sub-cutaneous

## D. LAIA DOSING & PHARMACOKINETICS

| LAIA | Dosing Options | Dosing interval (weeks) | Oral overlap needed (weeks) | Onset | Time to Cmax♦ (days) | Half-life (days) |
|---|---|---|---|---|---|---|
| Aripiprazole (Abilify Maintena®) | 400 mg, but can reduce dose to 300 mg if needed | 4 | 2 | ≈ 4-7 days | 4 D (Cmax ↑ 31%) 5-7 G | 29.9-46.5 |
| Aripiprazole lauroxil (Aristada®) | 441, 662, 882 & 1064 mg | 4-8 | 3 | 3-4 weeks | 24.4-35.2 | 53.9-57.2 |
| Aripiprazole lauroxil (Aristada Initio®) | 675 mg + 30 mg oral x 1 | 1 time | 0 | 3 days to 4 weeks | 27 (4 if with 30 mg oral on day 1) | 15-18 |
| Fluphenazine decanoate (Prolixin® Decanoate) | Initial dose: 1.25 x total daily p.o. dose. Adjust dose in increments of 12.5 mg | 2-5 ❂ | 0-1 | ≈ 24hr & again in 8-12d | 0.3-1.5 | 9.7-14 |
| Haloperidol decanoate (Haldol® Decanoate) | Initial dose: 15-20 x total daily p.o. dose; NTE 100 mg for 1st time dose (Max dose – 450 mg) | 2-4 | 1-3 | ≈ 3-9 days | 6-9 | 21 |
| Olanzapine pamoate (Zyprexa Relprevv®) | 10 mg p.o. QD = 150 mg q2w or 300 mg q4w 15 mg p.o. QD = 210 mg q2w or 405 mg q4w 20 mg p.o. QD = 300 mg q2w | 2 or 4 | 0 | ≈ 1-7 days | 2-7 | 30 |
| Paliperidone palmitate (Invega Sustenna®) | Initial dose: 234 mg in D 1 week later: 156 mg; Maintenance: 117 mg q4w (3w after 2nd dose) | 4 | 0 | ≈ a few hours | 13 | 25-49 |
| Paliperidone palmitate (Invega Trinza®) | 273, 410, 546 & 819 mg | 12 | N/A | ≈ a few hours | 30-33 | 84-95 D 118-139 G |
| Risperidone (Risperdal Consta®) | 2 mg p.o. QD = 25 mg 4 mg p.o. QD = 50 mg 6 mg p.o. QD = 75 mg[1094] | 2 | 3 | ≈ 3 weeks | 21-28 | 3-6 |
| Risperidone (Perseris™) | 3 mg p.o. QD = 90 mg 4 mg p.o. QD = 120 mg | 4 | 0 | ≈ a few hours | 4-6 hours | 9-11 |

♦ Cmax is the time until maximum plasma concentration is reached   D=Deltoid   G=Gluteal
❂ Q 5 week dosing in some unique cases

## E. QUICK REFERENCE ON HOW TO HANDLE MISSED DOSES OF LAIAs

| LAIA | SUPPLEMENTATION NEEDED IF LAST DOSE WAS ___ TIME AGO |
|---|---|
| Aripiprazole (Abilify Maintena®) | > 5 to 6 weeks – Give 2 weeks of oral |
| Aripiprazole Lauroxil (Aristada®) | > 6 to 12 weeks – Give 1 week of oral >12 weeks (or >7 if on 441 mg Q 4 weeks) – Give 3 weeks of oral |
| Fluphenazine (Prolixin®) decanoate | **Not specified***  If > 2 to 4 weeks (based on kinetics) resume injection ASAP |
| Haloperidol (Haldol®) decanoate | **Not specified***  If > 4 to 7 weeks (based on kinetics) resume injection ASAP If > 7 weeks, resume injection ASAP + supplement with 2 weeks of oral |
| Olanzapine pamoate (Zyprexa Relprevv®) | **Not specified***  If > 2 to 3 months (based on kinetics) resume injection ASAP |
| Paliperidone palmitate (Invega Sustenna®) | Missed 2nd dose of initiation: < 4 weeks – give 156 mg ASAP 4 to 7 weeks – give 156 mg + 156 mg (1-week later) > 7 weeks – Restart with 234 mg loading dose + 156 mg a week later -------------------------------------------- Missed regular maintenance dose: 4 to 6 weeks – resume at same dose 6 weeks to 6 *months* – resume at same dose (unless if on 234 mg dose, then give 156 mg + 156 mg 1-week later) > 6 *months* – Restart at beginning dose |

| LAIA | SUPPLEMENTATION NEEDED IF LAST DOSE WAS ___ TIME AGO |
|---|---|
| Paliperidone palmitate (Invega Trinza®) | 3.5 to 4 *months* – resume at same dose<br>4 to 9 *months* – re-initiate loading + 2nd dose in a week, then 1 *month* later, restart at previous Trinza® dose<br>> 9 *months* – Restart Invega Sustenna® for 4 months before using Trinza® |
| Risperidone (Risperdal Consta®) | **Not specified**\*<br>If > 2 to 5 weeks (based on kinetics) resume injection ASAP<br>If > 6 weeks, resume injection ASAP + give 2 weeks of oral |
| Risperidone (Perseris™) | **Not specified**\*<br>If > 4 to 7 weeks (based on kinetics) resume injection ASAP<br>If > 7 weeks, resume injection ASAP + may supplement with 2 weeks of oral |

\* = *Recommendations provided are based solely on clinical judgement and are subject to change as new information becomes available*

### F. ADVANTAGES & DISADVANTAGES OF LAIAs

| LAI | ADVANTAGES | DISADVANTAGES |
|---|---|---|
| Aripiprazole (Abilify Maintena®) | •SGA<br>•Q 4 week dosing<br>•Approved for maintenance of Bipolar I | •Reconstitution needed<br>•2 week oral overlap |
| Aripiprazole lauroxil (Aristada®) | •SGA<br>•Premixed<br>•Up to 2 month duration | •3 week oral overlap |
| Fluphenazine decanoate (Prolixin® Decanoate) | •SQ or IM dosing<br>•No oral overlap needed<br>•Short-acting IM available | •FGA<br>•↑ EPS<br>•↑ Prolactin<br>•Sesame allergy<br>•Oil deposits left in muscle tissue<br>•Q 2-3 week dosing |
| Haloperidol decanoate (Haldol® Decanoate) | •Q 3-4 week dosing<br>•If loaded<br>•No oral overlap needed<br>•Short-acting IM available | •FGA<br>•↑ EPS<br>•↑ Prolactin<br>•Sesame allergy<br>•Oil deposits left in muscle tissue<br>•1-3 week oral overlap recommended |
| Olanzapine pamoate (Zyprexa Relprevv®) | •SGA<br>•2-4 week duration<br>•Short-acting IM available<br>•No oral overlap needed | •Reconstitution needed<br>•REMS program for PDSS (0.07% per injection) – 3 hour observation needed |
| Paliperidone palmitate (Invega Sustenna® / Trinza®) | •SGA<br>•Premixed<br>•No oral overlap needed<br>•4 weeks to 3 month duration<br>•Approved for Schizoaffective Disorder | •↑ Prolactin<br>•No short-acting IM available |
| Risperidone (Risperdal Consta®) | •SGA | •Refrigeration & reconstitution needed<br>•(room temperature up to 7 days / use within 6 hours of mixing)<br>•3 week oral overlap<br>•Q 2 week dosing<br>•↑ Prolactin<br>•No short-acting IM available |
| Risperidone (Perseris™) | •SGA<br>•SQ 4 week dosing<br>•No oral overlap needed | •Refrigeration & reconstitution needed (room temperature up to 7 days)<br>•↑ Prolactin |

### I. BACKGROUND
A. Approximately 10% of the population will experience a seizure at some time
B. Each year, 300,000 people experience a first-time seizure (120,000 under the age of 18)
  1. Of these, 200,000 new cases of epilepsy are diagnosed (45,000 are children younger than 15)
  2. Incidence is highest with children < 2-years-old and increases with age $\geq$ 65
C. According to the CDC, epilepsy affects approximately 2.5-3 million people in the U.S.
  1. Between 0.5-1% of the general population has epilepsy
D. 70% have no apparent cause ("idiopathic")
E. Each year accounts for up to $20 billion in direct (medical) and indirect costs
F. With anticonvulsant medication(s), 60-70% will achieve seizure-free remission in > 5 years and
    may be able to be weaned off their medication
G. Comorbid mental illness is greatly $\uparrow$ in those with seizure disorders (bi-directional relationship)
  1. Particularly in postictal state
  2. Antidepressants may prevent future seizures in epileptics, or may increase the incidence,
     because they lower the seizure threshold
    i. $\uparrow$ intracellular 5HT concentrations in the hippocampus protect against seizures
H. American Epilepsy Society guidelines - http://www.aesnet.org/go/practice/guidelines
I. Risk of unexpected sudden death from a seizure is 0.22/1000 patient-years for children and
    1.2/1000 patient-years for adults (risk is highest with increase in generalized tonic-clonic seizures)

### II. PATHOPHYSIOLOGY
A. Small number of neurons fire abnormally
B. A breakdown of normal membrane conductance and inhibitory mechanisms leads to the spread of
    the excitability either to a local area or widespread generalized area

### III. ETIOLOGY
A. Drug-induced ("iatrogenic")      E. Metabolic disorders / Electrolyte imbalances
B. High fevers in children      F. Heredity
C. Stroke, brain lesion, or Alzheimer's disease    G. CNS tumor
D. Severe head trauma (i.e., penetrating) with loss of consciousness

### V. DIAGNOSIS
A. Seizure: A sudden, abnormal electrical activity in the brain
  1. An event in which there is a temporary change in behavior resulting from a sudden, abnormal
     burst of electrical activity in the brain
  2. If the electrical disturbance is limited to only one area of the brain, the result is a partial seizure
B. Epilepsy: A chronic condition that is characterized by recurrent seizures
  1. **2** or more unprovoked seizures occur that can't be explained by a medical condition (e.g., fever)

### VI. DIAGNOSTIC TESTS
A. EEG      E. Electrolyte concentration
B. MRI or CT Scan      F. CNS Culture & Sensitivity
C. History      G. Temperature
D. Glucose levels      H. PET (positron emission tomography) scan

### VII. CLASSIFICATION
A. Partial (seizure activity in one part of the brain)
  1. Simple partial or Focal seizures
    i. Onset: any age
    ii. Motor, spatial, sensory, autonomic, and/or psychic symptoms
    iii. No loss of consciousness
  2. Complex partial
    i. Psychomotor seizures
    ii. Onset: age 3 and up
    iii. Impaired consciousness at onset with or without automatisms
B. Generalized (seizure activity in entire brain)
  1. Absence seizures
    i. Formerly called *petit mal* seizures, "lapses," or "staring spells"
    ii. Onset: ages 4-12
    iii. Characterized by sudden, brief lapses of consciousness (i.e., stare blankly for 5-10 seconds)
      without loss of postural control and no postictal confusion
    iv. The seizures can be mistaken for daydreaming or inattentiveness
  2. Atonic seizures
    i. Also known as drop attack
    ii. Onset: ages 2-5
    iii. Characterized by sudden loss of postural muscle tone lasting 1-2 seconds, causing abrupt falls
    iv. Consciousness is briefly impaired, but there is usually no postictal confusion
  3. Clonic seizures
    i. Jerking movements of the entire body as muscles undergo rhythmic tightening and relaxation
    ii. Clonic events last fewer than 100 ms at a repetitive rate of 1 to 3 Hz
    iii. Consciousness is usually lost or impaired
    iv. Postictal phase is usually short
    v. Mainly affects infants and very young children

4. Myoclonic seizures
   i. Sudden muscle jerks, usually affecting the person's neck, shoulders, and upper arms
   ii. Single or non-rhythmic irregularly recurrent events
5. Tonic seizures
   i. Stiffening of the body, upward deviation of the eyes, dilation of the pupils, and altered respiratory patterns
6. Tonic-Clonic seizures
   i. Formerly known as grand mal seizures; affects the entire brain
   ii. Onset: any age
   iii. Most widely recognized epileptic seizure
   iv. Person loses consciousness, body stiffens, & falls to the ground, followed by jerking movements
      a. After a minute or two, the jerking movements usually stop, and consciousness slowly returns
      b. Postictal period - time between end of seizure and return of lucid consciousness
7. Lennox-Gastaut Syndrome
   i. Occurs in children < 4-years-old
   ii. Multiple seizure types, usually including generalized
      a. Tonic–clonic, atonic, and atypical absence seizures
8. Secondarily generalized seizures
   i. Observed following simple partial seizures

## VIII. MEDICATIONS THAT CAN CAUSE SEIZURES
A. Anticholinergics
B. Anticholinesterase inhibitors
C. Antidepressants (esp. milnacipran, MAOIs, clomipramine, bupropion, amoxapine, & maprotiline)
D. Antiemetics (phenothiazines)
E. Antihistamines
F. Anti-infective agents (e.g., antibiotics, antifungals, anti-parasitic agents)
   1. Particularly mefloquine, penicillins, and quinolones (e.g., ciprofloxacin) – esp. in high doses
G. Antipsychotics - but especially clozapine (has a **BBW** on this)
H. Carisoprodol (Soma®)
I. CNS stimulants - caffeine, decongestants, amphetamines, cocaine, ecstasy, street drugs
J. Dronabinol (Marinol®/Syndrose®)
K. Lithium toxicity
L. Opiates – but particularly buprenorphine, hydrocodone, hydromorphone, meperidine, morphine, oxycodone, oxymorphone, pentazocine, tapentadol, tramadol
M. Sodium oxybate (Xyrem®)
N. Sudden discontinuation of anticonvulsants
O. Sumatriptan
P. Withdrawal from alcohol, benzodiazepine, muscle-relaxants, and other drugs that affect GABA

## IX. TREATMENT GUIDELINES[1101-1109]
A. From the American Academy of Neurology and the American Epilepsy Society and the National Institute for Health and Care Excellence (NICE)[1113]
B. 21-45% risk of a second seizure within 2 years after a first-time unprovoked seizure
C. Starting medication after a first-time unprovoked seizure is likely to reduce recurrence, but not likely to improve quality of life (QOL)
D. Medication should be reserved until after a second seizure has occurred
E. Monotherapy is preferred over polypharmacy, unless refractory seizures occur
F. For new onset focal (partial) or generalized tonic-clonic (GTC) seizures in *adults* (*in preferred order if ">" is placed between medications*)
   1. Valproate > lamotrigine > Levetiracetam > Zonisamide / or carbamazepine, oxcarbazepine
   2. Adjunctive treatment for refractory GTC seizures: clobazam, levetiracetam, or topiramate
   3. For treatment-resistance: eslicarbazepine, pregabalin or perampanel
      i. If absence or myoclonic seizures are suspected, carbamazepine, gabapentin, oxcarbazepine, phenytoin, pregabalin, tiagabine or vigabatrin are _not recommended_
G. New onset focal (partial) or generalized tonic-clonic seizures in *children*
   1. Carbamazepine ER, lamotrigine, levetiracetam, oxcarbazepine, or valproate
   2. Adjunctive treatment for refractory focal seizures: carbamazepine, clobazam, gabapentin, lamotrigine, levetiracetam, oxcarbazepine, valproate or topiramate
H. Myoclonic seizures: valproic acid > levetiracetam or topiramate
I. Tonic or atonic seizures: valproate > levetiracetam or topiramate
J. Juvenile myoclonic epilepsy: lamotrigine, levetiracetam, topiramate, valproic acid
K. Absence seizures in children
   1. Ethosuximide > valproate (may cause attention disturbances) > lamotrigine
L. Lennox–Gastaut syndrome: valproate
M. Dravet syndrome: valproate or topiramate

---

*NEVER abruptly discontinue **ANY** anticonvulsant, as rebound seizures can occur*

# X. PHARMACOLOGIC TREATMENT

A. General side effects common to anticonvulsants
   1. Drowsiness, dizziness, loss of coordination, cognitive impairment, psychiatric effects
   2. Potential for dermatologic reactions: rash, **SJS** (Steven-Johnson Syndrome), **TEN** (Toxic Epidermal Necrolysis), or **DRESS** (Drug Reaction with Eosinophilia and Systemic Symptoms)
   3. Monitor for *suicidal thoughts* or behaviors (could be twice as frequent as placebo)
   4. All side effects can be compounded when using more than one anticonvulsant concomitantly
   5. Behavioral dysregulation can occur with any anticonvulsant
      i. **BBW** for perampanel (**Fycompa**®) - 0.07% incidence of aggression and homicidal ideation
      ii. Aggressive-type behavior (in order of most to least severe) most frequently seen with topiramate, tiagabine, clobazam, levetiracetam, vigabatrin, and perampanel
      iii. Psychosis most often observed with topiramate, zonisamide, and levetiracetam
      iv. Hyperactivity/restlessness most frequently seen with phenobarbital, clobazam, and vigabatrin
      v. Over 1/3 of people initiated on levetiracetam stop the drug due to irritability & aggression[1110]

# XI. ANTICONVULSANT FDA-APPROVED INDICATIONS (AS OF 1/2020)

| SEIZURE TYPE | MONOTHERAPY | ADJUNCT THERAPY | |
|---|---|---|---|
| Generalized Tonic–Clonic | barbiturates; fos-/phenytoin; carbamazepine; topiramate ($\geq$ 2 y.o.); ethotin | gabapentin (> 12 y.o.) lamotrigine ($\geq$ 2 y.o.) levetiracetam ($\geq$ 6 y.o.) lorazepam | perampanel (> 12 y.o.) phenytoin primidone topiramate ($\geq$ 2 y.o.) |
| Partial (focal) | barbiturates; valproic acid; brivaracetam ($\geq$ 4 y.o.); carbamazepine; phenytoin; eslicarbazepine ($\geq$ 4 y.o.); ethotin; felbamate; lacosamide ($\geq$ 4 y.o.); lamotrigine (as crossover only); oxcarbazepine ($\geq$ 4 y.o.); topiramate ($\geq$ 2 y.o.); | brivaracetam ($\geq$ 4 y.o.) eslicarbazepine ($\geq$ 4 y.o.) felbamate gabapentin (> 3 y.o.) lacosamide ($\geq$ 4 y.o.) lamotrigine ($\geq$ 2 y.o.) levetiracetam (> 1 mo. old) lorazepam oxcarbazepine ($\geq$ 2 y.o.) | perampanel (> 12 y.o.) phenytoin pregabalin (> 1 mo. old) primidone tiagabine ($\geq$ 12 y.o.) topiramate ($\geq$ 2 y.o.) valproic acid vigabatrin (refractory only $\geq$ 10 y.o.) zonisamide |
| Absence | ethosuximide; valproic acid; clonazepam; methsuximide or trimethadione (refractory only) | valproic acid clonazepam | |
| Clonic | phenobarbital | | |
| Tonic | phenobarbital | | |
| Atonic Seizures | clonazepam | clonazepam lorazepam | |
| Myoclonic | clonazepam; phenobarbital | clonazepam lorazepam levetiracetam ($\geq$ 12 y.o.) | |
| Lennox-Gastaut Syndrome (LGS) | cannabidiol; clonazepam | cannabidiol clonazepam clobazam ($\geq$ 2 y.o.) felbamate | lamotrigine ($\geq$ 2 y.o.) rufinamide ($\geq$ 1 y.o.) topiramate ($\geq$ 2 y.o.) |
| Dravet syndrome | cannabidiol | cannabidiol stiripentol (as adjunct to clobazam $\geq$ 2 y.o.) | |
| Mixed types | carbamazepine | diazepam valproic acid | |
| Infantile Spasms | vigabatrin (1 mo. – 2 y.o.) | | |

# XII. ENZYMATIC INTERACTIONS

A. **EIAEDs** = Enzyme-inducing antiepileptic drugs
   1. Barbiturates
   2. Carbamazepine
   3. Oxcarbazepine
   4. Phenytoin
   5. Topiramate (weak)
   6. Rifampin
B. Enzyme inhibitors
   1. Eslicarbazepine (CYP2C19)
   2. Rufinamide (CYP2E1)
C. Medications that are mostly renally eliminated (usually adjust dose in renal failure patients)
   1. Gabapentin, levetiracetam, and topiramate
D. Intravenous/intramuscular formulations available
   1. Lacosamide, levetiracetam, phenytoin (as phenytoin and fosphenytoin), phenobarbital, valproic acid (Depacon®), and various benzodiazepines (e.g., clonazepam, lorazepam)
E. Birth control for women of child-bearing age
   1. *Most anticonvulsants interact with oral contraceptives, making them less effective*
   2. Most anticonvulsants are not safe in pregnancy or with breastfeeding
   3. TWO methods of birth control are recommended (e.g., intrauterine device, barrier method, depot medroxyprogesterone given Q 2 months instead of Q 3 months)
   4. Most of the anticonvulsants are teratogenic
   5. If patient becomes pregnant while on an anticonvulsant, it is recommended to continue it if the risk of seizures outweighs the risk to the fetus

## XIII. SPECIFIC PHARMACOTHERAPY

A. Benzodiazepines - C-IV Controlled Substances
  1. SEs: Sedation, dry mouth, constipation, cough, UTI, aggression, insomnia, dysarthria, fatigue, memory impairment, withdrawal seizures
    i. BBW on all BZDs: risks from concomitant use with opioids
  2. Clobazam (Onfi®)[125]
    i. Indicated as **adjunctive** therapy in patients >2 y.o. with *Lennox-Gastaut syndrome* (LGS)
    ii. Half-life of 10-50 hours
    iii. Side effects: somnolence/sedation, dysarthria, drooling, aggression or other behavioral changes
      a. Rare cases of Stevens-Johnson syndrome & toxic epidermal necrolysis have been reported
    iv. Interactions
      a. Adjust dose of clobazam with strong or moderate CYP2C19 inhibitors
      b. Alcohol increases blood levels of clobazam by about 50%
    v. Compared to other benzodiazepines, it is much less effective on anxiety and less sedating
    vi. Available as: 10 and 20 mg tablets and 2.5 mg/mL in 120 mL bottles oral suspension
      a. Dose: 5 mg/d at HS, titrated to a maximum of 40 mg/d (divide BID if >30mg)
  3. Clonazepam (Klonopin®)[38]
    i. Indications: **Monotherapy** or **adjunct** in the treatment of the *Lennox-Gastaut syndrome (petit mal type)*, *akinetic* and *myoclonic seizures*
      a. *Absence seizures* who have failed to respond to ethosuximide
      b. Drug of choice for myoclonic seizures and subcortical myoclonus
    ii. Half-life of 20-80 hours
    iii. Availability: 0.5, 1, & 2 mg tablets, orally disintegrating tablets, and an IV solution
    iv. Dose: Start 0.25 mg BID and ↑ slowly until seizures are controlled (Max. 20 mg/d ÷TID)
  4. Diazepam (Valium®/Diastat®/Valtoco®)[40,41,42]
    i. Indicated as adjunctive therapy for "*convulsive disorders*"
    ii. Dose: 2-10 mg I.V. every 5-10 minutes given at ≤ 5 mg/minute (max dose: 30mg)
    iii. Diastat: Dosage: 0.2 mg/kg in patients > 12-years-old (0.3-0.5 mg/kg in younger children)
      a. Indicated in the management of refractory seizure patients
      b. Rectal gel available in 2.5, 10, & 20 mg pre-filled syringes, with a dose-dialing mechanism
    iv. Valtoco® nasal spray available in blister packs of 5, 7.5, and 10 mg devices (approved 1/2020)
      a. Indicated for acute treatment of intermittent episodes of frequent seizure activity (i.e., seizure clusters, acute repetitive seizures) in patients > 6-years-old
      b. Dosage: 1 spray (5-10 mg) into 1 nostril. May repeat in 4 hours. Max 2 doses for one seizure episode or one use every 5 days, and no more than 5 episodes a month.
  5. Lorazepam (Ativan®)[45]
    i. **Adjunctive** therapy for *myoclonic* & *atonic seizures*; *focal* & *generalized tonic-clonic seizures*
    ii. Dose: 4 mg slow I.V. (max rate: 2 mg/min); may repeat in 5-10 minutes if needed
  6. Midazolam (Versed / Nayzilam[141] nasal spray - BZD C-IV Controlled Substance
    i. Same indication as Valtoco® patients > 12-years-old (approved 5/17/19)
    ii. BBW: risks from concomitant use with opioids
    iii. Contraindicated in patients with acute narrow-angle glaucoma
    iv. Side effects: somnolence, headache, nasal discomfort, throat irritation, and rhinorrhea
    v. Dosage: 1 spray (5 mg in 0.1 mL) into 1 nostril. Repeat in 10 minutes if patient is still seizing.
      a. If patient's seizures persist, use alternative medications
      b. A full treatment should not be used more than once every 3 days or 5 times a month
    vi. Tmax from 7.8 to 28.2 minutes
    vii. Metabolized by CYP3A4
    viii. Concomitant use with moderate or strong CYP3A4 Inhibitors may result in prolonged sedation
    ix. T½ from ~ 2 to 7 hours
    x. Available in boxes of 2 nasal sprays
B. Brivaracetam (Briviact®)[123]
  1. Oral dosage forms approved for the treatment of partial-onset seizures in patients > 4-y.o.
    i. *Injection* approved for treatment of partial-onset seizures in patients > 16-years-old
  2. MOA: May be from a highly selective affinity for CNS synaptic vesicle protein 2A (SV2A)
  3. Dose for 4 to 15-year-olds:
    i. If weight is 11-20 kg: 0.5 mg/kg to 1.25 mg/kg BID (up to 2.5 mg/kg BID)
    ii. If weight is 21-49 kg: 0.5 mg/kg to 1 mg/kg BID (up to 2 mg/kg BID)
    iii. If weight is > 50 kg: 25 to 50 mg BID (up to 100 mg BID)
    iv. For patients > 16-years-old: 100 mg a day (divided BID), titrated up to 200 mg a day (÷ BID)
    v. Dose of *injectable* is equivalent to oral doses, administered over 2-15 minutes IV
    vi. ↓ dose with hepatic impairment & CYP2C19 inhibitors and ↑ dose when used with EIAEDs
  4. Availability: 10, 25, 50, 75 & 100 mg tablets; 10 mg/mL oral solution; 50 mg/5 mL vial for injection
  5. Metabolized by hydrolysis and CYP2C19
  6. T½ is approx. 9 hours
  7. Side effects: somnolence/sedation, dizziness, fatigue, and nausea/vomiting
  8. Safety data in pregnancy and lactation is lacking
C. Cannabidiol (Epidiolex®)[124] oral solution (C-V Controlled Substance)
  1. Indicated for treatment of Lennox-Gastaut syndrome or Dravet syndrome in patients > 2-y.o.
  2. WARNING: Can cause liver damage (especially if given with valproate)
  3. Must obtain serum transaminases (ALT and AST) & total bilirubin levels prior to starting drug

4. Side effects: somnolence, decreased appetite, diarrhea, transaminase elevations, fatigue, malaise, asthenia, rash, insomnia, and infections
5. Dose is 2.5 mg/kg p.o. BID; ↑ after 1 week to 5 mg/kg p.o. BID (max of 20 mg/kg/day)
   i. Adjust dose in moderate to severe hepatic impairment
6. Available as a 100 mg/mL oral solution
7. >94% protein bound
8. Metabolized by CYP2C19 & CYP3A4 enzymes, and UGT1A7, UGT1A9, & UGT2B7 isoforms
9. T½ of 56 to 61 hours
10. Reduce dose with moderate or strong CYP3A4 or CYP2C19 inhibitors or substrates of UGT1A9, UGT2B7, CYP2C8 and CYP2C9 (increase dose with strong CYP3A4 or CYP2C19 inducers)
11. Substrates of CYP1A2 and CYP2B6 may also require dose adjustment

D. Carbamazepine (Tegretol® Equetro®, Carbatrol®, Epitol®, Carnexiv (injection))[113-115,116,]
1. See *Bipolar Disorder* section for more details
2. Indicated as **monotherapy** to treat *complex partial seizures*, *generalized tonic-clonic seizures*, and *mixed seizure* patterns
3. MOA: Enhances fast inactivation of voltage gated $Na^+$ channels; interacts with L-type $Ca^{2+}$ & $K^+$ channels
4. **BBW: SJS and TEN (must test for HLA-B*1502 in Asians and other high risk ancestries), aplastic anemia and agranulocytosis**[541]
   i. Those who also have HLA-A*3101 and HLA-A*2404 polymorphisms also at risk of rash
5. SEs: Rash, constipation, nausea, vomiting, xerostomia, ataxia, dizziness, *hyponatremia*, bone marrow suppression
   i. Must monitor WBCs and neutrophils, because of rare aplastic anemia, agranulocytosis, and thrombocytopenia
6. Drug interactions as a <u>potent</u> inducer of CYP3A4 (lowers blood levels of other drugs)
7. Available as: 100 mg chewable tablet, 200 mg tablet, 100, 200, & 300 mg ER capsules, 100, 200, and 400 mg ER tablets, and 100 mg/5 mL suspension
8. Dose: 200 mg BID (children < 6-years-old: 10-20 mg/kg/day divided BID or TID)
   i. After 4-5 weeks, autoinduction takes place, so may need to ↑ dose according to blood levels
   ii. Maintenance: May increase 200 mg/d weekly in 3-4 divided doses (Max dose: 1200mg)
9. Serum level range: 4-12 mcg/mL

E. Eslicarbazepine (Aptiom®)[126]
1. Indicated for **adjunctive** or **monotherapy** treatment of *partial-onset seizures* in those ≥ 4-y.o.
2. *Prodrug:* Eslicarbazepine and oxcarbazepine share the same main active metabolite (S-licarbazepine or S-MHD)
   i. Do not use *with* oxcarbazepine
3. Half-life is 13-20 hours
4. Weak inducer of CYP3A4 and uridine diphosphate-glucuronosyltransferase (UGT) 1A1 and a moderate inhibitor of CYP2C19
   i. UGT inducers (e.g., carbamazepine, phenytoin) can ↓ drug levels
   ii. It can ↓ drug levels of CYP3A4 substrates, oral contraceptives and warfarin
5. Available as: 200 mg, 400 mg, 600 mg, 800 mg tablets
6. Dose: In adults: 400 mg/d, titrated slowly to 800 mg/d. Max dose of 1600 mg/d
   i. Pediatric patients:

| Weight | Initial dose (mg/day) | Maintenance dose (mg/day) |
|---|---|---|
| 11 to 21 kg | 200 | 400 to 600 |
| 22 to 31 kg | 300 | 500 to 800 |
| 32 to 38 kg | 300 | 600 to 900 |
| more than 38 kg | 400 | 800 to 1200 |

   ii. Reduce dose by 50% in moderate to severe renal impairment
   iii. Not recommended in patients with severe liver impairment
   iv. Increase dose if given with EIAEDs
7. Common side effects are dizziness, drowsiness, nausea, headache, diplopia, fatigue, vertigo, ataxia, blurred vision, and tremor
   i. Rare PR interval prolongation, ↑ LFTs, hyponatremia, and DRESS reported
8. May have cross-sensitivity with oxcarbazepine and carbamazepine for rash occurrence

F. Ethosuximide (Zarontin®)[128]
1. MOA: Inhibits T-type $Ca^{2+}$ channels
2. Indicated for the control of *absence (petit mal) epilepsy* (**monotherapy**)
3. SEs include N&V, dizziness, sleep disturbance, drowsiness, HA, ↓ appetite, and hyperactivity
4. Warnings of blood dyscrasias, changes to liver and kidneys, and potential Lupus induction
5. Metabolized by CYP3A4
6. Half-life: 30 hours in children / 60 hours in adults
7. May ↓ VPA levels and phenytoin ↑ levels
8. Conversely, VPA may ↑ and phenytoin may ↓ ethosuximide levels
9. Available in 250 mg liquid-filled capsules and 250 mg/5 mL oral solution
10. Dose: 500 mg/d (≥ 6-years-old), titrated to an optimal dose of 20 mg/kg (divided up to TID)
   i. Max dose: 20-30 mg/kg; Should not exceed 1.5 g daily unless under strict supervision

G. Ethotoin (Peganone®)[127]
1. Structurally related to phenytoin

2. Indicated for the control of tonic-clonic (grand mal) and complex partial (psychomotor) seizures
3. <u>NOT</u> a first-line agent
4. Contraindicated in patients with hepatic abnormalities or hematologic disorders
5. Pediatric dose starts at 750 mg/d (divided every 4-6 hours) with FOOD
   i. Avg pediatric dose is 500-1000 mg/d (up to 2 grams a day) divided every 4-6 hours with FOOD
   ii. Avg adult dosage is 2-3 grams a day (divided every 4-6 hours) with FOOD
6. Available in 250 mg tablets
7. Side effects: chest pain, nystagmus, diplopia, fever, dizziness, diarrhea, headache, insomnia, fatigue, numbness, skin rash, and SJS
   i. Rare cases of lymphadenopathy and systemic lupus erythematosus have been reported
8. T½ of 6-9 hours
9. Caution in patients on warfarin or other drugs that affect the hematopoietic system
10. Recommended monitoring includes monthly CBC and urinalysis, as well as LFTs

H. Ezogabine (Potiga®)[1111] – *Discontinued by GSK in April 2017*[1112]
I. Felbamate (Felbatol®)[129]
1. MOA: Blocks N-methyl-D-aspartate (NMDA) synaptic response & modulates $GABA_A$ receptors
2. Indicated as a last-line treatment as **monotherapy** or **adjunctive therapy** in the treatment of *partial seizures, with and without generalization* and as **adjunctive** therapy in the treatment of *partial and generalized seizures* associated with *Lennox-Gastaut syndrome* in children
3. BBW: Aplastic Anemia (100 times greater than general population) and Hepatic Failure
   i. Requires WRITTEN informed consent
4. 40-49% renally eliminated (dose adjustments may be needed in renal impairment)
5. Half-life: 20-23 hours (with EIAEDs: 13-14 hours)
6. SEs: Photosensitivity, weight loss, pancytopenia, insomnia, GI disturbances
7. Drug interactions: moderate CYP3A4 inducer, BBW, hepatotoxicity
8. Available in 400 mg & 600 mg tablets and 600 mg/5 mL oral suspension
9. In patients $\geq$ 14-years-old, start with 400 mg TID
   i. Slowly titrate up to 3,600 mg/d as needed (divided TID)
10. Therapeutic range has not been established

J. Fosphenytoin sodium (Cerebyx®)[130] – *Also see phenytoin*
1. Indicated for the treatment of generalized tonic-clonic status epilepticus (also to prevent seizures during neurosurgery)
2. BBW: Cardiovascular risk associated with rapid infusion rates
   i. Fosphenytoin – a prodrug that is metabolized to phenytoin *in vitro*
      a. 1.5 mg of Fosphenytoin = 1 mg of phenytoin equivalents (PEs)
      b. Available in 50 mg PE/mL
   ii. Rate N.T.E. 150 mg PE per minute in adults and 2 mg PE/kg/min (or 150 mg PE/min, if less) in pediatric patients
      a. Risk of severe hypotension and cardiac arrhythmias
      b. Cardiac monitoring required during and after administration
3. For **status epilepticus**: loading dose is 15 to 20 mg PE/kg in adults and peds
   i. Dose and rate can be reduced for non-emergency use
   ii. Compatible with D5W and NS 0.9% at a maximum concentration of 25 mg PE/mL
4. Available as 2 mL or 10 mL single-dose vials at a concentration of 50 mg PE/mL
5. Contraindications: Sinus bradycardia, sino-atrial block, 2º or 3º A-V block, Adams-Stokes syndrome, or a history of prior acute hepatotoxicity attributable to fos-/phenytoin
6. Side effects and interactions are the same as for phenytoin

K. Gabapentin (Neurontin®)[131] / Other brands not indicated for seizures: Gralise™, Horizant®[132,133]
1. Attenuates voltage gated $Ca^{2+}$ channels at the $\alpha 2\delta$ (*alpha-2-delta*) sub-unit to decrease the release of excitatory neurotransmitters, such as glutamate
2. Indicated for **adjunctive** therapy in the treatment of *partial seizures* (ages 3-12) *with and without secondary generalization* (>12-years-old)
3. American Academy of Neurology (AAN) guidelines state it may also be used as initial monotherapy in newly diagnosed partial epilepsy
4. Zero protein binding and mainly renal elimination (adjust dose in renal impairment)
5. Half-life: 5-9 hours
6. Available as 100, 300, & 400 mg capsules; 600 mg & 800 mg tablets; 250 mg/5 mL oral solution
7. Dose: 300 mg QD (titrate up to TID over 3 days). Average dose: 1800-3600 mg/d divided TID
   i. Maximum dose: 4800 mg/d divided TID
8. Therapeutic range has not been established, but suggested at 4-20 μg/mL
9. No significant drug interactions

L. Lacosamide (Vimpat®)[134] - C-V controlled substance
1. Indicated for the treatment of *partial seizures* in patients $\geq$ 4-years-old
   i. Injection is for short-term replacement when oral administration not feasible in patients $\geq$ 17 y.o.
2. MOA: selectively enhances slow inactivation of voltage-dependent $Na^+$ channels
   i. Also binds to the collapsin response mediator protein 2 (CRMP2)
3. WARNING: *cardiac arrhythmias* and rare dose-dependent PR interval prolongations on EKG
   i. Recommended to obtain an EKG before starting and after titration to steady-state
   ii. Caution in those with known conduction problems (e.g., AV block, sick sinus syndrome without a pacemaker, Brugada Syndrome), severe ischemic or structural heart disease, or concomitant use of medications that prolong the PR interval

4. Side effects: Dizziness, nausea, vertigo, diplopia, abnormal coordination and ataxia
5. Low protein binding (< 15%)
6. ~ 40% renally eliminated unchanged (must supplement with 50% of daily dosage after dialysis)
7. 30-50% metabolized by CYP3A4, CYP2C9, & CYP2C19
8. Half-life: 13 hours
9. Dose: 50 mg BID (as adjunct therapy in pediatric patients) or 100 mg BID (monotherapy) in adults
   i. Increase slowly up to a maximum of 400 mg/d
   ii. Pediatric patients weighing < 50 kg: 1 mg/kg BID up to a maximum of 8-12 mg/kg/day
   iii. Adjust dose in severe renal or mild to moderate hepatic impairment
   iv. Not recommended for use in severe hepatic impairment
   v. Patients on strong inducers or inhibitors of CYP3A4 or CYP2C9 may have to adjust the dosage
      a. *In vivo* and *in vitro* studies did not show any clinically significant drug interactions
10. Available as 50, 100, 150 & 200 mg tablets, 10 mg/mL oral solution, & 200 mg/20 mL injection
M. Lamotrigine (Lamictal®/XR)[117,118]
   1. Indicated for **adjunctive therapy** ($\geq 2$ y.o. for RR (regular-release) / $\geq 13$ y.o for XR) with *partial-onset seizures, primary generalized tonic-clonic seizures, generalized seizures of Lennox-Gastaut syndrome,* and as **monotherapy** ($\geq 16$ y.o. for RR / $\geq$ 13 y.o. for XR) for *partial-onset seizures when crossing over from another anticonvulsant*
      i. Also effective in *primary generalized seizures* (i.e., *absence seizures* and *primary generalized tonic-clonic seizures*), *atypical absence seizures,* and *tonic/atonic seizures*
   2. MOA: Inhibits voltage dependent $Na^+$ channels & high voltage activated $Ca^{2+}$ channels; attenuates release of glutamate, GABA & DA
   3. NICE guidelines suggest that lamotrigine can exacerbate myoclonic seizures[1113]
   4. BBW: Risk of life-threatening rash (possible **SJS** or **TEN** - toxic epidermal necrolysis)
      i. Incidence: 0.8% of pediatrics / 0.3% of adults
      ii. Usually within 2-8 weeks of initiation
      iii. *Discontinue lamotrigine at the first sign of any rash*
   5. See *Bipolar Disorder* section for more details and dosing titration schedule
   6. Therapeutic range has not been established, but suggested at 1-20 mcg/mL
N. Levetiracetam (Keppra®/Keppra XR®/ Elepsia XR™/ Roweepra & XR® / Spritam®)[135-138]
   1. MOA: Binds to synaptic vesicle protein 2A (SV2A); may indirectly modulate GABA and glycine activity; partially inhibits N-type $Ca^{2+}$ currents
   2. Approved indications (as **adjunctive therapy**)

| Brand name | Indication |
|---|---|
| Keppra / Roweepra | Partial-onset seizures (ages $\geq$ 1-month-old) |
| Elepsia XR / Spritam | Partial-onset seizures (ages $\geq$ 4-years-old) |
| Elepsia XR / Keppra XR | Partial-onset seizures (ages $\geq$ 12-years-old) |
| Keppra / Roweepra / Spritam | Myoclonic seizures (ages $\geq$ 12-years-old) |
| Keppra / Roweepra / Spritam | Primary generalized tonic-clonic seizures (ages $\geq$ 6) |

   3. Dosage:

| Indication | Dosage |
|---|---|
| Partial-onset seizures (ages 1 to 6-months-old) | 7 mg/kg po BID (max. 42 mg/kg/d) |
| Partial-onset seizures (ages 6 mo. to < 4-years-old) | 10 mg/kg po BID (max. 48 mg/kg/d) |
| Partial-onset seizures (4 to 16-years-old) | 10 mg/kg po BID (max. 60 mg/kg/d) |
| Primary generalized tonic-clonic seizures (6 to 16-y.o.) | 10 mg/kg po BID (max. 60 mg/kg/d) |
| Partial-onset seizures (ages > 16-years-old) | 500 mg po BID (max. 3000 mg/d) |
| Myoclonic seizures (ages > 12) | 500 mg po BID (max. 3000 mg/d) |

   Note: Intravenous dosing is the same as oral dosing
   4. 66% renally eliminated (MUST adjust dose in mild renal impairment)
      i. Not recommended in moderate to severe renal impairment
   5. Half-life: 6-8 hours
   6. Adverse events (usually mild) include fatigue, somnolence, dizziness, loss of appetite, mood swings, cough, rare anaphylaxis & angioedema
      i. Rare: behavior problems - increased agitation & aggression, and psychotic reactions reported
      ii. Requires slow titration to minimize CNS side effects
   7. Availability
      i. Keppra / Roweepra: 250, 500, 750, & 1000 mg scored tablets
      ii. Spritam: 250, 500, 750, & 1000 mg ODT (can also be put into a liquid > 15 mL)
      iii. Keppra: 100 mg/mL grape-flavored oral solution
      iv. Keppra XR: 500 mg & 750 mg extended-release tablets
      v. Elepsia XR: 1000 mg & 1500 mg extended-release tablets (max dose 3000 mg/d)
      vi. Single-dose 100 mL bags for injection:
         a. 500 mg/100 mL in 0.82% NaCl
         b. 1,000 mg/100 mL in 0.75 % NaCl
         c. 1,500 mg/100 mL in 0.54% NaCl
   8. Therapeutic range has not been established, but suggested at 5-60 mcg/mL
   9. No CYP drug interactions

O. **Methsuximide (Celontin)**[140]
1. Approved for *refractory* absence (petit mal) seizures
2. Dosage: 300 mg QD x 1 week, and then ↑by 300 mg QD each week to a target of 1.2 gm/d
3. Available in 300 mg capsules
4. Side effects similar to other anticonvulsants (GI, blood dyscrasias, CNS effects, & skin reactions)
   i. CBC monitoring is highly recommended due to rare blood dyscrasias
5. Because of the potential to melt, it should NEVER be exposed to *temperatures over 104ºF*
6. Methsuximide may ↓ lamotrigine levels and ↑ phenytoin & phenobarbital levels

Q. **Oxcarbazepine (Trileptal®, Oxtellar XR™)**[142,143]
1. MOA: Block voltage-sensitive $Na^+$ channels, increase $K^+$ conductance and modulate the activity of high-voltage activated $Ca^{2+}$ channels
2. Shares the same main active metabolite as eslicarbazepine (S-licarbazepine or S-MHD)
3. Approved as **monotherapy** (ages ≥4) or **adjunctive therapy** (ages ≥2) for *partial seizures*
4. Half-life: 8-10 hours
5. FDA suggests testing for the HLA-B*1502 allele in genetically at risk populations (i.e., those with Asian ancestry) before initiating treatment with oxcarbazepine
6. SEs: GI, sedation, headache, dizziness, rash, vertigo, ataxia, hyponatremia, & diplopia
   i. Rare angioedema, anaphylaxis, Stevens-Johnson syndrome (**SJS**), toxic epidermal necrolysis (**TEN**), and multi-organ hypersensitivity
   ii. Cross-sensitivity with rash for carbamazepine
7. Induces CYP3A4, CYP3A5, and CYP2C19
8. Available in 150 mg, 300 mg, & 600 mg tablets, 300 mg/5 mL plum-lemon flavored oral suspension, and 150 mg, 300 mg, & 600 mg extended-release tablets (Oxtellar XR™)
9. Dose in children: 8-10 mg/kg (divided BID) initially & ↑ weekly (max of 600 mg/d or 60 mg/kg/d)
   i. Adults: 150-300 mg BID, ↑ weekly, up to max dose of 2400 mg/d
10. Therapeutic range not established, but suggested at 10-40 mcg/mL (measure S-MHD)

R. **Perampanel (Fycompa®)**[144] - C-III controlled substance
1. Approved as **adjunctive** treatment for *partial-onset seizures (with or without 2º generalized seizures)* & for *primary generalized tonic-clonic seizures* in adults or children ≥ 12-years-old
2. MOA: non-competitive AMPA glutamate receptor antagonist
3. BBW: Serious or life-threatening psychiatric and behavioral adverse reactions including aggression, hostility, irritability, anger, and homicidal ideation/threats have been reported
4. Metabolized primarily via CYP3A4, CYP3A5, and glucuronidation
   i. May induce the metabolism of Progestin-containing contraceptives
5. Long half-life of 105 hours
6. Concomitant EIAEDs ↓ perampanel's blood levels by 50-67% (may need to double the dose)
7. SEs observed in randomized trials include dizziness, somnolence, headache, fatigue, irritability, gait disturbance, falls, nausea and weight gain
8. Available in 2, 4, 6, 8, 10, & 12 mg tablets
9. Dose: 2 mg QHS (4 mg with concomitant EIAEDs)
   i. Max dose of 12 mg/d (can go higher with concomitant EIAEDs)
   ii. Use lower doses in patients with hepatic impairment

S. **Phenobarbital (Luminal®)**[145] (PHB) - C-IV Controlled Substance
1. Indicated for the treatment *of all types of seizure disorders*, including *partial seizures, clonic seizures, myoclonic seizures, tonic seizures*, or *tonic-clonic seizures* not responding to other anticonvulsants
2. MOA: Increase seizure threshold by facilitating intrinsic $Cl^-$ channel function, blocks high voltage activated $Ca^{2+}$ channels, blocks AMPA & kainate receptors
3. Not a first-line drug any more due to toxicity in overdose and cognitive impairment
4. SEs: Somnolence, liver damage, psychomotor slowing, poor concentration, depression, irritability, ataxia, and decreased libido
   i. High doses can cause severe respiratory depression (especially with other CNS depressants)
   ii. Long-term use of PHB may be associated with coarsening of facial features, osteomalacia, and Dupuytren's contractures
   iii. Recommended to give Folic Acid supplementation with phenobarbital therapy
5. Metabolized by CYP2C19 (major), CYP2C9 (minor), and CYP2E1 (minor)
6. T½ in adults: 53-118 hours (mean 79 hours) / T½ in pediatrics: 60-180 hours (mean 110 hours)
7. Induces CYP1A2 (weak), CYP2A6/2B6 (weak), CYP2C9 (weak), CYP3A4 (strong), UGT1A1
8. Significant drug interactions: ↑ clearance of other drugs metabolized by CYP2C-family enzymes, CYP3A-family enzymes, CYP1A2, and UGT (UDP-glucuronosyltransferase)
9. 20-50% is removed in dialysis
10. Dose:
    i. Adults: 60-200 mg/d divided up to TID (max 400 mg/d)
    ii. Pediatrics: 1-6 mg/kg/day divided up to TID
    iii. For status epilepticus: 15 mg/kg x 1 dose
11. Available in 15, 16.2, 30, 32.4, 60, 64.8, 97.2, & 100 mg tablets; elixir (20 mg/5 mL); and injection (65 and 130 mg/ml)
12. Therapeutic serum levels: 15-40 mcg/mL
13. Pregnancy Category D

T. Phenytoin (Dilantin®, Phenytek®)[146,147]
   1. MOA: Inhibits voltage dependent $Na^+$ channels
   2. Indicated as **monotherapy** or **adjunctive treatment** of *tonic-clonic (grand mal)* and *complex partial (psychomotor, temporal lobe) seizures* and prevention and treatment of *seizures* occurring during or following neurosurgery
     i. Also used for Lennox-Gastaut syndrome, status epilepticus, & childhood epileptic syndromes
   3. HLA-B*1502 genetic allele variants are at higher risk of serious rash
     i. Occurs mostly in patients of Asian ancestry, including South Asian Indians
     ii. Genetic testing highly recommended
   4. Side effects: Drug-induced gingival hyperplasia, rash, folic acid deficiency, hirsutism, ↓ bone density, SJS, agranulocytosis, myelosuppression, nephrotoxicity, liver damage, confusion, slurred speech, double vision, ataxia, and neuropathy (with long-term use)
     i. Folic acid supplementation (0.5 mg/d) also recommended to reduce incidence of gingival hyperplasia and anemia
     ii. Calcium & Vit D supplementation, as well as bone mineral density testing, are suggested
   5. NOTE: Non-linear kinetics translates to blood levels much higher than proportional dose ↑s
   6. Highly protein bound - can be competitively displaced by other drugs
   7. Metabolized by CYP2C9 and CYP2C19 (inducers or inhibitors will affect phenytoin levels)
   8. Half-life of 22 hours (range 7-42 hours) / IV half-life is 10-15 hours
   9. Phenytoin is a broad-spectrum *inducer* of CYP enzymes and UGT-glucuronidation (most problematic of all anticonvulsants)
     i. Contraindicated with delavirdine due to virologic resistance[1114]
     ii. If given with fosamprenavir alone may ↓ the levels of amprenavir (the active metabolite)
   10. Oral loading dose – 1 gm divided as 400 / 300 / & 300 mg given 2 hours apart on first day
     i. Adult dose: 100 mg TID or 300 mg QD (ER capsules) up to a max dose of 600 mg/d
     ii. Pediatric dose: 5 mg/kg/d (divided TID) (range of 4-8 mg/kg/d) up to a max of 300 mg/d
   11. Available in:
     i. Dilantin: 50 mg chewable Infatabs, 125 mg Kapseals, 100 mg capsules & 125 mg/5 mL suspension
     ii. Phenytek: 200 & 300 mg extended-release capsules
   12. Therapeutic serum levels: 10-20 mcg/mL total phenytoin (1-2 mcg/mL *unbound* phenytoin)
     i. If patient's albumin < 3.5 mg/dl, you can calculate a corrected true phenytoin level
     ii. Sheiner-Tozer Method:
     `Corrected total phenytoin = [measured phenytoin (µg/mL)] / {[0.2 x albumin] + 0.1}`
     iii. Second method:
     `Corrected total phenytoin = [measured phenytoin (µg/mL)] / {[(albumin (g/dL)/4.4) ×0.9) +0.1}`
U. Pregabalin (Lyrica® / Lyrica CR®)[148,149] - C-V Controlled Substance
   1. Approved for **adjunctive therapy** for *partial seizures* in patients ≥ 1 month of age (& for treatment of neuropathic pain, fibromyalgia, and postherpetic neuralgia)
   2. Chemically related to gabapentin
   3. MOA: Inhibits voltage gated $Ca^{2+}$ channels at the α2δ (*alpha-2-delta*) sub-unit to decrease the release of excitatory neurotransmitters
     i. Similar to gabapentin, but at much greater potency
   4. ≥ 90% renally eliminated
   5. Half-life is 6.3 hours
   6. SEs: Somnolence, dizziness, ataxia, peripheral edema, visual distortions, tremor, asthenia, impaired concentration, weight gain, constipation, xerostomia, jaundice, euphoria
     i. Rare: angioedema, CPK elevations, and cardiac PR interval prolongation
   7. Available as 25, 50, 75, 100, 150, 200, 225, & 300 mg capsules, and 20 mg/mL oral solution
     i. Extended-release (CR) tablets: 82.5 mg, 165 mg, and 330 mg
     ii. 75 mg/d (total) of regular-release (RR) = 82.5 mg of CR (i.e., RR + 10% = CR)
   8. Dosing:
     i. Pediatric pts weighing < 30 kg: 3.5 mg/kg/d up to a max dose of 14 mg/kg/d (÷ BID or TID)
     ii. Pediatric pts weighing ≥ 30 kg: 2.5 mg/kg/d up to a max dose of 10 mg/kg/d (÷ BID or TID)
     iii. Adults: 75 mg BID, titrated slowly up to a max dose of 600 mg/d (÷ BID or TID)
     iv. Reduce dose to 1/2 if CrCl is 30-60, by 1/4 if CrCl is 15-30, and by 1/8 if CrCl < 15 ml/min
     v. Lyrica CR® should be dosed after an evening meal
   9. No CYP interactions or metabolism
V. Primidone (Mysoline®)[150] - C-IV Controlled Substance
   1. MOA: Decreases neuron excitability to increase seizure threshold
   2. Approved as **monotherapy/adjunctive treatment** of *grand mal, psychomotor* & *focal seizures*
   3. Metabolized to phenobarbital and phenylethylmalonamide (PEMA)
   4. SEs: Ataxia, vertigo, megaloblastic anemia, thrombocytopenia
   5. Available as 50 mg and 250 mg (scored) tablets
   6. Dosing (≥ 8-years-old): 100-125 mg at bedtime with slow titration to 250 mg TID
     i. 250 mg of primidone is equivalent to 60 mg of phenobarbital
     ii. Average dose: 500-1500 mg/d, up to a max of 2g/day
   7. Serum levels: 5-12 mcg/mL (can also measure phenobarbital)
   8. Same drug interactions as phenobarbital

W. **Rufinamide (Banzel®)**[151]
1. MOA: Prolongs inactivation of voltage-gated Na⁺ channels to suppress neuronal hyperexcitability
   1. MOA: Prolongs inactivation of voltage-gated $Na^+$ channels to suppress neuronal hyperexcitability
2. **Adjunctive treatment** for seizures associated with *Lennox-Gastaut syndrome* in those $\geq$ 1-y.o.
   i. May have efficacy in partial epilepsy as well
3. Metabolized by non-CYP enzymes to inactive metabolites
   i. Not recommended in severe hepatic impairment
4. Half-life: 6-10 hours
5. SEs: Headache, dizziness, nausea, somnolence, fatigue, suicidal behavior/ideation
   i. Rare Shortened QT interval, leukopenia, and DRESS
6. Enzyme inducers can ↑ its clearance
   i. Rufinamide may reduce the effectiveness of oral hormonal contraceptives
   ii. Weak inhibitor of CYP2E1 and weak inducer of CYP3A4
7. Dosing: Children: 10 mg/kg (divided BID) up to maximum of 45 mg/kg/day
   i. Adults: 400-800 mg/d (divided BID), up to a maximum of 3200 mg/d (divided BID)
   ii. Take with food to ↑ absorption
8. Available in 200 mg & 400 mg tablets (crushable), and 40 mg/mL oral suspension

X. **Stiripentol (Diacomit®)**[152]
1. Indicated as adjunct therapy to clobazam for seizures with Dravet syndrome in patients $\geq$ 2-y.o.
2. MOA: possibly has direct effects on $GABA_A$ receptors
   i. Also ↑ levels of clobazam and norclobazam through CYP3A4 and CYP2C19 inhibition
3. Side effects: insomnia, decreased appetite, agitation, ataxia, weight loss, hypotonia, nausea, tremor, dysarthria, and somnolence (if severe, decrease dose of clobazam)
   i. Rare: Neutropenia and thrombocytopenia – obtain CBC w/diff at baseline & every 6 months
4. 99% protein bound
5. T½ of 4.5 to 13 hours
6. Not recommended in moderate or severe renal impairment
7. Metabolized by CYP1A2, CYP2C19, and CYP3A4
8. An inhibitor and inducer of CYP1A2, CYP2B6, and CYP3A4 (adjust doses of their substrates)
9. Potent inhibitor of CYP2C8, CYP2C19, CYP3A4, P-gp and BCRP (reduce doses as needed)
10. Avoid use with rifampin, EIAEDs, and strong inducers of CYP1A2, CYP3A4 or CYP2C19 (alternately, consider using a higher dose)
11. Dose: 50 mg/kg/day (divided BID or TID) up to a max of 3000 mg/d
12. Availability: 250 mg & 500 mg capsules; 250 mg & 500 mg pale pink, fruit-flavored powder for suspension in packets (contains phenylalanine – caution in patients with phenylketonuria)
13. Mix powder in water. Should be taken immediately after mixing during a **meal**

Y. **Tiagabine (Gabitril®)**[153]
1. MOA: GABA Reuptake Inhibitor
2. Indicated as **adjunctive therapy** of *partial seizures* in patients $\geq$12-years-old
3. 96% protein bound (watch for protein-binding interactions)
4. Mostly metabolized by CYP3A4 (adjust dose with hepatic insufficiency)
5. Half-life: 7-9 hours (↓ by 50-65% with EIAEDs)
6. Side effects include dizziness, nervousness, emotional lability, lack of energy, somnolence, nausea, nervousness, tremor, difficulty concentrating, and abdominal pain
   i. Rare multi-organ hypersensitivity syndrome has been reported
   ii. Avoided in patients with short QT syndrome
7. Available as 2 mg, 4 mg, 12 mg, and 16 mg tablets
8. Dosing: 4 mg daily, titrated to 32-56 mg/d in 2-4 divided doses
   i. Max dose: 56 mg/d (32 mg in patients $\leq$ 18-years-old) in 2-4 divided doses
   ii. Take with **food** to ↑ absorption
9. Therapeutic range has not been established
   i. Effective median plasma level of 23.7 ng/mL seen in study

Z. **Topiramate (Topamax®, Trokendi XR™, Qudexy® XR / Topiragen®)**[154-156]
1. MOA: Blocks voltage dependent Na⁺ channels, increases GABA activity, antagonizes kainate/AMPA subunits
   1. MOA: Blocks voltage dependent $Na^+$ channels, increases GABA activity, antagonizes kainate/AMPA subunits
2. Approved as **adjunctive** or **monotherapy** in patients $\geq$ 2*-years-old with *partial onset* or *primary generalized tonic-clonic seizures* and **adjunctive therapy** for *seizures associated with Lennox-Gastaut syndrome (LGS)* in patients $\geq$ 2*-years-old (*Trokendi XR is $\geq$ 6-years-old)
3. Per American Academy of Neurology (AAN) guidelines, it may be used as monotherapy for refractory generalized tonic-clonic convulsions and partial seizures in adults and children
4. 70% eliminated unchanged in urine
5. Half-life: 18-23 hours (XR half-life is 56 hours)
6. Weak inhibitor of CYP2C19 and a mild inducer of CYP3A4
7. Drug interactions:
   i. EIAEDs (e.g., phenytoin and carbamazepine) can ↓ topiramate levels by 50%
   ii. Topiramate can lower oral contraceptive levels by up to 30%
   iii. Hyperammonemia risk with concomitant valproic acid
8. SEs: Dizziness, weight loss, somnolence, impaired cognition & expressive language, behavioral dysregulation, paresthesia, and depression
9. Rare: metabolic acidosis (↓$CO_3^-$, periodic monitoring required), decreased sweating (particularly in children), acute myopia, secondary angle glaucoma, kidney stones
   i. Hyperammonemia and hypothermia (↑ risk with valproic acid use), SJS, liver failure

10. Pregnancy Category D: associated with an ↑ risk of oral clefts and low birth weight
11. Dosing: 25-50 mg/d, with slow titration to a maximum dose of 400 mg/d (divided BID)
    i. Reduce dose by half with renal impairment
    ii. Dialysis significantly reduces levels
12. Available as
    i. Topamax: 25, 50, 100, & 200 mg tablets and 15 mg & 25 mg sprinkle caps formulations
    ii. Qudexy XR & Topamax XR: 25, 50, 100, 150, & 200 mg ER capsules (can be opened and sprinkled on food)
    iii. Trokendi XR: 25, 50, 100, & 200 mg capsules (should <u>not</u> be opened)
13. Therapeutic range has not been established, but suggested from 2 to 25 µg/mL

AA. **Trimethadione (Tridione)**[157]
1. Indicated for the control of petit mal (absence) seizures refractory to treatment with other drugs
2. A rare, exfoliative dermatitis or severe forms of erythema multiforme is possible
    i. Discontinue at the first sign of a cutaneous reaction
    ii. Blood dyscrasias, hepatic and renal dysfunction, ocular effects, and Lupus/Myasthenia-like syndromes require baseline labs and periodic monitoring
3. Adult Dose: 300 to 600 mg TID-QID and ↑ weekly as needed or until toxic symptoms appear
4. Pediatric Dose: 75 to 150 mg TID-QID and increase weekly as needed
5. Available in 150 mg chewable Dulcet® sweetened tablets

AB. **Valproic acid/valproate/divalproex sodium (Depakote®/ER, Depacon®, Stavzor®, Depakene®)**[122] See *Bipolar Disorder* section for more details
1. Approved as **monotherapy** or **adjunctive therapy** of *complex partial, simple and complex absence seizures*, and *mixed seizure* types that include *absence seizures*
    i. Drug of choice in idiopathic generalized epilepsy and juvenile myoclonic epilepsy
    ii. First-line drug in photosensitive epilepsy and Lennox-Gastaut syndrome
    iii. Second-line choice in the treatment of infantile spasms
2. MOA: Alters synthesis & degradation of GABA; potentiates post-synaptic GABA responses
3. BBW: *Hepatotoxicity* (especially < 2 y.o. and within first 6 months)
    i. 5-10% of patients develop transient LFT ↑s
    ii. *Pancreatitis*
    iii. *Teratogenic* Fetal Risk (neural tube defects, other major malformations, and decreased IQ)
4. >85-95% protein bound (watch for interactions with other protein bound drugs)
5. SEs: Alopecia, rash, increase appetite, GI disturbances, asthenia, headache, dizziness, dose-related, palpations, thrombocytopenia, hematemesis
    i. *Hyperammonemia* - mild & transient in 25-30% of patients, but rare <u>encephalopathy</u> can occur
    a. Higher risk with concomitant topiramate
6. Drug interactions:
    i. ↑ plasma levels of free fractions of phenytoin, phenobarbital, carbamazepine epoxide, and lamotrigine
    ii. ↓ the total phenytoin level (bound & unbound)
    iii. EIAEDs ↓ levels of valproate
    iv. Felbamate and clobazam ↑ valproate plasma levels
7. Available as 125 mg, 250 mg, & 500 mg delayed-release tablets (Stavzor is capsules); 125 mg & 250 mg sprinkle capsules; 250 mg & 500 mg extended-release tablets; 250 mg/5 mL syrup; and parenteral 500 mg/ 5mL preparation for IV injection (Depacon®)
8. Dosing: 10-20 mg/kg/day (divided up to TID), with slow titration to a max dose of 60 mg/kg/day
9. Serum levels: 50-100 mcg/mL (NOTE: for Bipolar Disorder, the range is 50-125 mcg/ml)

AC. **Vigabatrin (Sabril® / Vigadrone®)**[158,159] – *NOT A FIRST-LINE AGENT*
1. Indicated for **adjunctive therapy** of *refractory complex partial seizures* in patients ≥ 10-years-old, and as **monotherapy** for *Infantile Spasms* (ages 1 month to 2-years-old)
2. Selective irreversible GABA transaminase inhibitor and a close structural analogue of GABA
3. BBW: Permanent vision loss (risk increases with total dose and duration of use)
    i. 30-50% incidence by 5 years into treatment
    ii. Only available through restricted distribution program (Vigabatrin REMS program)
    iii. Baseline and periodic vision assessments are recommended
    iv. General warning: neurotoxicity
4. 95% renally eliminated (adjust dose in renal impairment)
5. Half-life: 5.7-10.5 hours
6. Drug interactions: Inducer of CYP2C9 / may ↓ phenytoin (by 25%) and ↑ clonazepam levels
7. SEs: Rash, anemia, ↑ weight, somnolence, fatigue, infections, HA, vision problems, liver failure
8. Available as *Sabril:* 500 mg tablets and *Sabril/Vigadrone:* 500 mg packets (powder for oral mixture in 10 mL liquid)
9. Dosing: 500 mg BID (children: 25 mg/kg BID) up to a max of 6 gm/d (children: 75 mg/kg BID)
10. Adjust dose in renal failure
11. Therapeutic range has not been established, but suggested as 20–160 mcg/mL

AD. **Zonisamide (Zonegran®)**[160]
1. FDA-approved for **adjunctive therapy** for adult patients with *partial seizures*
2. Also effective in partial and generalized seizures (children & adult) and myoclonic seizures
3. MOA: Inhibits slow Na+ channels, blocks T-type Ca2+ channels, inhibits glutamate release, weak carbonic anhydrase inhibitor
4. NOTE: this is a **sulfonamide** (<u>do not use if allergic!</u>)

5. Metabolized by CYP3A4 (inducers of CYP3A4, such as phenytoin, carbamazepine, or phenobarbital, will lower zonisamide blood levels
  i. Weak inhibitor of P-gp (MDR1)
6. Half-life of 63 hours (with EIAEDs, is 27-38 hours)
7. SEs: Somnolence, ataxia, headache, anorexia (with weight loss or gain), confusion, abnormal thinking, nervousness, fatigue, and dizziness, cognitive and psychiatric side effects (including depression, psychosis, and aggression)
  i. Rare kidney stones (1.5% incidence), ↓ sweating (in children), and SJS/TEN skin reactions
8. Available as 25 mg or 100 mg capsules
9. Dosing: 100 mg QD (or divided BID), with slow titration to a max. of 600 mg QD (or ÷ BID)
10. Therapeutic range has not been established, but suggested at 10-40 mcg/mL

## XIV. NON-PHARMACOLOGIC TREATMENTS
A. Ketogenic diet
B. Surgery
C. Vagus nerve stimulation

## XV. MECHANISM OF ACTION FOR VARIOUS ANTICONVULSANTS

| DRUGS THAT AFFECT SODIUM CHANNEL FUNCTIONS | | | |
|---|---|---|---|
| ◆ Carbamazepine | ◆ Felbamate | ◆ Oxcarbazepine | ◆ Topiramate |
| ◆ Eslicarbazepine | ◆ Lacosamide | ◆ Phenytoin | ◆ Valproic acid |
| ◆ Ethotoin | ◆ Lamotrigine | ◆ Rufinamide | ◆ Zonisamide |
| **DRUGS THAT AFFECT CALCIUM CHANNEL FUNCTIONS** | | | |
| ◆ Carbamazepine | ◆ Gabapentin | ◆ Phenobarbital | ◆ Valproic acid (?) |
| ◆ Clobazam (?) | ◆ Lamotrigine | ◆ Phenytoin (?) | ◆ Zonisamide |
| ◆ Ethosuximide | ◆ Levetiracetam (?) | ◆ Pregabalin | |
| ◆ Felbamate (?) | ◆ Oxcarbazepine | ◆ Topiramate (?) | |
| **DRUGS THAT AFFECT GABA ACTIVITY** | | | |
| ◆ Cannabidiol (?) | ◆ Gabapentin | ◆ Primidone | ◆ Vigabatrin |
| ◆ Clobazam | ◆ Lamotrigine (?) | ◆ Tiagabine | ◆ Zonisamide (?) |
| ◆ Clonazepam | ◆ Levetiracetam | ◆ Topiramate | |
| ◆ Felbamate | ◆ Phenobarbital | ◆ Valproic acid | |
| **DRUGS THAT AFFECT GLUTAMATE RECEPTORS** | | | |
| ◆ Carbamazepine (?) | ◆ Levetiracetam (?) | ◆ Phenobarbital | ◆ Valproic acid (?) |
| ◆ Felbamate | ◆ Oxcarbazepine (?) | ◆ Pregabalin (?) | ◆ Zonisamide |
| ◆ Lamotrigine | ◆ Perampanel | ◆ Topiramate | |
| **CARBONIC ANHYDRASE INHIBITORS** | | | |
| ◆ Topiramate | ◆ Zonisamide | | |
| **DRUGS THAT BIND TO SYNAPTIC VESICLE PROTEIN 2A (SV2A)** | | | |
| ◆ Brivaracetam | ◆ Levetiracetam | | (?) = Suspected MOA |

## XVI. DRIVING AND EPILEPSY
A. Each state has laws regulating the licensure of drivers who have a diagnosis of epilepsy. The interval of time a person has to go without having a seizure to qualify for licensure varies from 6 months to 2 years depending on the state and the specific driver' s condition or type of seizures.
  1. Driver Licensing Laws. Epilepsy Foundation website. Available at: http://www.epilepsy.com/search/site/driving?f[0]=bundle%3Adriving_laws
  2. Driving When You Have Had Seizures. U.S. Department of Transportation National Highway Traffic Safety Administration website. Available at: http://www.nhtsa.gov/people/injury/olddrive/Seizures%20Web

## XVII. PROPOSED ANTICONVULSANT THERAPEUTIC RANGES (EXTRAPOLATED)[1103,1115-1117]

| 1st Generation antiepileptics | | 2nd Generation antiepileptics | | 3rd Generation antiepileptics | |
|---|---|---|---|---|---|
| Drug | Therapeutic range (µg/mL) | Drug | Therapeutic range (µg/mL) | Drug | Therapeutic range (µg/mL) |
| Carbamazepine | 4-12 | Felbamate | 30-140 | Brivaracetam | Not known |
| Clonazepam | 20-70 ng/mL | Gabapentin | 4-20 | Clobazam | 30-300 |
| Ethosuximide | 40-100 | Lamotrigine | 1-20 | Eslicarbazepine | 3-35 |
| Ethotoin | 15-50 | Levetiracetam | 5-60 | Lacosamide | 1-15 |
| Phenobarbital | 15-40 | Oxcarbazepine | 10-40 | Perampanel | Not known |
| Phenytoin | 10-20 | Pregabalin | 2-5 | Rufinamide | 5-30 |
| Primidone | 5-12 | Tiagabine | 5-7 ng/mL | Vigabatrin | 20-160 |
| Valproic acid | 50-100 | Topiramate | 2-25 | | |
| | | Zonisamide | 10-40 | | |

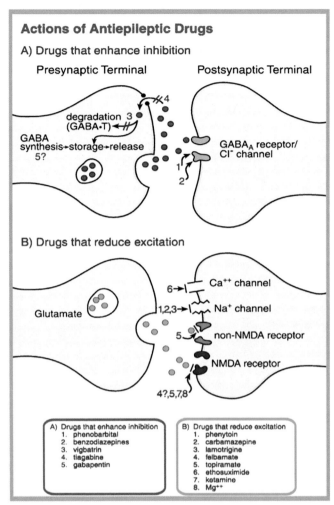

**Actions of Antiepileptic Drugs**

A) Drugs that enhance inhibition

Presynaptic Terminal                    Postsynaptic Terminal

degradation 3
(GABA·T)

GABA
synthesis→storage→release
5?

GABA$_A$ receptor/
Cl$^-$ channel

B) Drugs that reduce excitation

Glutamate

6→ Ca$^{++}$ channel

1,2,3→ Na$^+$ channel

5. non-NMDA receptor

NMDA receptor

4?,5,7,8

| A) Drugs that enhance inhibition | B) Drugs that reduce excitation |
|---|---|
| 1. phenobarbital | 1. phenytoin |
| 2. benzodiazepines | 2. carbamazepine |
| 3. vigbatrin | 3. lamotrigine |
| 4. tiagabine | 4. felbamate |
| 5. gabapentin | 5. topiramate |
| | 6. ethosuximide |
| | 7. ketamine |
| | 8. Mg$^{++}$ |

*Adapted from: http://pedsinreview.aappublications.org/content/19/10/342/F6.large.jpg*

XVIII. FUTURE POTENTIAL THERAPIES FOR SEIZURE DISORDERS
A. ADX71149 by Janssen Pharmaceuticals
  1. A novel, first-in-class potent, oral, small molecule positive allosteric modulator (PAM) of metabotropic glutamate receptor 2 (mGlu2)
    i. A Family C class of G Protein Coupled Receptor (GPCR).
  2. Acts synergistically with levetiracetam in preclinical models of epilepsy
    i. https://www.addextherapeutics.com/en/pipeline/researches/adx71149/
B. Deep brain stimulation targeting the anterior nucleus of the thalamus, the Entorhinal cortex, Fornix, and Hippocampus of the brain[1118]
C. Finteplar® (fenfluramine/ZX008) – by Zogenix Pharmaceuticals https://www.zogenix.com/pipeline
  1. Phase III study for Lennox-Gastaut Syndrome
  2. Post-Phase III study for Dravet Syndrome
    i. 64% reduction in seizures (Dravet Syndrome)[1119]
D. Ganaxolone (CCD-1042) from Marinus Pharmaceuticals
  1. GABA receptor positive allosteric modulator
  2. Phase III for Epilepsy

→ Benefits of medication must always outweigh risks!!!

## I. BACKGROUND
A. Baseline risk in the US for congenital malformations is 3-4%
1. 49% of pregnancies are unintended[1132]
2. 80-98% of teen pregnancies are unintended
B. At least 70% of pregnant women take at least 1 prescription medication[1133]
C. On 12/3/14, FDA established new standards for drug labeling on pregnancy and breastfeeding which replaces the current product letter categories – A, B, C, D and X (from 1979)[1134]
1. Went into effect on June 30, 2015, and applies retroactively to drugs approved after 6/30/01
2. Must have 3 sections labeled:
   i. *"Pregnancy,"* *"Lactation"* and *"Females and Males of Reproductive Potential"*
   ii. Each section has 3 subheadings: *"Risk summary,"* *"clinical considerations"* and *"data"*
D. Mental illness poses a great risk to an unborn child and mother such as suicide, accidents, substance abuse, medical disorders, placental abnormalities, antepartum hemorrhaging, prematurity, low birth weight, neonatal hypoglycemia, intrauterine growth retardation in the fetus, and ↑ likelihood of cesarean delivery[502]
1. Postpartum period is high risk time for first-onset or recurrent depression, bipolar, or psychosis
2. Bipolar women have a 25% risk for relapse following delivery
E. Excess weight gain and gestational diabetes - risk factors for congenital malformations
F. Useful resources:     http://www.motherisk.org/women/drugs.jsp
1. National Pregnancy Registry for Psychiatric Medications - 1-866-961-2388 or
   http://womensmentalhealth.org/clinical-and-research-programs/pregnancyregistry
2. Australian (PPMIS) Perinatal Psychotropic Medicines Information Service at:
   http://www.ppmis.org.au/
3. Canadian Centre for Addiction and Mental Health handbook available at: **Error! Hyperlink reference not valid.**
G. **Time Frame for Congenital Malformations During Gestation**

| Weeks | Body part or organ(s) involved | Possible birth defects |
|-------|-------------------------------|------------------------|
| 2-38 | Brain / spine | Neural tube defect |
| 3-9 | Heart | Ebstein's Anomaly / ventricle issues |
| 4-9 | Arms and legs | Lack of limb formation |
| 6-20 | Face, ears, eyes, cranium, and palate | Cleft lip / cleft palate / craniofacial anomalies |

## II. PREGNANCY CATEGORIES (USURPED BY NEW CLINICAL EVIDENCE CATEGORIES)
A. Category A
1. Animal and controlled human studies show no fetal risks; these drugs are considered the safest
B. Category B
1. Animal studies show no fetal risk, but controlled human studies have not been conducted, or
2. Animal studies show a risk to the fetus, but well-controlled human studies do not
C. Category C
1. No adequate animal or human studies have been conducted, or
2. Adverse fetal effects have been shown in animals, but human data is not available
D. Category D
1. Evidence of human fetal risk exists, but *benefits could outweigh risks in certain situations*
E. Category X
1. Proven fetal risks outweigh any possible benefit

## III. ANTIDEPRESSANTS
A. 55-85% relapse rates of non-treatment of depression in pregnancy
B. Most antidepressants are Category C, but maprotiline is Category B
1. Bupropion is very safe (absolute risk of an abnormality of 0.2%)
   i. It does cross the placenta and enters the fetal circulation, but significance is unknown[1135]
2. Paroxetine is Category D due to risk of CV malformations (right ventricular obstructions)
C. Brexanolone (Zulresso™) FDA-approved for Postpartum Depression (*see page 55 for details*)
D. SSRIs have small risk of Persistent Pulmonary Hypertension in the Newborn (PPHN)
1. FDA reports that the SSRI link to PPHN is unclear because some studies say yes, but others say no, or risk is small[1136]
   i. Meta-analysis showed SSRI-use in 2nd or 3rd trimester ↑ risk of PPHN by up to 6x [1137,1138]
   ii. 2016 Swedish study found 1.5x risk for newborn admission to the NICU (Neonatal ICU)[1139]
   a. NICU & PPHN risk was higher if SSRI used in late pregnancy (for PPHN, NNH was 285)
   b. Neonates also had more respiratory problems, CNS disorders, and hypoglycemia
2. 7-year study (2014) of depressed pregnant women: SSRIs <u>not</u> related to cardiac defects[1140]
3. SSRIs may ↑ pre-term birth risk & ↓ fetal head growth more than untreated depression[1141,1142]
4. In a 2017 review, SSRIs ↑ # of newborns who required minor respiratory support by 15.2%[1143]
   i. An ↑ of 5.3% of mothers also experienced hypertensive diseases during pregnancy
5. Up to 30% of infants exposed to an SSRI *in utero* experience withdrawal symptoms[1144]
6. Small study of 63 children found ↑ risk of Chiari Malformation, attributed to duration of SSRI exposure, SSRI exposure at conception, and family history of depression[1145]

7. SSRI-discontinuation during early pregnancy or 3-12 months before pregnancy are associated with a small ↑ risk of miscarriage[1146]
8. Recommended to continue SSRIs during pregnancy
9. Some birth defects may occur 2-3.5 X more frequently with paroxetine and fluoxetine[1147]
10. Overall, SSRIs do not increase risk of Autism Spectrum Disorder (ASD)[1148,1149]
    i. Some conflicting data shows that 1st trimester exposure in boys ↑ risk of ASD[1150]
    ii. 2017 meta-analysis did find an absolute increase in risk of ASD, but it was not statistically significant after adjusting for maternal mental illness[1151]
11. Retrospective study of Finnish mothers who filled at least 2 prescriptions for an SSRI during pregnancy revealed a significant 37% ↑ risk of speech/language disorders in their offspring[1152]
12. Long-term data shows no significant differences in neurobehavioral development in children of mothers who used antidepressants
13. Paroxetine: anencephaly, atrial septal defects, right ventricular outflow tract obstruction (5x normal)[1153], gastroschisis, and omphalocele
14. Fluoxetine: right ventricular outflow tract obstruction defects (2x normal) and craniosynostosis
15. Citalopram: neural tube defects (2.5 x normal)
E. Lactation
1. Most antidepressants can be used in breastfeeding with little problems if mother's need outweighs risk to infant[1154]
2. One open study found women taking SSRIs at time of birth were less likely to breastfeed than mothers where were not taking SSRIs[1155]
3. SSRIs and most TCAs considered safe, with rare infant side effects reported as reduced weight gain, ↑ crying, ↓ sleep, gastrointestinal distress, and irritability
4. 5-9% of mother's dose of fluoxetine is excreted in breast milk, so not 1st-line
5. Citalopram and escitalopram are not 1st-line and if used, high doses should be avoided
6. Doxepin should not be used (because of high concentrations of its metabolite)
7. Nefazodone should be avoided if possible
IV. ANXIOLYTICS / BZDs ("like EtOH in a pill") – Category D and X
A. Small risk of cleft palate (controversial)
B. BZD use early in pregnancy increases risk of spontaneous abortion by approx. 1.8 times[1156]
C. Lactation - low concentrations appear in breast milk
1. The more lipophilic the BZD, the higher the milk concentration (e.g., diazepam)
V. ANTIPSYCHOTICS - All considered relatively safe in pregnancy[1157]
A. No major congenital malformations seen vs. no medication treatment
1. Infrequent cases do exist, where reports of major malformations, gestational metabolic complications, poor pregnancy outcome, and perinatal adverse reactions have occurred
2. Risperidone is associated with a 26% ↑ risk in cardiac overall and malformations[1158]
    i. May be due to high levels of prolactin induced by risperidone
B. Most are Category C
C. Population-based study showed side effects = placebo on infant[1159]
D. No higher risk of gestational diabetes, HTN, venous thromboembolism, preterm birth, or change in birth weight found
E. Observational study found respiratory distress (37%) and drug withdrawal symptoms (15%) at birth with no permanent sequelae[1160]
F. National Pregnancy Registry for Atypical Antipsychotics (NPRAA)[1161]
1. At Massachusetts General Hospital
G. Watch for transient EPS (abnormal muscle movements), seizures, respiratory distress, feeding difficulties, tachycardia, and low BP in newborns
1. FGAs may cause EPS in the infant or other rare effects
2. FGAs have significantly ↑ rate of preterm birth vs. untreated women with schizophrenia[1157]
3. Avoid loxapine, thioridazine, thiothixene if possible
H. Significantly lower neuromotor-performance scores may also be seen[502]
I. Due to increased volume of distribution during pregnancy, higher doses may be needed[1162,1163]
J. ↑ risk of gestational diabetes seen
K. Clozapine and Lurasidone are Category B
1. Some reports of serious congenital anomalies and intellectual delays with clozapine[1160]
L. Lactation - little information available. SGAs considered relatively safe
1. Avoid iloperidone & ziprasidone (because of cardiac risks)
M. Postpartum psychosis occurs in 1-2 out of 1000 pregnancies
1. Suspect underlying bipolar disorder
2. High risk of harm to self and infant (4% infanticide rate)
VI. MOOD STABILIZERS (*See Bipolar Disorders for more information*)
→ Lithium, valproic acid, carbamazepine, lamotrigine
A. Risks with medications below are greatest in 1st trimester, when the heart and neural tube form
B. Pregnancy with untreated Bipolar Disorder incurs many risks, from mental to physical[502]
1. Higher risk of obesity, substance abuse, smoking, low birth weight, cesarian delivery, neonatal hypoglycemia, smaller infant head circumference, antepartum hemorrhaging
2. 25% risk of postpartum *psychosis*, mania and depression
3. 40% of time pregnant woman is ill without a mood stabilizer vs. 8.8% of time if on medication
C. Meta-analysis of 68 trials showed that antipsychotics were significantly more effective than mood stabilizers for acute mania (haloperidol was the best, but has risks of EPS)[502]

1. *Atypical antipsychotics* are preferred during pregnancy to classic mood stabilizers
2. Monotherapy at lowest effective doses preferred over polytherapy
D. Most mood stabilizers are Category D (known teratogenic effects) esp. in 1$^{st}$ trimester
E. Folic Acid supplementation reduces the risk of neural tube malformations
F. Lithium
  1. Avg. risk is 2.2- 2.41% for cardiac malformations during *first trimester* lithium exposure[1164,1165]
  2. Risk was found to be dose-dependent
    i. Risk ↑ 1.11 x normal at daily doses ≤ 600 mg
    ii. Risk ↑ 1.6 x normal for daily doses between 601 to 900 mg
    iii. Risk ↑ 3.22 x normal at daily doses > 900 mg
  3. Ebstein's anomaly
    i. Right ventricular outflow tract obstruction defect (displacement of the tricuspid valve leaflets)
    ii. Occurs in ≈ 6 in 1000 lithium-exposed births vs. 1.8 in 1000 in unexposed infants
      a. Risk ↑ 2.66 x normal
  4. Lithium effectively controls bipolar up to 80% of time while pregnant
  5. Volume of distribution and clearance increase, so must ↑ dose
  6. Transient hypotonicity, muscle twitching, breathing and feeding difficulties, cardiac arrythmias, and lethargy have been reported in lithium-exposed infants
  7. Lithium should be temporarily held for 1-2 days before birth (if possible)
  8. Lactation
    i. Infant serum concentration up to 40-50% of mother's concentration
    ii. Up to 30% of mother's lithium dose is excreted in breast milk[1166] (?? risk of infant toxicity)
      a. 2019 systematic review unable to conclude in concrete recommendations[1167]
      b. Decision must be personalized based on individual risk to benefit assessment
G. Valproic acid
  1. 5-11% overall risk of major congenital malformations
  2. Craniofacial defects, spina bifida (5-20X general population), cleft palate, pulmonary valve atresia, hypoplastic left heart syndrome, anorectal atresia, atrial/ventricular septal defects, hypospadia, and polydactyly
  3. Children may have a 10 point lower IQ and an increased risk of having autism[537,538,1168]
  4. Children also show ↓ gross motor skills, ↓ comprehension and expressive language abilities[1169]
  5. Lactation - Low concentrations in milk. Rare anemia and thrombocytopenia reported
    i. If it must be dosed, keep dose <1000 mg/d and give folic acid[502]
H. Carbamazepine
  1. 2-6% overall risk of major congenital malformations
    i. Cleft palate; also neural tube, cardiovascular, hypospadia & urinary tract defects noted
  2. Lactation - Low concentrations in milk. Rare transient hepatic dysfunction reported.
I. Lamotrigine - Category C
  1. 2-6% overall risk of major malformations
  2. Reports to the FDA of up to 25X higher risk of cleft palate, hypospadia, and other malformations have been seen
  3. Still the safest option for seizure control
  4. Pregnancy ↑ lamotrigine clearance > 50% (need ↑ dose)
  5. Lactation - Risks are unknown
VII. ANTICONVULSANTS[1170]
A. French study of over 1.8 million pregnancies and births looking at 23 specific malformations
B. All risks of malformations are increased with higher doses
C. Clonazepam (↑ risk of microcephaly (odds ratio 10.2) as well as atrial/ventricular septal defects)
D. Phenobarbital (↑ risk of ventricular septal defects (odds ratio 10.5))
E. Topiramate (↑ risk of cleft lip with or without cleft palate (odds ratio 6.8))
F. Pregabalin (↑ risk of coarctation of the aorta (odds ratio 5.8))
G. No significant association of malformations with lamotrigine, levetiracetam, oxcarbazepine and gabapentin found in study
H. Other anticonvulsants were not reported
VIII. CONTRACEPTION AND PSYCHOTROPICS[1121,1124]
A. Two methods of contraception are advised: hormonal and mechanical
B. Combined oral contraceptives with high dose progestin if taking an enzyme-inducing drug
C. Patients should take their pill continuously ("long cycle therapy")
D. Avoid progestin-only pills and subdermal progestogen implants because likely to be ineffective if used with an enzyme inducing antiepileptic drug (EIAED)[1171]
E. Depot medroxyprogesterone acetate (MPA) should be effective, but may have serious side effects, such as delayed return to fertility and impaired bone health
  1. Giving injection every 2 months (as opposed to every 3 months) is more effective
F. Levonorgestrel intrauterine system is effective, even with enzyme-inducing drugs
G. IUDs and condoms avoid drug-drug interactions

**I. INTRODUCTION**
A. Psychotropic use in the elderly has more than doubled in the last 15+ years[1172]
B. Many prescriptions do not match a formal diagnosis
C. The more medications a patient receives, the more likely an interaction is to occur
D. Drug interactions lead to hospitalizations and increase morbidity and mortality
E. Elderly are more sensitive to the cognitive side effects of drugs
F. Many psychotropics increase the risk of bone turnover and falls in the elderly
  1. Over half of elderly in the community are on a psychotropic that can lead to a fall[1173]
G. 15-25% of nursing home residents are receiving antipsychotics for various indications, many of which are not psychiatric[1174]
H. Antipsychotic use in the elderly significantly increases risk of death[1175]
I. All antipsychotics have a Black Box Warning for use in dementia patients
**II. POTENTIALLY INAPPROPRIATE MEDICATIONS USED IN OLDER ADULTS[1176,1177]**
A. 10-30% of hospital visits in older adults can be attributed to ADRs[1178]
B. **Beers List** / Criteria Compendium
  1. 2019 update is available - See https://onlinelibrary.wiley.com/doi/10.1111/jgs.15767 for full-text
  2. Printable pocket card (free for members) available at:
    i. https://geriatricscareonline.org/ProductAbstract/beers-criteria-pocketcard-2019/PC007
  3. Summary of drugs to be avoided in the elderly
    i. Anticholinergics & antihistamines with anticholinergic side effects
      a. Includes GI antispasmodics, TCAs, FGAs and antiparkinson medication
    ii. Benzodiazepines, barbiturates, non-BZD hypnotics ("Z-drugs"), and other CNS depressants
    iii. Synthetic hormones (estrogens & testosterone) unless need outweighs ↑ the risk of cancer
  4. Drugs to avoid in patients with a history of falls or fractures
    i. Antidepressants (TCAs, SSRIs, and *especially* SNRIs[1179])
    ii. Opiates, anticonvulsants, and antipsychotics
    iii. Mood stabilizers (lithium, valproate, carbamazepine, gabapentin, pregabalin)[1180]
    iv. Benzodiazepines, Z-drugs (zaleplon, zolpidem, eszopiclone)
  5. Also listed are drugs to avoid in renal dysfunction patients, list of drug-drug interactions, and drugs that are highly anticholinergic
  6. Drugs removed since the last 2015 list was published
    i. H2-receptor antagonists
    ii. Stimulants (amphetamines, decongestants, caffeine, etc.)
C. **START** (Screening Tool to Alert to Right Treatment) and **STOPP** criteria (Screening Tool of Older People's Potentially Inappropriate Prescriptions)[1181,1182]
  1. Available free at: http://ageing.oxfordjournals.org/content/44/2/213
  2. More stringent than BEERS criteria and identifies more inappropriate medications
  3. Includes drug-disease interactions and tries to reduce adverse drug effects
  4. As an intervention applied within 72 h of hospitalization, it can significantly reduce ADRs
    i. Over 40% of ADRs in long-term care of the elderly are preventable[1183]
D. BZDs ↑ risk of hip fractures, delirium, cognitive impairment, auto accidents, & death[1184,1185]
  1. Data shows that in the community, up to 30% of elderly with Alzheimer's and 26% without Alzheimer's are prescribed long-term BZDs (>180 days)[337-340]
  2. Risk of re-hospitalization within 30 days is statistically ↑ for patients on BZDs[1186]
  3. Rapid inpatient discontinuation of BZDs very successful & results in shorter length of stays[1187]
E. Long-term and higher cumulative dosing of anticholinergic drugs almost doubles the risk for dementia and Alzheimer's Disease later in life[1188]
F. Case-control study found that compared with nonuse, anticholinergics ↑ the risk of dementia[1189]
  1. Adjusted odds ratios ranged from 1.16 to 2 times increased risk
    i. Antidepressants -- 1.29 times increased risk
    ii. Antiparkinson drugs -- 1.52 times increased risk
    iii. Antipsychotics -- 1.70 times increased risk
    iv. Bladder antimuscarinics -- 1.65 times increased risk
    v. Antiepileptic drugs -- 1.39 times increased risk
G. Study of > 5000 geriatric patients found 37% received 1 anticholinergic drug and 11% received 2 or more[1190]
H. Anticholinergic effects
  1. Quantifiable using the Anticholinergic Cognitive Burden Scale (ACB)[1191-1194]
  2. Sample scale at: www.agingbraincare.org/uploads/products/ACB_scale_-_legal_size.pdf
  3. ACB score of ≥ 3 = definite/high anticholinergic activity of medication
  4. ACB score of ≥ 3 may ↑ the risk of cognitive impairment by 46% over 6 years
  5. For each point increase in the ACB total score:
    i. Decline of 0.33 points in MMSE score of over 2 years is possible
    ii. Correlated with a 26% ↑ in the risk of death
  6. Almost 50% of community-dwelling elderly have medications ≥3 on ACB[1195]
  7. One observational study of hospitalized patients with acquired brain or spinal injury found a direct correlation of a higher ACB score on discharge, (compared with on admission) was associated with a longer length of stay (lower ACB = shorter length of stay)[1196]

## I. ANTICHOLINERGIC ACTIVITY OF FREQUENTLY USED MEDICATIONS[1197-1199]

| | | | |
|---|---|---|---|
| + Amantadine | + Dicyclomine | + Meclizine | + Propantheline |
| + Atropine | + Digoxin | + Mepenzolate | + Ranitidine |
| + Benztropine | + Dimenhydrinate | + Methscopolamine | + Scopolamine |
| + Chlorpheniramine | + Diphenhydramine | + Nifedipine | + Solifenacin |
| + Chlorpromazine | + Diphenoxylate | + Olanzapine | + Theophylline |
| + Cimetidine | + Disopyramide | + Orphenadrine | + Thioridazine |
| + Clozapine | + Fesoterodine | + Oxybutynin | + Tolterodine |
| + Cyclizine | + Furosemide | + Paroxetine | + Tricyclic antidepressants |
| + Cyclobenzaprine | + Glycopyrrolate | + Prednisone | + Trihexyphenidyl |
| + Cyproheptadine | + Hydroxyzine | + Prochlorperazine | + Trimethobenzamide |
| + Dantrolene | + Hyoscyamine | + Promethazine | + Trospium |

## J. DRUGS THAT MIMIC OR CAUSE COGNITIVE IMPAIRMENT

| | | | |
|---|---|---|---|
| + *Alpha2* agonists | + Antihistamines | + Corticosteroids | + Lithium |
| + Anticholinergics | + Antiparkinsonian agents | + Digoxin | + Narcotics |
| + Anticonvulsants | + Antipsychotics | + Disopyramide | + Sedative/hypnotics |
| + Antidepressants | + Cimetidine | + Indomethacin | |
| + Antiemetics | + Skeletal Muscle Relaxants | | |

## III. NEUROCOGNITIVE DISORDERS
A. Higher rates of depression and suicide, due to medical comorbidities and declining function[1200]
  1. Includes: Delirium, Dementia, Traumatic Brain Injury, Alzheimer's, and others

## IV. DELIRIUM
A. DELIRIUM occurs suddenly and is usually caused by another factor, such as drugs/medications, drug withdrawal, physical trauma, or infections (e.g., urinary tract, respiratory)
B. Delirium develops quickly, and symptoms may fluctuate during the day
  1. May resolve within hours or last months
C. Resolving any underlying causes is imperative
  1. Refer to Schizophrenia Chapter (*see page 82*) -
    "Underlying Triggers of Delirium and Psychosis"
  2. Can be drug-induced or medically-induced
    (e.g., UTI, hypoglycemia)
  3. Delirium is usually correctable by fixing the cause
  4. UTIs, respiratory infections, and dehydration: can induce psychosis/delirium

| DELIRIUM CAUSES | |
|---|---|
| **I** | Infections |
| **W** | Withdrawals (drug & alcohol) |
| **A** | Age / elderly |
| **T** | Trauma |
| **C** | Cardiac (post-surgery) / CNS |
| **H** | Hypoxia |
| **D** | vitamin Deficiencies |
| **E** | Electrolyte imbalances (burn patients) |
| **A** | Acute metabolic changes |
| **T** | Toxins |
| **H** | HIV / Heavy metal |

## V. DEMENTIA
A. DEMENTIA is termed in the DSM-5 as a major Neurocognitive Disorder (NCD)
B. Symptoms usually appear gradually, as in Alzheimer's disease
C. Trauma, Vascular, Parkinson's, or Huntington's onset may be abrupt or gradual, but persistent
D. Dementia has a *slow* onset over many years or decades
E. Types:
  1. Alzheimer's, Creutzfeldt-Jakob disease, Frontotemporal, Lewy Body, Multi-infarct, normal pressure hydrocephalus, Parkinson's disease, tertiary syphilis, vascular, frontotemporal, & others
F. Common symptoms
  1. Abnormal motor movements, agitation, anger, anxiety (20%), apathy, balance problems, changes in sleep or appetite, crying, delusions (i.e., theft), depression (20-30%), disinhibition, elated mood, hallucinations, impulsivity, irritability, memory problems, restlessness, speech and language difficulty, tremor, trouble eating or swallowing, wandering

## VI. TRAUMATIC BRAIN INJURY (TBI) AND TREATMENTS[1201-1203]
A. *Brain Trauma Foundation* guidelines[1204] (https://www.braintrauma.org/coma/guidelines)
B. 1.7-2.8 million brain injuries occur each year
  1. Mostly in children, adolescents, men and seniors (highest in those > 75 y.o.)
  2. 80% are mild / 10% are moderate / 10% are severe (overall incidence: 14/100,000 people)
C. Head injuries have multiple causes
  1. Falls (#1 cause of brain injuries), followed by assaults and car accidents
  2. Closed head: stroke, hematoma, contusions (brain bruise), concussions (have loss of consciousness)
  3. Diffuse axonal injury (DAI) can occur from concussive forces (i.e., explosion) or sudden acceleration-deceleration
  4. Penetrating - skull fracture from trauma
D. Highest risk of mortality in the first 9 hours
E. Cerebral edema peaks between 48 & 96 hours
F. Tranexamic acid (loading dose 1 g over 10 min then infusion of 1 g over 8 h) within 3 hours of TBI was associated with a 20% $\downarrow$ in deaths among those with mild to moderate (but not severe) TBI[1205]
G. Medications to decrease intracranial pressure (ICP)
  1. Mannitol
  2. Hypertonic saline (50:50 mix of NaCl to Na+ acetate to $\downarrow$ hyperchloremic metabolic acidosis)
  3. Albumin is not recommended

H. To decrease oxygen demand of the brain, use pentobarbital or propofol (or extreme cooling)
I. N-acetylcysteine given in the hours after a TBI may ↓ oxidative damage and speed healing[1206]
J. Some patients develop seizures, increased (ICP), emotional changes, sensitivity to noise and light, dementia, headaches, and movement disorders
K. Prophylactic anticonvulsants (phenytoin, levetiracetam, carbamazepine) recommended within 7 days
  1. Valproate and phenobarbital are not recommended
L. Even mild TBI can double the risk of dementia later in life
M. Approx. 30% develop depression within 1st year
  1. Prophylactic antidepressant therapy can reduce that incidence four-fold
N. Other medication management

| Medication[1207-1211] | Target symptoms |
|---|---|
| Beta-blockers: propranolol, pindolol | Agitation |
| Buspirone | Anxiety |
| CDP (cytidine diphospheryl) choline | Cognition, executive function and inattention |
| Cholinesterase inhibitors: donepezil, rivastigmine | Cognitive impairment, executive function deficits, inattention, memory deficits, difficulty learning new information |
| Dopamine agonists: amantadine, bromocriptine | Cognitive deficits |
| Methylphenidate | Apathy, amotivation, arousal, attention, and processing speed and general cognitive function |
| Modafinil or armodafinil | Persistent daytime sleepiness |
| NMDA antagonists: memantine, amantadine | General neuroprotective effects: cognition, executive function, improves coma scores/arousal, attention, visuospatial function, social inappropriateness, lack of judgement & insight |
| • Amantadine | Impulsivity, disinhibition and poor motivation |
| • Memantine | Significantly reduces serum neuron-specific enolase levels after injury |
| Prazosin (Minipress®) | Persistent nightmares |
| Quetiapine (1st-line), risperidone (2nd-line), lithium (3rd-line) | Acute mania, aggression |
| Quetiapine, lurasidone, or risperidone (1st-line) Clozapine, ziprasidone (2nd-line) | Psychosis, agitation, aggression |
| Ramelteon | Significantly affects total sleep time and improves cognition |
| SSRIs/SNRIs – preferred 1st-line agents (less drug interactions): sertraline, escitalopram, citalopram, venlafaxine 2nd-line: fluoxetine, mirtazapine *Avoid benzodiazepines!* | Depression (and prevention of), PTSD, Panic and anxiety |
| Triptans, NSAIDs, acetaminophen & other non-narcotic analgesics | Headaches, migraines |
| Valproic acid (1st-line), carbamazepine (2nd-line) | Bipolar/mania maintenance |
| Zolpidem, zopiclone, melatonin, amitriptyline (2nd-line), lorazepam (last-line) | Insomnia |

O. Medications that are not recommended:
  1. Typical antipsychotics, benzodiazepines, and anticholinergics can worsen symptoms
  2. Avoid phenytoin and lithium if possible due to neurotoxicity
P. **POTENTIAL FUTURE THERAPIES FOR TBI IN STUDY**[1212]
  1. AVP-786/AVP-923 (deuterium-modified dextromethorphan + quinidine) by Otsuka/Avanir
   i. Sigma-1 (σ1) receptor agonist, SNRI, and NMDA receptor antagonist
   ii. Phase II for Disinhibition Syndrome in neuro-degenerative disorders
  2. NeuroSTAT® (Ciclosporin-A) - targets cellular mitochondria to counteract the emergence of neurological and functional secondary brain damage
   i. In Phase II STUDY - Decreased brain injury volume by 35%
    a. https://www.liebertpub.com/doi/10.1089/neu.2018.6369
   ii. In July 2019, NeuroSTAT received Fast Track designation from the FDA

# 33. ALZHEIMER'S DISEASE AND OTHER DEMENTIAS

I. Background
   A. Named after Alois Alzheimer, the neuropathologist who discovered the disease in 1906
   B. 60-70% of dementias are Alzheimer's
   C. Involves progressive synthesis of diffuse and neuritic plaques with an aggregation of β-amyloid (aβ), a proteolytic fragment derived from amyloid precursor protein (aPP)
   D. Intracellular neurofibrillary tangles from hyperphosphorylated microtubule-associated protein tau (τ) with subsequent neurodegeneration
   E. May also involve Lewy bodies (abnormal *alpha*-synuclein accumulation)
   F. **Mini-mental Status Exam (MMSE)**
      1. Used to thoroughly assess mental status – can be used repeatedly and routinely
      2. 11-questions test five areas of cognitive function
      i. Orientation, registration, attention and calculation, recall, and language.
      3. Maximum score is 30 (a score of $\leq$ 23 indicates cognitive impairment
      4. Estimated annual *decrease* in MMSE is 4-5 with all types of dementia
II. Behavioral interventions are 1st-line treatments
III. Cholinesterase inhibitors (donepezil, galantamine, rivastigmine) and NMDA antagonist (memantine)
   A. In moderate-to-severe disease, the combination of a cholinesterase inhibitor with memantine was no different than without memantine[1213]
   B. Anticholinergic drugs can counteract the benefits of cholinesterase inhibitors (e.g., donepezil) or cause confusion and memory loss
   C. Altogether, may delay progression of cognitive decline by approx. 3 months and $\uparrow$ MMSE 1 point[1214]
      1. Effects are greater in Lewy Body & Parkinson's Dementia than Alzheimer's and vascular dementia
IV. **Black Box Warning** for ALL typical and atypical antipsychotics' use in dementia
   A. 1.6-1.7x $\uparrow$ risk of death (CV, infection, other)[1071,1073]
      1. Atypicals still preferred over typical antipsychotics if patient is psychotic
   B. Adjusted absolute mortality risk difference[1215]
      1. 3.8% for haloperidol (higher at higher doses)
      2. 3.7% for risperidone (higher at higher doses)
      3. 2.5% for olanzapine
      4. 2.0% for quetiapine
      i. American Psychiatric Association advises against using antipsychotics for behavioral issues in dementia, unless patient is psychotic, manic, or violent[452]
   C. Psychosis & agitation are more highly correlated with earlier death in elderly vs. antipsychotics[1216]
V. To date, no medications are <u>proven</u> to help with Alzheimer's apathy
   A. Methylphenidate may have therapeutic benefits[1217]
VI. **ALZHEIMER'S MEDICATIONS**
   A. Acetylcholinesterase Inhibitors (AchEIs)
      1. Meta-analysis of 80 trials revealed AchEIs 2 x as effective in Parkinson's & Lewy body dementia[1218]
      2. Common side effects: Anorexia, weight loss, nausea, vomiting, diarrhea, headache, dizziness, dyspepsia, asthenia, muscle cramps, fatigue, and ecchymosis
      3. Cautions: bradycardia, heart block, GI bleeding, bladder outflow obstructions, seizures
      i. Asthma or COPD – prescribe with caution
      ii. NOTE: Tacrine (Cognex®) removed from the market in 2013 due to severe hepatotoxicity
      4. Donepezil (Aricept®)[87]
      i. Indicated for treatment of mild, moderate, and severe Alzheimer's disease
      ii. Additional effects: inhibits various aspects of glutamate-induced excitotoxicity, reduces early expression of inflammatory cytokines and reduces oxidative stress-induced effects[1219]
         a. Highly selective for AChE (acetylcholinesterase) compared with butyrylcholinesterase (BChE)
      iii. Adult Dose: 5 mg QD; may $\uparrow$ to 10 mg QD after 4 to 6 weeks
         a. Dose may be $\uparrow$ to 23 mg once daily after use of 10 mg dose for at least 3 months
         b. No dose adjustments are indicated for renal or hepatic impairment
      iv. Available in 5, 10, & 23 mg tablets and 5 & 10 mg orally disintegrating tablets (ODT)
      v. 96% protein bound with a t½ of 70 hours
      vii. Metabolized by CYP2D6 and CYP3A4
      5. Galantamine (Razadyne®, Razadyne ER®)[89]
      i. Indicated for mild to moderate Alzheimer's disease
      ii. Derived from an alkaloid naturally present in many plants, including daffodil bulbs[1219]
         a. Used as a medicine in Russia and eastern European countries for the treatment of myopathy, myasthenia, and sensory and motor deficits of the CNS
         b. Also binds to nicotinic cholinergic receptors
      iii. Adult Dose: 4 mg BID (or 8 mg ER QD); may $\uparrow$ by 8 mg Q 4 weeks, up to a max of 24 mg/d
         a. Max dose for moderate hepatic or renal impairment (CrCl 9-59 mL/min) is 16 mg/d
         b. Do not use in severe hepatic or renal impairment
      iv. Available in 4 mg, 8 mg, and 12 mg IR tablets, 8 mg, 16 mg, and 24 mg ER capsules, and 4 mg/mL oral solution
      v. Side effects: highest incidence of GI side effects of the acetylcholinesterase inhibitors
      vi. 18% protein bound
      vii. Half-life: 7 hours
      viii. Metabolized by CYP2D6 and CYP3A4

6. Rivastigmine tartrate (Exelon® / Exelon Patch®)[97]
   i. Indicated for mild to moderate Alzheimer's disease and Parkinson's-related dementia
     a. Patch indicated for *severe* Alzheimer's and *mild to moderate* Parkinson-related dementia
   ii. A reversible inhibitor of both AChE and butyrylcholinesterase (BChE)
   iii. Adult oral dose
     a. Slow dose titrations suggested for low body weight (less than 50 kg)
     b. 1.5 mg BID with **FOOD** and may ↑ by 1.5 mg BID in 2 week intervals (max of 6 mg BID)
     c. Adjust doses for moderate to severe renal or mild to moderate hepatic impairment
   iv. Transdermal patch
     a. 4.6 mg/24 hours once daily; may ↑ to 9.5 mg/24 hours QD after 4 weeks
       1. Can ↑ to 13.3 mg/24 hours QD if decline in efficacy of 9.5 mg patch occurs
     b. Mild to moderate hepatic impairment: maximum dose 4.6 mg/24 hours
       1. Not studied in severe hepatic impairment
   v. Available in 1.5 mg, 3 mg, 4.5 mg, and 6 mg capsules and 4.6 mg/24 hours, 9.5 mg/24 hours, and 13.3 mg/24 hours transdermal patches
     a. Oral solution (2 mg/mL) was supposedly discontinued in 2014, but still in its package insert
   vi. Concomitant metoclopramide (↑ risk of EPS side effects), cholinomimetics (synergistic effects), *beta*-blockers (↑ risk of syncope), or anticholinergic medications (antagonistic effects) is not recommended
   vii. Watch for disseminated allergic contact dermatitis
   viii. 40% protein bound
   ix. Half-life - Oral: 1.5 hours / Transdermal patch: 3 hours (after removal)
   x. Metabolized by cholinesterase-mediated hydrolysis in the brain

B. NMDA Antagonists
  1. Memantine (Namenda®, Namenda XR®)[92]
   i. A noncompetitive NMDA receptor antagonist of moderate affinity
   ii. Indicated for moderate to severe Alzheimer's disease
   iii. Adult Dose: 5 mg/d IR (7 mg/d XR); may ↑ by 5 mg/d IR (7 mg/d XR) at weekly intervals to a target dose of 20 mg/d IR (28 mg/d XR)
     a. Doses above 5 mg/d should be divided BID (immediate-release tablets)
     b. Max of 5 mg BID (or 14 mg XR) in severe renal impairment (CrCl 5-29 mL/min)
   iv. Available in 5 mg and 10 mg IR tablets, 7 mg, 14 mg, 21 mg, and 28 mg XR capsules, and 10 mg/5 mL oral solution (titration packs are available)
   v. Side effects similar to AchEIs
   vi. 45% protein bound
   vii. Half-life: 60-80 hours
   viii. Only partially metabolized (not by CYP system!); about 50% renally eliminated
   ix. Alkaline urine with increase plasma levels (e.g., use of carbonic anhydrase inhibitors or $NaCO_2$
  2. Memantine XR + donepezil (Namzaric™)[93] combination capsules taken each evening
   i. Patients on memantine 10 mg BID and donepezil 10 mg/d → Namzaric 28 mg/10 mg
     a. Available in combination tablets of <u>10 mg donepezil</u> + 7, 14, 21, or 28 mg memantine
   ii. In severe renal impairment, do not exceed 14 mg/10mg
  3. Selegiline (MAO-B inhibitor) has antioxidant properties (*see page 137 in Parkinson's Disease*)
C. Ineffective or unproven therapies[1220]
  1. Estrogen, gingko biloba, anti-inflammatories, statin drugs, Vitamin B, and Omega-3 fatty acids
D. Kinetics of Alzheimer's Disease Medications

| Generic | Brand | Average Adult Dose | Half-life | CYP450 Substrate |
|---|---|---|---|---|
| Donepezil | Aricept® | 10 mg/d | 70 hours | 2D6 and 3A4 (minor) |
| Rivastigmine | Exelon® | 6 mg/d (oral)<br>9.5 mg/d (patch) | 1.5 hours (oral)<br>3 hours (patch) | N/A |
| Galantamine | Razadyne®<br>Razadyne ER® | IR: 8 mg twice daily<br>ER: 16 mg once daily | 7 hours | 2D6 and 3A4 (minor) |
| Memantine | Namenda®<br>Namenda XR® | IR: 20 mg/d<br>XR: 21 mg/d | 60-80 hours | N/A |

## VII. COMPLEMENTARY AND ALTERNATIVE THERAPIES
A. Naturally occurring Lithium in drinking water may reduce the incidence of developing dementia[1221]
B. Cerefolin NAC caplets (L-methylfolate calcium (Metafolin®) 6 mg, Algae-S powder (schizochytrium is an algae that produces DHA (Docosahexaenoic Acid)) 90.314 mg, methylcobalamin (Vitamin B12) 2 mg, and N-acetylcysteine 600mg
  1. A "medical food" approved for mild cognitive impairment taken once a day
  2. Made by Alfasigma USA, Inc.
  3. Interactions with concomitant nitrates → increased risk of headaches
    4. Adverse Reactions: N/V/D, allergic reactions, itching, rash, fever, flushing, edema, GI pain
C. Vitamin E (alpha-tocopherol) at > 2000 international units daily
D. Bacopa monnieri/Brahmi (Water hysop)[360]
  1. Commonly used in Ayurvedic (traditional Indian) medicine to improve memory and cognition
  2. Benefits are thought to be from triterpenoid saponins known as bacosides
  3. Common side effects: nausea, increased gastrointestinal motility and gastrointestinal upset
E. Huperzine (Hup) - a lycopodium alkaloid isolated from the Chinese club moss herb, *Huperzia serrata*

1. More effective than rivastigmine and galantamine at inhibiting AChE
2. **Huperzine A** is currently in Phase II & III trials for Alzheimer's and Schizophrenia

## VIII. POTENTIAL FUTURE THERAPIES FOR ALZHEIMER'S AND OTHER DEMENTIAS IN STUDY

A. AC-1204 by Cerecin in Phase II/III for mild to moderate Alzheimer's Disease (NCT01741194)
   1. Contains 20 g of caprylic (octanoic acid) triglyceride, given QD
B. ACE inhibitor + calcium channel blocker + exercise (ClinicalTrials.gov Identifier: NCT02913664)
   1. The University of Texas Southwestern Medical Center is evaluating if exercise + losartan + amlodipine reduces the risk of cognitive decline in AD (Phase II/III)
C. Aducanumab (BART/ BIIB 037) by Biogen/Neurimmune Therapeutics
   1. Anti-beta amyloid monoclonal antibody
   2. In Phase III trials, but Biogen plans to apply for FDA approval in early 2020
D. AGB101 by AgeneBio (https://www.agenebio.com/pipeline)
   1. A GABA$_A$ α5 Positive Allosteric Modulator (PAM)
   2. A proprietary once-daily, low-dose, extended-release formulation of levetiracetam (220 mg)
   3. Also being studied for Autism and Schizophrenia
   4. In Phase III study (HOPE4MCI) for mild cognitive impairment (MCI) is expected to complete in late 2022
E. Alfoatirin® (choline alphoscerate 400 mg bid) with donepezil 10 mg qd for 24 weeks
   1. By Yuhan Corporation in Phase IV trials
   2. Will measure cognitive performance on the Alzheimer's Disease Assessment Scale-cognitive subscale (ADAS-cog) (ClinicalTrials.gov Identifier: NCT03441516)
F. ALZT-OP1 by AZTherapies, Inc. in Phase III study for early Alzheimer's
   1. ALZT-OP1a (cromolyn) for inhalation plus ALZT-OP1b (ibuprofen) tablet vs. placebo
   2. ClinicalTrials.gov Identifier: NCT02547818
G. Amilomotide (CAD106) by Novartis in Phase II & III trials
   1. *Beta*-amyloid-protein therapy
H. Antidepressants show promise in reducing incidence of Alzheimer's[1222]
   1. In mice and humans, antidepressants significantly reduce amyloid beta protein production, which, in excess, clump and cause plaques in the brain
I. AVN-101 by Avineuro Pharmaceuticals (Phase II for Alzheimer's)
   1. 5HT$_6$ receptor antagonist
J. AVP-786/AVP-923 (deuterium-modified dextromethorphan + quinidine) by Otsuka/Avanir Pharma
   1. Sigma-1 (σ1) receptor agonist, SNRI, and NMDA receptor antagonist
   2. Phase III for agitation associated with dementia of the Alzheimer's type
K. AXS-05 - (bupropion/dextromethorphan fixed-dose combination) by Axsome Therapeutics for agitation in Alzheimer's (Phase II/III)
L. Azeliragon (TTP488) by VTV Therapeutics (http://vtvtherapeutics.com/pipeline/azeliragon)
   1. An orally bioavailable small molecule that inhibits the receptor for advanced glycation end-products (RAGE) (ClinicalTrials.gov Identifier: NCT02080364)
   2. In Phase II/III clinical trials for treatment of mild-AD in patients with type 2 diabetes
M. BAN2401 by BioArctic Neuroscience/Biogen/Eisai Co Ltd in Phase III study
   1. Amyloid beta-protein inhibitor (ClinicalTrials.gov Identifier: NCT03887455)
   2. Evaluating efficacy in early AD on the change from baseline in the Clinical Dementia Rating-Sum of Boxes (CDR-SB)
   3. 18-month study is projected to be complete in 2024
N. BI-409306 (SUB-166499) by Boehringer Ingelheim
   1. A phosphodiesterase 9A inhibitor in Phase II (also for Schizophrenia)
O. Blarcamesine (ANAVEX2-73) by Anavex Life Sciences Corp. (https://www.anavex.com)
   1. Sigma-1 and muscarinic receptor agonist which blocks tau hyperphosphorylation in Phase IIb/III
   2. An aminotetrahydrofuran derivative - ClinicalTrials.gov Identifier: NCT03790709
   3. "High dose" vs. "Mid dose" vs. placebo capsules QD for 48 weeks in early AD
   4. Also being studied for Parkinson's disease, Angelman Syndrome and Rett Syndrome
P. BNC-210 (IW-2143) by Bionomics and Ironwood Pharmaceuticals
   1. "GABA modulator" – a negative allosteric modulator (antagonist) of the α7 nicotinic Ach receptor
   2. Doses of 150 mg, 300 mg and 600 mg BID for 12 weeks studied for agitation in dementia
   3. Also in Phase II trials for PTSD and Generalized Anxiety Disorder
Q. Brexpiprazole (Lu AF41156, OPC-34712; Rexulti) by Otsuka/Lundbeck
   1. Phase III, but Fast tracked by the FDA for Agitation associated with Alzheimer's dementia
   2. Doses studied: 2 mg and 3 mg po QD (NCT03594123)
R. Carvedilol Being studied by Johns Hopkins University in Phase IV
   1. To measure decline in episodic memory in participants with early AD (NCT01354444)
S. COR388 by Cortexyme Inc. in Phase II/III study (ClinicalTrials.gov Identifier: NCT03823404)
   1. A peptide hydrolase inhibitor
   2. 40 mg or 80 mg given po BID vs. placebo
T. Crenezumab (MABT5102A, R 5490245, RG 7412, RO5490245, RG7412)
   1. By Roche/AC Immune/Genentech/Universidad-de-Antioquia
   2. Amyloid beta-protein antibody
   3. Phase III done 2018 - data presented at 2018/2019 Alzheimer's Association International Conferences
U. DB105 / ORM-12741 by Denovo Biopharma
   1. Two Phase II trials completed with positive results on quality of memory
   2. An α$_{2C}$ (*alpha* adrenergic-2C) receptor antagonist
V. Deep brain stimulation of the Fornix and nucleus basalis of Meynert[1118]
W. BNC375 by Bionomics and Merck & Co.

    1. An $\alpha_7$ (*alpha*-7) nicotinic acetylcholine receptor modulator
    2. In Phase I trials for cognitive disorders
X. D-Cycloserine[357]
Y. Elenbecestat (E2609) by Eisai Co., Ltd. and Biogen
    1. In Phase III trials for safety and efficacy of 50 mg QD
    2. ClinicalTrials.gov Identifiers: NCT02956486 and NCT03036280
    3. Expected completion in November 2023
Z. Gantenerumab R-1450; RG-1450; RO-4909832 by Roche and Chugai Pharmaceutical
    1. An amyloid beta-protein inhibitor
    2. Phase III trials completed in 2018 and data presented at the 2018 & 2019 Alzheimer's Association International Conferences
AA. Ginkgo Biloba ester dispersible tablets vs. donepezil vs. both combined
    1. In Phase II/III study in China by The First Affiliated Hospital with Nanjing Medical University
    2. ClinicalTrials.gov Identifier: NCT03090516
AB. Hydromethylthionine mesylate (TRx0237) as leuco-methylthioninium bis(hydromethanesulphonate) (LMTX®) - ClinicalTrials.gov Identifier: NCT03446001
    1. TauRx Pharmaceuticals' second-generation tau aggregation inhibitor (TAI)[1223,1224]
    2. Also being studied for Behavioral Variant Frontotemporal Dementia (bvFTD) – Pick's disease
    3. Doses of 8 and 16 mg/d (divided BID) and 150-250 mg/day vs. placebo
AC. Inhaled intranasal insulin is being explored[1225]
AD. Ladostigil hemitartrate – Phase II by Avraham Pharma
    1. Inhibits AChE, BChE, and MAO-B
    2. Neuroprotective (anti-apoptotic and anti-inflammatory) properties and reduces oxidative stress
    3. Only being studied for mild cognitive impairment, not Alzheimer's
AE. Levomilnacipran (Fetzima®)
    1. Found to inhibit β-amyloid plaque formation and reduce the progression of Alzheimer's[677]
AF. Lithium by the National Institute on Aging (NIA) and the University of Pittsburgh Medical Center
    1. Study of its ability prevent cognitive decline in people diagnosed with Mild Cognitive Impairment
    2. "Lithium treatment has been associated with neurogenesis in the hippocampus, up-regulation of important neurotrophic factors such as B-cell lymphoma 2 (Bcl-2) and brain-derived neurotrophic factor (BDNF), and inhibition of glycogen synthase kinase 3 (GSK-3) isoforms α and β."
    3. ClinicalTrials.gov Identifier: NCT03185208 – Estimated completion in 2022
    4. Lithium will be slowly titrated to a blood level between 0.6 and 0.8 mEq/L for 2 years
AG. Masupirdine (SUVN-502) by Suven Life Sciences in Phase II study
    1. A potent, orally active, $5HT_6$ receptor antagonist with CNS penetration
    2. http://www.suven.com/drugdiscoveryresearch.aspx#clinical-pipeline-section
AH. Nabilone by Sunnybrook Health Sciences Centre in Phase II/III study
    1. For the treatment of outpatients with moderate to severe AD and agitation
    2. A Δ9-tetrahydrocannabinol (THC) analogue
AI. NBTX-001 (the noble gas xenon) by Nobilis Therapeutics[430]
    1. Antagonist of NMDA, AMPA, nicotinic ACh (α4β2), $5HT_3$, & plasma membrane $Ca^{2+}$ ATPase
    2. Currently in Phase III trials using the Zephyrus™ inhalational Device
    3. Also in Phase II for Irritable Bowel Syndrome (IBS), Autism, & Parkinson's Disease
AJ. NeuroAD™ Therapy System by Neuronix Ltd. (https://www.fda.gov/media/122847/download)
    1. Neuro-stimulation via transcranial direct current stimulation (tDCS) given concurrently with cognitive training for mild to moderate dementia (ClinicalTrials.gov Identifier: NCT02772185)
    2. Dramatic benefits seen in ~1/3 of patients, and some benefit for an additional 1/3 of the population
    3. In Phase II/III trials in Brazil, but trials are also being conducted in Israel, the U.S., and Korea
AK. NNI-362 by Neuronascent, Inc. in Phase Ia trials
    1. A novel class of drugs, called "Neuron Regenerative therapies"
    2. To reverse the cognitive deficit in AD patients by stimulating new neurons and protecting "nascent" neurons from further neurodegeneration" - https://www.neuronascent.com/
AL. Octohydroaminoacridine Succinate (an aminoacridine and acetylcholinesterase inhibitor)
    1. ClinicalTrials.gov Identifier: NCT03283059
    2. At the Shanghai Mental Health Center by Changchun Huayang High-tech
    3. Doses: 4 mg po TID tablet vs. donepezil 5 mg QD for Mild-to-Moderate Alzheimer's Disease
AM. Pimavanserin (Nuplazid; ACP-103; BVF-048) by ACADIA Pharmaceuticals
    1. In Phase III for Dementia-related Psychosis (*See page 96 for more information*)
AN. Piromelatine (Neu-P11) by Neurim Pharmaceuticals
    1. A melatonin receptor agonist and $5HT_{1A/1D}$ agonist and $5HT_{2B}$ receptor antagonist
    2. In Phase II trials for Alzheimer's, insomnia, ocular hypertension and open-angle glaucoma
AO. R-phenserine (Posiphen®) - ANVS-401 / ANVS-405
    1. Inhibits AChE, α-synuclein, amyloid β-protein precursor, Huntington's disease & tau protein
    2. Currently in Phase II by Annovis Bio.
    3. Also being studied for mild cognitive impairment and Parkinson's disease
    4. Other physostigmine derivatives investigated: *phenserine* & *eseroline* (metabolite of physostigmine)[1219]
AP. RVT-101 by Axovant Sciences Ltd. In Phase III NCT02586909
    1. Dose: 35 mg tablets
AQ. Semorinemab (MTAU-9937A/ RG6100 / RO 7105705) by AC Immune/Genentech/Roche
    1. An anti-tau monoclonal antibody
    2. For Alzheimer's disease - Phase II trial initiated in Feb. 2019

AR. Sodium oligomannurarate (GV-971/Hamput/Mannut Sodium) by Shanghai Green Valley Pharm.
   1. An amino acid modulator, Amyloid beta-protein inhibitor, and Microbiome modulator
   2. An oligosaccharide sugar derived from seaweed/brown algae[1226]
   3. Found to suppress certain bacteria in the gut which can cause neural degeneration and "dysbiosis-promoted neuroinflammation of the brain"
   4. Plans to launch Phase III clinical trials in the US and Europe in early 2020
AS. Solanezumab (LY2062430) by Eli Lilly and Company in Phase III study
   1. A monoclonal antibody and amyloid beta-protein inhibitor
   2. Drug is administered intravenously (IV) once every 4 weeks for up to 2 years
AT. SUVN-G3031 by Suven Life Sciences at the end of Phase I trials for Cognitive & Sleep Disorders
   1. An $H_3$ inverse agonist
AU. SUVN-D4010 by Suven Life Sciences the end of Phase I for Cognitive Disorders
   1. $5HT_4$ receptor partial antagonist
AV. SUVN-I6107 by Suven Life Sciences
   1. A muscarinic receptor-1 positive allosteric modulators (M1-PAM) for cognitive disorders that is devoid of cholinergic side effects
   2. Suven is working on another compound that is an M1/M4 agonist for both cognition & psychosis
   3. Still in pre-clinical stage, but Phase I studies planned soon
   4. http://www.suven.com/drugdiscoveryresearch.aspx#clinical-pipeline-section
AW. Troriluzole (BHV4157) by Biohaven Pharmaceutical and Yale University
   1. In Phase III trials for GAD and Phase II/III for Alzheimer's Disease and OCD
AX. Tulrampator (Ampakine-CX-1632 /CX-1632/ S47445) by RespireRx Pharmaceuticals/Servier
   1. AMPA receptor modulators; Nerve growth factor stimulants
   2. Phase II for Alzheimer's Disease & Major Depressive Disorder

# 34. PARKINSON'S DISEASE (PD)[1227-1229]

## I. BACKGROUND
A. Progressive neurodegenerative disorder from loss of DA neurons in the brain's substantia nigra
B. PD first described in detail by a London Member of the Royal College of Surgeons, James Parkinson, in 1817 in "An Essay on the Shaking Palsy"[1230]
   1. He wrote about six people that he never actually examined
   2. He just watched them walking down the street
C. Other names are Parkinson's syndrome, shaking palsy, *paralysis agitans*, and parkinsonism
D. Second most common neurodegenerative disorder after Alzheimer's disease

## II. PATHOPHYSIOLOGY
A. Ventral tier region of pars compacta in the substantia nigra is specifically affected
   1. An extrapyramidal motor system disorder
B. A marked loss and progressive degeneration of dopaminergic neural cells
C. Symptoms occur when 80-85% of substantia nigra neurons are lost
D. Presence of abnormal intracellular aggregates of alpha-synuclein inclusion bodies in substantia nigra, called "Lewy bodies" that kill the neuron
E. Most cases are idiopathic, but can also occur following encephalitis or exposure to certain toxins
   1. Manganese dust, carbon disulfide, severe carbon monoxide poisoning, and pesticides (e.g., paraquat or Agent Orange)
F. $D_1$ and $D_5$ receptors are generally associated with dyskinesias
G. $D_2$, $D_3$, and $D_4$ receptors are related to symptoms of movement disorders

## III. EPIDEMIOLOGY[1231-1233]
A. Peak age of onset = 55-65
B. Occurs in 1-2% of people over the age of 60 years, rising to 3.5% at age 85-89 years
C. About 0.3% of the general population is affected
D. Men > Women with a ratio of 1.5 to 1
E. Exercise, caffeine, NSAIDs, and anti-oxidants can reduce the incidence

## IV. COMMON EARLY PRODROMAL COMPLAINTS
A. Resting tremor
B. Writing smaller; difficulty fastening buttons
C. Slowness, "weakness", limb not working well, stiff or achy limb(s)
D. Stoop, shuffle-walk, "dragging" leg(s)
E. Trouble getting out of chairs or turning in bed
F. Low or soft voice
G. Anosmia (↓ smells), dream enactment, constipation, anxiety, depression, "passiveness"

## V. DIFFERENTIAL DIAGNOSIS OF PARKINSONISM
A. "Parkinson-plus" degenerations (dementia with Lewy bodies, progressive supranuclear palsy, corticobasal degeneration, multiple system atrophy)
B. Drug-induced parkinsonism (anti-dopaminergics)
   1. Antipsychotics / antiemetics: e.g., haloperidol, metoclopramide, promethazine, prochlorperazine
C. Rare but treatable in young people: Wilson disease and Dopa-responsive dystonia
D. Other: "vascular" parkinsonism, brain trauma, CNS infection

## VI. DIAGNOSIS
A. No absolute diagnostic criteria exist, although some proposed one have been suggested
   1. The International Parkinson and Movement Disorder Society (MDS)[1234]

2. UK Queen Square Brain Bank for Neurological Disorders (https://www.ucl.ac.uk/ion/research/departments/clinical-and-movement-neurosciences/centres-and-projects/queen-square-brain)
3. U.S. National Institute of Neurological Disorders and Stroke (https://www.ninds.nih.gov)

## VII. 4 CARDINAL MOTOR FEATURES
A. Postural Instability (imbalance, falls, stooped flexed posture)
B. Resting tremor
  1. Usually unilateral before it becomes generalized
  2. 4-6 Hz pill-rolling, often involving the thumbs
  3. Typically absent during activity
C. Rigidity / Dystonia - different from spasticity
  1. Cog-wheeling occurs when lead pipe rigidity is broken up by tremor
D. Akinesia/Bradykinesia = slow and small movements
  1. Reduced blink, face expression, and gesturing
  2. Difficulty getting out of chair, motor freezing
  3. *Festinant* gait (slow to start + small shuffling steps + difficult turns)
    i. Diminished arm swing = leads to recurrent falls
    ii. Reduction in amplitude of repetitive movements
    iii. Festination is an involuntary tendency to take short accelerating steps when walking
      a. As if the patient is continuously trying to catch up with their centre of gravity
  4. PD patients with more than 1 fall in previous year are likely to fall again within next 3 months
    i. Most falls occur during transfers and freezing of gait

## VIII. OTHER MAJOR PARKINSON'S DISEASE SYMPTOMS[1235,1236]
A. Motor symptoms
  1. Akathisia, drooling, dysphagia (Impaired swallowing – drooling, choking on food, aspiration)
  2. Fatigue, hypophonia (quiet voice progressing to dysarthria), mask-like face
  3. Micrographia (small + spidery writing)
B. Non-motor symptoms (because PD affects many parts of the nervous system)
  1. Earliest involvement is in gut nerve plexus, lower brainstem, and olfactory bulb
  2. Non-motor symptoms often predate motor symptoms
    i. E.g. anosmia, constipation, dream enactment, anxiety, apathy
  3. Autonomic symptoms: blood pressure dysregulation
    i. Causes orthostatic hypotension ("neurogenic orthostasis") and supine hypertension
    ii. Syncope can occur, sometimes with injury
    iii. Lower extremity edema may also reflect vascular dysregulation
  4. Cognitive decline with memory deficits = May be depression & dementia
    i. ~80% of patients will develop dementia (progressive mental decline)
    ii. 20-80% suffer from depression
      a. Levodopa can deplete S-adenosylmethionine (SAMe) in the CNS[358]
      b. SAMe supplementation can improve depression in Parkinson's
  5. Constipation, incontinence, sexual dysfunction, weight loss, hyperhidrosis (sweating)
  6. Slowed thinking, reaction time, and executive dysfunction
  7. Vision problems, impaired proprioception, oily skin, hallucinations - usually visual
  8. REM sleep behavior disorders
    i. Typically in men, often years before motor symptoms
    ii. Complex movements or fighting (Can injure patient or bed partner)
    iii. Usually early in the morning, varying frequency
    iv. Excessive daytime sleepiness and/or insomnia
  9. Overall 2-6 times increased risk of malignant melanoma vs. general population

## IX. PROGNOSIS
A. Disease is slowly progressive with variable severity
B. Earlier age of onset = poorer prognosis
C. Average life expectancy after diagnosis is 7-15 years
  1. Death is not from disease but usually from complications (e.g., pneumonia, aspiration)

## X. PARKINSON'S DISEASE (PD) TREATMENTS[1237] - *For more detail see page 87*
A. Levodopa, DA agonists, MAO-B inhibitors, COMT inhibitors, amantadine, anticholinergics, others
B. Drugs don't alter the natural progression – they just improve symptoms
  1. Delaying medication treatment is of no long-term benefit
    i. Meds are symptomatic treatments and are not neuroprotective or neurotoxic
  2. Patients will still experience "OFF" episodes ("end-of-dose wearing OFF" and unpredictable "ON/OFF" episodes) while on routine doses of medication
C. Levodopa (L-dopa) - (usually with carbidopa)
  1. Most effective for motor symptoms (bradykinesia, tremor, gait changes) and usually best tolerated
  2. It's discovery in the 1960's revolutionized the treatment of Parkinson's disease
  3. Crosses the BBB, enters the nigrostriatal neurons, and is converted to dopamine
    i. Usually given in combination with carbidopa (a *dopa-decarboxylase* inhibitor) to inhibit peripheral levodopa metabolism, so more can penetrate the CNS
      a. Also reduces nausea & vomiting
      b. Carbidopa does NOT cross the BBB
      c. Carbidopa 70-100 mg a day saturates peripheral *dopa-decarboxylase*
        1. Less carbidopa = more nausea and vomiting
        2. **Carbidopa (Lodosyn)**[81] 25 mg tablets are available to augment any levodopa therapy

4. Half-life of levodopa is about 50 minutes (about 1.5 hours with carbidopa)
5. Common side effects include nausea/vomiting, orthostasis, sleepiness or trouble sleeping (insomnia or strange dreams), hallucinations (visual/auditory), dyskinesias, "ON-OFF" phenomena (switch between mobility and immobility) and urinary symptoms (urgency/UTI)
   i. Rare: Hyperpyrexia, Neuroleptic Malignant Syndrome (NMS) and confusion
6. Typical daily l-dopa dose range: 300 mg to 1500mg
7. Most common preparation is regular 25/100 mg (carbidopa/levodopa) dosed at 1 po TID, increased to 1.5 po TID, and increased again to 2 po TID or QID (with FOOD to reduce nausea)
   i. Need 2 weeks between steps to appreciate effect.
   ii. If no response is seen with maximum tolerated doses, then it may not be actual PD
   iii. Some patients need QID or more frequent dosing (even Q3H in advanced disease)
8. Pyridoxine (vitamin B6) 10-25 mg may reverse the effects of levodopa by increasing the rate of aromatic amino acid decarboxylation (carbidopa negates this effect)
9. Drug interactions
   i. Levodopa is absolutely contraindicated when using a MAOI
     a. Concomitant selegiline use may cause severe orthostatic hypotension
   ii. Dopamine antagonists (i.e., antipsychotics) will reduce the effectiveness of L-dopa
   iii. VMAT2 inhibitors (*see page 88*) used for tardive dyskinesia are not recommended
   iv. Caution with iron supplements (or multivitamins with iron) which can chelate L-dopa
10. Warnings and precautions
   i. Contraindicated in patients with narrow-angle glaucoma
   ii. Advise patients that urine, sweat, or saliva may be discolored (e.g., red, brown, black)
   iii. Levodopa may activate a malignant melanoma
   iv. May cause somnolence and "falling asleep during activities of daily living"
   v. May increase impulsive/compulsive behaviors
   vi. Taking with a high fat or high protein meal may result in lower serum concentrations
11. Duopa[®85] (carbidopa/levodopa enteral suspension)
   i. Administered into the jejunum through a percutaneous endoscopic gastrostomy with jejunal tube (PEG-J) using a portable infusion pump (CADD®-Legacy 1400) for 16 continuous hours
     a. Patients still need to take their RR levodopa at night
   ii. Dosing requires a conversion to RR carbidopa/levodopa
   iii. Calculate morning dose by first totaling up a usual day's 1st morning dose of RR levodopa
     a. Converting to mL by multiplying the totaled 1st morning dose by 0.04 and add 3
     b. Morning dose is administered over 10-30 minutes
   iv. Calculate the Continuous Dose by adding up all levodopa doses taken after the 1st morning's dose (from above) until bedtime (16 waking hours)
     a. Convert to mL by dividing the total waking dose by 20
   v. Adjust doses as needed based on response or side effects
     a. Extra "bolus" doses of 20 mg L-dopa can be administered Q2h (max 2000 mg/d = 1 cassette)
   vi. Available in cassettes containing 100 mL of 4.63/20 mg (carbidopa/levodopa) per mL
     a. Cassettes need to be refrigerated, but brought to room temp for 20 minutes before using
   vii. Side effects include surgical site complications, infections, and GI upset
   viii. Shown in clinical trial to ↓ "OFF" periods by 2 out of 16 hrs compared to oral RR levodopa
     a. Also increased "ON" time without bothersome dyskinesias
12. Inbrija[™91] (levodopa inhalation powder)
   i. Indicated for prn use of "OFF" episodes (up to 5 times a day)
   ii. Dosage: 2 capsules (2 x 42 mg = 84 mg) via the oral Inbrija inhaler
13. Parcopa[®83]ODT (carbidopa/levodopa orally disintegrating tablet)
   i. Brand name discontinued – only generic available
   ii. Available in 25/100, 10/100, and 25/250 mg tablets (carbidopa/levodopa)
   iii. Contains phenylalanine – caution in Phenylketonuric patients
   iv. Dosing and pharmacokinetics are the same as regular-release carbidopa/levodopa
14. Rytary[®84] (extended-release carbidopa/levodopa)
   i. Contains special beads designed to dissolve at different rates within the stomach and intestines
   ii. Capsules can be opened and sprinkled on applesauce or other soft food
   iii. Available in: 23.75/95, 36.25/145, 48.75/195, 61.25/245 mg extended-release capsules
   iv. Converting from regular levodopa to Rytary is difficult (use chart below)
     a. First, total up RR (regular-release) levodopa doses for one day of existing therapy

| b. Total daily levodopa dose | Dose of Rytary |
|---|---|
| 400-549 mg | 3 capsules of 23.75/95 mg taken TID |
| 550-749 mg | 4 capsules of 23.75/95 mg taken TID |
| 750-949 mg | 3 capsules of 36.25/145 mg taken TID |
| 950-1249 mg | 3 capsules of 48.75/195 mg taken TID |
| ≥ 1250 mg | 4 capsules of 48.75/195 mg taken TID *or* 3 capsules of 61.25/245 mg taken TID |

     c. Max recommended daily dose - 612.5/2450 mg (10 of the highest dosage capsules a day)
   v. Peak concentration in 1 hour, which lasts for 4-5 hours before declining
15. Sinemet[®] (regular-release (RR)) and Sinemet CR[®] (controlled-release)[82]
   i. RR available in 25/100, 10/100, and 25/250 mg tablets (carbidopa/levodopa)
   ii. CR available in 25/100 and 50/200 mg tablets (SR carbidopa/levodopa)

iii. CR peaks in about 2 hours, compared to ½ hour with RR
iv. Serum trough levels with CR are approx. double the RR levels
v. Giving CR with **FOOD** ↑ L-dopa bioavailability by 50% and ↑ peak serum concentrations by 25%
vi. RR can be dosed up to Q3h / CR is usually dosed BID-TID
16. Stalevo[®86] (carbidopa, levodopa and entacapone)
i. Combination tablet of carbidopa/levodopa and a Catechol-O-Methyltransferase (COMT) inhibitor
ii. Available as 200 mg of entacapone + a 1:4 ratio of carbidopa to levodopa, where the dose of levodopa is the Stalevo dose
iii. Stalevo 50 (12.5/50/200), Stalevo 75 (18.75/75/200), Stalevo 100 (25/100/200), Stalevo 125 (31.25/125/200), Stalevo 150 (37.5/150/200), and Stalevo 200 (50/200/200)
iv. Dosing is the same as for RR carbidopa/levodopa
a. Max daily dose of levodopa is 1200 mg
b. Do not split, crush or chew tablets, because the components may not be equally divided

D. Dopamine agonists
1. Two classes: **ergoline** (derivatives of an alkaloid called ergot) and **non-ergoline** agonists
i. **Ergoline** agonists (e.g., bromocriptine, cabergoline, and pergolide) are $1^{st}$ generation agents
ii. **Non-ergolines** (e.g., pramipexole, ropinirole, rotigotine, and apomorphine) are $2^{nd}$ generation
2. May be monotherapy in early disease – save L-dopa for mid to late disease
3. Can add to L-dopa to reduce "OFF" time
4. Common side effects and warnings of dopamine agonists are similar to those of levodopa
i. Confusion, DAWS (Dopamine Agonist Withdrawal Syndrome), dizziness, hallucinations, impulse control problems & compulsive behaviors, lower limb edema, nausea, orthostatic hypotension, sleep attacks and prolactin suppression
5. Best to wean dose gradually than abruptly discontinue
6. Bromocriptine mesylate (Parlodel[®])[79]
i. Post-synaptic dopamine receptor agonist
ii. Also approved for Hyperprolactinemia-Associated Dysfunctions and Acromegaly
a. Another brand of bromocriptine (Cycloset[®])[78] is approved to improve glycemic control in adults with type 2 diabetes at a dose of 0.8 to 4.8 mg QAM with food (contraindicated with strong CYP3A4 inhibitors)
iii. Dosage: start with a ½ tablet to 1 full tablet of 2.5 mg po BID with FOOD
a. Increase as needed every 2-4 weeks in 2.5 mg increments
b. Max dose is 100 mg/d, but average is usually under 40 mg a day (divided)
c. Available in 2.5 scored "SnapTabs[®]" and 5 mg capsules
iv. Peak plasma concentrations in 2.5 hours ± 2 hours
v. Metabolized by (and an inhibitor of) CYP3A4
vi. T½ = 4.85 hours
vii. Levels ↑ by inhibitors of CYP3A4
viii. 90-96% protein bound
ix. Pregnancy Category B (but may cause hypertension – monitor for CV complications)
x. Do not use while breastfeeding - it reduces milk production
7. Pergolide mesylate (Permax[®])[94]
i. $D_1$ and $D_2$ post-synaptic receptor agonist
ii. 10 to 1000 times more potent than bromocriptine
iii. BBW: Cardiac Valvulopathy and Fibrotic Complications (pleural, retroperitoneal)
a. Rare pleuritis, pleural effusion & fibrosis, pericarditis, pericardial effusion, cardiac valvulopathy involving one or more valves, or retroperitoneal fibrosis, and arrhythmias (atrial premature contractions and sinus tachycardia)
iv. Initiate with dose of 0.05 mg QD for 2 days, then increase by 0.1-0.15 mg Q 3 days for 12 days
a. Increase dose by 0.25 mg Q 3 days until optimal therapeutic response seen
b. Average dose is 3 mg/d divided TID / Max dose is 5 mg/d divided TID
c. Available in 0.05, 0.25 and 1 mg tablets
v. 90% protein bound
vi. Mostly eliminated renally
vii. Pregnancy Category B
8. Pramipexole dihydrochloride (Mirapex[®])[95]
i. Potent $D_3$ agonist, as well as a lesser $D_2$ & $D_4$ agonist
ii. Also indicated in moderate to severe RLS (restless leg syndrome)
a. Dosing for RLS is at HS only (0.125 to 0.5 mg)
iii. Dosage: 0.375 up to 4.5 mg a day divided TID
a. Start low and titrate dose weekly
b. Reduce doses with moderate to severe renal impairment (not recommended in ESRD)
c. Renal clearance is 30% lower in patients > 65 y.o. (t-1/2 ≈ 12 hours)
d. Available in 0.125, 0.25, 0.5, 0.75, 1 and 1.5 mg scored tablets
iv. Peak concentrations in approx. 2 hours
v. Little metabolism, so elimination is mostly renal
vi. Adult average t½ is 8.5 hours
vii. Pramipexole extended-release (Mirapex ER[®])[95]
a. Dosing is QD (with or without food) at <u>same total daily dose</u> as the RR version
b. ER is <u>not</u> indicated for RLS
c. Available in 0.375, 0.75, 1.5, 2.25, 3, 3.75 and 4.5 mg tablets

       d. Do not crush or divide tablets
       e. Peak concentrations in approx. 6 hours
       f. Pharmacokinetics are similar to the RR version dosed TID
       g. Ghost tablet (or fragments) may appear in patient's stool
   9. Ropinirole (Requip®)[98]
     i. $D_2$ receptor agonist within the caudate-putamen in the brain
     ii. Also indicated in moderate to severe RLS (restless leg syndrome)
       a. Dosing for RLS is at HS only (0.25 to 4 mg) given 1-3 hours before bedtime
       b. Max dose for RLS is 3 mg/d in those with ESRD on dialysis
     iii. Initiate dosing at 0.25 mg po TID
       a. Titrate to a max dose of 24 mg a day (divided TID) and 18 mg/d in those with ESRD on dialysis
       b. Available in 0.25, 0.5, 1, 2, 3, 4 and 5 mg tablets
     iv. Peak concentrations in approx. 1-2 hours
     v. Metabolized by CYP1A2
     vi. T½ is approx. 6 hours
     vii. Inhibitors or inducers of CYP1A2 will ↑ or ↓ levels, respectively
       a. Smoking will induce ropinirole metabolism
     viii. Not safe in pregnancy – may cause fetal harm
     ix. Ropinirole extended-release (Requip XL®)[98]
       a. XL is not indicated for RLS
       b. Dosing is QD (with or without food), starting at 2 mg QD and titrated as needed Q 1-2 weeks
         1. Available in 2, 4, 6, 8 and 12 mg tablets
       c. Peak concentrations in 6 to 10 hours
  10. Rotigotine (Neupro®)[99] transdermal system
     i. Also indicated in moderate to severe RLS (restless leg syndrome)
     ii. Start with 2-4 mg/24 hour patch QD, and titrate weekly up to 8 mg/24 hour patch
       a. Available in 1, 2, 3, 4, 6 and 8 mg/24 hours transdermal patches (individually wrapped)
     iii. Caution: Sulfite sensitivity (contains sodium metabisulfite) – patch also contains aluminum
     iv. May cause weight gain, peripheral edema, and patch site reactions
     v. Peak plasma levels occur from 4 to 27 hours (avg. 15-18) after patch placement
     vi. Primarily eliminated renally (plasma levels double in those with CrCl $\leq$ 30 ml/min
       a. Has a bi-phasic t½ of 3 hours and 5-7 hours after patch removal
     vii. Rotate application site daily and avoid external heat sources (↑ absorption 7 fold)
     viii. Patches should not be cut – can be held in place with bandage if necessary
     ix. Risks in pregnancy and breastfeeding are unknown
  11. Apomorphine (Apokyn®)[77] subcutaneous injection
     i. $D_2$, $D_3$, $D_4$ and $D_5$ receptor agonist, and adrenergic $\alpha_{1D}$, $\alpha_{2B}$, $\alpha_{2C}$ receptor agonist
     ii. Indicated for acute, intermittent treatment of hypomobility, in advanced PD (i.e., OFF periods)
     iii. **Contraindicated** for use with **5HT3 antagonists**, such as newer antiemetics due to severe
       hypotension and loss of consciousness
       a. However, pre-treatment with a D2-blocking antiemetic to reduce N&V is recommended for 3
         days before starting therapy (i.e., trimethobenzamide (Tigan®))
     iv. Starting dose is 0.2 mL (2 mg) subQ titrated up to the max recommended dose of 0.6 mL/d (6
       mg) given > 2 hours apart (a test dose should be given under medical supervision to monitor
       blood pressure and pulse)
       a. May cause QT-prolongation in doses > 6 mg a day
       b. Reduce dose by half in those with renal impairment
       c. Available in a 30 mg/3 mL multi-dose glass cartridge with pen injector (not for IV use)
     v. Peak plasma concentrations in 10-60 minutes
     vi. T½ is 40 minutes
     vii. Risks in pregnancy and breastfeeding are unknown
  12. Cabergoline (Dostinex®)[80]
     i. $D_2$ receptor agonist
     ii. *Not approved Parkinson's Disease* - approved for hyperprolactinemia
     iii. Dosage is 0.25 to 1 mg **twice a week** (titrated Q 4 weeks)
       a. Available in 0.5 mg tablets in bottles of 8 tablets
       b. Caution in those with severe hepatic insufficiency (Child-Pugh score > 10)
     iv. T½ = 63-69 hours
E. Monoamine Oxidase B (MAO-B) inhibitors
  1. Irreversibly inhibits MAO-B, the enzyme that breaks down/metabolizes dopamine
     i. After discontinuing a MAO-B inhibitor, it may take 7 days to replenish this enzyme – must wait 2
       weeks to initiate any contraindicated medications
  2. Used in conjunction with other medications
  3. Motor symptom improvement is mild to modest
  4. Common class side effects for MAO-B inhibitors
     i. Hypertension, hypotension/orthostatic, dyskinesia, hallucinations/psychosis, impulsive or
       compulsive behaviors, sudden sleep attacks, nausea, falls, insomnia
  5. **Contraindicated** with meperidine, tramadol, methadone, propoxyphene dextromethorphan, St.
     John's wort, cyclobenzaprine, or another (selective or non-selective) MAO inhibitor
  6. Concomitant antidepressant use may cause serotonin syndrome
  7. Tyramine-restricted diet is not necessary (as with non-selective MAOIs)

8. Rasagiline (Azilect®)[96]
  i. Initiate dose at 0.5-1 mg QD (or lower if used with adjunct L-dopa)
    a. Max dose is 1 mg QD
    b. Patients on CYP1A2 inhibitors or with mild hepatic impairment – half usual dose
    c. Do not use in those with moderate to severe hepatic impairment
    d. Available in 0.5 and 1 mg tablets
  ii. Can cause severe hypo- or hypertension, arthralgia, depression, dyspepsia, N&V, dry mouth, abdominal pain, constipation, rash, abnormal dreams, falls, and tenosynovitis
  iii. Metabolized mostly by CYP1A2
  iv. T½ = 3 hours
9. Selegiline (Eldepryl®[101], Emsam®[103] transdermal system, Zelapar®[102] ODT)
  i. Also called "*l-deprenyl*"
  ii. 85-90% protein bound
  iii. Metabolized by CYP2A6, 2B6, 2C9, and 3A4/5 to methamphetamine and amphetamine
  iv. Eldepryl is dosed at 5 mg BID (at breakfast and lunch)
    a. Bioavailability is increased 3 to 4 fold when it is taken with FOOD
    b. Oral doses > 10 mg/d will non-selectively inhibit other MAO enzymes, thus making dietary restrictions necessary
  v. Emsam patch's starting and target dose is 6 mg/24 hour
    a. Increases to 9 or 12 mg/24 hr (max dose) can be made Q 2 weeks per patient response
    b. Dietary restrictions are necessary with the 9 & 12 mg/24 hr doses
    c. Because Emsam is an antidepressant, it is not approved for PD
      1. Additional warnings are suicidal ideation and bipolar mania
    d. Avoid external heat on the patch and do NOT cut patches
  vi. Zelapar ODT is dosed at 1.25 mg QD x 6 weeks, with an increase to 2.5 mg QD
    a. With mild or moderate hepatic impairment, reduced dose to 1.25 mg
    b. Not recommended with severe hepatic (Child-Pugh score >9) or renal (CrCl < 30 ml/min) impairment
    c. Caution Phenylketonurics (PKU): contains aspartame
  vii. Availability: Eldepryl® 5 mg capsules / Emsam® 6, 9 & 12 mg/24 hr patches / Zelapar® 1.25 mg orally disintegrating tablets
  viii. Eldepryl t½ = 10 hours / Zelapar ODT t½ = 10 hours / Emsam patch t½ = 18-25 hours
  ix. Not recommended in pregnancy or breastfeeding
10. Safinamide (Xadago®)[100]
  i. Initiate with 50 mg QD and increase to 100 mg po QD after 2 weeks if required
    a. With moderate hepatic impairment – Max 50 mg/d
    b. Contraindicated with severe hepatic impairment (Child-Pugh C: 10-15)
    c. Available in 50 and 100 mg tablets
  ii. May cause *retinal damage* – patients must be regularly monitored for visual changes
  iii. Inhibits intestinal breast cancer resistance protein (BCRP) and ↑ levels of substrates (e.g., imatinib, methotrexate, mitoxantrone, irinotecan, lapatinib, rosuvastatin, sulfasalazine & topotecan)
  iv. Primarily metabolized by non-microsomal enzymes (cytosolic amidases/MAO-A)
    a. Minor metabolism by CYP3A4
  v. T½ = 20-26 hours
F. COMT (catechol *O*-methyl transferase) Inhibitors
  1. Indicated as adjunctive therapy to levodopa/carbidopa in PD
  2. Selectively and reversibly inhibits the enzyme that *peripherally* breaks down of DA & NE
  3. Prolongs the elimination half-life of levodopa (from ≈ 1.3 to 3.5 hours)
  4. A reduction in the dose of levodopa may be necessary
  5. Do not use with a non-selective MAOI
  6. Common side effects: somnolence, sudden sleep attacks, hypotension/syncope, diarrhea, vomiting, dry mouth, hallucinations/psychosis, dyskinesia/hyperkinesia, impulsive or compulsive behaviors, anorexia, sweating and urine discoloration
  7. Use in pregnancy and breastfeeding must weigh the potential risks against the benefits
  8. Entacapone (Comtan®)[88]
    i. Recommended dose is one 200 mg tablet taken concomitantly with each levodopa/carbidopa dose to a maximum of 8 times daily (1600 mg)
      a. Available in 200 mg tablets
    ii. Exhibits biphasic elimination with t½ of 0.4-0.7 hour and 2.4 hours
    iii. 98% protein bound
  9. Tolcapone (Tasmar®)[104]
    i. BBW: Potentially fatal, acute fulminant liver failure (1%)
      a. Requires baseline & frequent monitoring of LFTs (every 2-4 weeks for > 6 months)
      b. Patients are required to sign a waiver with their physician concerning potential liver failure
    ii. Dosage is 100 mg po TID – increases to 200 mg po TID can be made if required
    iii. Peak concentrations in 2 hours
    iv. >99.9% protein bound
    v. Some metabolism by CYP3A4 and CYP2A6
    vi. T½ = 2-3 hours

G. Amantadine
  1. *See page 87 for detailed information*
  2. Anti-viral medication
  3. Weak antagonist of NMDA-type glutamate receptor, ↑ dopamine release, and blocks DA reuptake
  4. Can help PD symptoms in general, and in particular dyskinesias and freezing of gait
  5. Side effects: nausea, orthostasis, levido reticularis, hallucinations, nightmares
H. Anticholinergics
  1. Benztropine mesylate (Cogentin®) and trihexyphenidyl (Artane®)
    i. *See page 87 for detailed information*
  2. Procyclidine (Kemadrin®) and biperiden (Akineton®) are no longer available in the US
I. Adenosine A$_{2A}$ Receptor Antagonist
  1. Istradefylline (Nourianz™)[90]
    i. Indicated as adjunctive treatment in PD and for those experiencing OFF episodes
    ii. **Warnings** include Dyskinesia, Hallucinations/psychosis, and Impulsive/compulsive Behaviors
    iii. Dosage is 20 mg QD, but can be increased to a max of 40 mg QD
      a. Max dose in moderate hepatic impairment or with concomitant CYP3A4 inhibitors is 20 mg
      b. Avoid in severe hepatic impairment or with concomitant CYP3A4 inducers
      c. Cigarette smokers will need higher doses
      d. Available in 20 and 40 mg tablets
    iv. Common side effects: dyskinesia, dizziness, constipation, nausea, hallucinations and insomnia
    v. Peak concentration in 4 hours
    vi. 98% protein bound
    vii. Metabolized by CYP1A1 & 3A4, with minor metab. from CYP1A2, 2B6, 2C8, 2C9, C18, & 2D6
    viii. A weak CYP3A4 & P-glycoprotein (P-gp) inhibitor
    ix. T½ = 83 hours
    x. Not recommended in pregnancy or breastfeeding
J. Over-the-counter medications
  1. Coenzyme Q10 - mitochondria health
  2. Vitamin E, Vitamin C & Health foods – to evaluate their oxidative properties
  3. Creatine - increases levels of phosphocreatine (energy source in muscle & brain)
XI. RESIDUAL SYMPTOMS
  A. Some motor symptoms may not respond to med adjustments
  B. Postural instability and falls, freezing of gait, some tremors
  C. Fatigue, dysarthria, dysphagia
  D. Resting tremor
  E. Motor complications as PD progresses
    1. Medication wears off before next dose, so OFF periods get worse as disease progresses
    2. Dyskinesias (usually at the peak of ON)
XII. TREATMENT OF ORTHOSTASIS
  A. Worse with dopamine agonists and higher doses of L-dopa
  B. Fludrocortisone: retains body sodium (beware of hypokalemia)
  C. Midodrine: raises BP (beware supine hypertension)
  D. Droxidopa (Northera®)[1238]
    1. Turns to norepinephrine, raises BP (beware supine hypertension)
    2. Was FDA approved for management of Neurogenic orthostasis in 2014
    3. Used to treat orthostatic hypotension that can occur from the disease itself or PD medications
XIII. REM SLEEP BEHAVIOR DISORDER
  A. Melatonin 3 - 12 mg QHS helps mild to moderate symptoms
  B. Clonazepam 0.25-1 mg QHS may be needed for more severe symptoms
  C. Trazodone
  D. Mirtazapine (do not use with apomorphine, because it has 5HT$_3$ antagonist properties)
XIV. HALLUCINATIONS AND DEMENTIA IN PD
  A. Assess medical comorbidities, B12, TSH
  B. Simplify medication regimen
    1. Prioritize eliminating anticholinergics and dopamine agonists
    2. Reduce L-dopa as a last resort
  C. Rivastigmine (cholinesterase inhibitor) - FDA approved in PD dementia – treats apathy
  D. Antipsychotics (off label)
    1. Quetiapine and clozapine least likely to worsen parkinsonism
    2. Caution: D$_2$ blockers will worsen PD
  E. Pimavanserin (Nuplazid) – (*See page 96 for detailed information*)
    1. FDA-approved for hallucinations and delusions associated with Parkinson's Disease psychosis
    2. Not a dopamine antagonist, so shouldn't exacerbate parkinsonism
XV. NON-PHARMACOLOGIC TREATMENTS OF PD
  A. Deep Brain Stimulation (DBS) of the nucleus basalis of Meynert, subthalamic nucleus, and pedunculopontine nucleus[1118]
    1. St. Jude – Received FDA approval for the **Brio DBS** system in 2015
  B. Surgery - Pallidotomy involves surgical destruction of the globus pallidus to control dyskinesia
  C. Stem Cell Therapy – very expensive and complicated

# XVI. POTENTIAL FUTURE THERAPIES FOR PARKINSON'S DISEASE IN STUDY

A. **Alpha-synuclein therapies**
  1. α-synuclein is the abnormal protein that accumulates in the brain in PD
  2. Two different strategies:
    i. Vaccine against the protein
    ii. Intravenous infusion of antibodies directly targeting this protein
B. **AXO-Lenti-PD** by Axovant Gene Therapies https://www.axovant.com/pipeline-overview
  1. Investigational one-time gene therapy that delivers three genes via a single lentiviral vector
    i. Delivered directly into the putamen, a neurosurgical procedure that does not require the use of intraoperative MRI
  2. Encodes a set of critical enzymes required for dopamine synthesis
  3. Preliminary results expected in late 2019 from Phase II trial (SUNRISE-PD)
C. **Blarcamesine** (ANAVEX2-73) in Phase II by Anavex Life Sciences Corp. (www.anavex.com)
  1. Sigma-1 and muscarinic receptor agonist which blocks tau hyperphosphorylation
  2. An aminotetrahydrofuran derivative
D. **BTRX-246040** (LY-2940094) - BlackThorn Therapeutics and Eli Lilly and Company
  1. Nociceptin receptor antagonist
  2. Phase II trial completed
  3. Also being studied in Major Depression (Phase II trial completed)
E. **Bumetanide (Bumex)** by B&A Therapeutics in Phase II clinical trials
  1. A "loop" diuretic
F. **Cannabidiol** (GWP42003) by GW Pharmaceuticals in Phase II
G. **Dipraglurant-IR** (mGlu5 NAM) by Addex Therapeutics
  1. NAM=Negative Allosteric Modulator in Phase II
H. **"DopaFuse"** by SynAgile (http://www.synagile.com/dopafuse.html)
  1. Continuous oral levodopa infusion using the OraFuse® technology[1239]
  2. Currently undergoing Phase II trials
  3. DopaFuse Delivery System consists of a custom-made retainer, drug container, and a case
  4. Retainer holds a small drug container that continuously releases drug in the back of the mouth
I. **Dronabinol**
J. **Eltoprazine** by Amarantus Bioscience (Elto Pharma)
  1. MOA: $5HT_{1A}$ and $5HT_{1B}$ partial agonist, as well as a and $5HT_{2C}$ receptor antagonist
  2. A phenylpiperazine, similar to aripiprazole, brexpiprazole, and cariprazine
  3. Originally developed as an anti-aggressive agent (serenic) to ↓ aggressive impulses & behaviors
  4. In Phase II clinical trials for the treatment of levodopa-induced dyskinesia in Parkinson's disease
K. **Gene therapies** (various)
L. **Lisuride** – not available in the US
  1. Transdermal System in Phase II study because oral dosing has low bioavailability and short t½
M. **MCC950** – Small molecule drug developed by Inflazome LTD in Ireland/UK to halt progression of PD by blocking NLRP3 activation in the brain and reducing inflammation (in pre-clinical trials)[1240]
N. **NBTX-001** (the noble gas xenon) by Nobilis Therapeutics[430]
  1. Antagonist of NMDA, AMPA, nicotinic ACh (α4β2), $5HT_3$, & plasma membrane $Ca^{2+}$ ATPase
  2. Currently in Phase III trials using the Zephyrus™ inhalational Device
  3. Also in Phase II for Irritable Bowel Syndrome (IBS), Autism, & Alzheimer's Disease
O. **NNI-362 and NNI-370** by Neuronascent, Inc.
  1. Part of a novel class of drugs, called Neuron Regenerative therapies to stimulate neuroplasticity & protect neurons from degeneration
  2. Both are currently in pre-clinical study in animal models
  3. https://www.neuronascent.com/r&d-parkinsons.htm
P. **Ongentys®** (opicapone)[1241]
  1. Approved in Europe in 2016
  2. NDA submitted by Neurocrine Biosciences to the FDA in July 2019 for adjunctive treatment to levodopa/carbidopa in PD patients
  3. FDA has to make a determination by April 26, 2020
  4. Selective Catechol-O-Methyltransferase (COMT) inhibitor
  5. Significantly reduced OFF time without troublesome dyskinesia
  6. Dose: 25-50 mg QD
Q. **Prasinezumab** (RG7935) by Roche in Phase II
R. **Rotigotine** extended-release (LY03003) by Luye Pharma Group in Phase III trials
S. **R-phenserine (Posiphen®)** - ANVS-401 or ANVS-405
  1. Inhibitor of AChE, α-synuclein, amyloid β-protein precursor, Huntington's disease protein and Tau
  2 Currently in Phase II by Annovis Bio.
T. **Zonisamide** for PD with Lewy Body Dementia
  1. Adding 25-50 mg to levodopa improves parkinsonism[1242]
U. **Zuranolone** (SAGE-217/S812217) - SAGE Therapeutics
  1. A synthetic, orally active, inhibitory pregnane neuro-steroid, that acts as a positive allosteric modulator of the $GABA_A$ receptor
  2. Developed as an improvement of allopregnanolone (brexanolone/Zulresso™) with high oral bioavailability and a biological half-life suitable for once-daily administration
  3. Currently in Phase III trials for Major depressive disorder, Postnatal depression, and Insomnia
  4. In Phase II trials for Bipolar Depression, Essential Tremors, and Parkinson's Disease

# 35. SPECIAL TOPICS IN PSYCHIATRY

## I. SUICIDE AND SUICIDE RISKS[374,377,378]
A. People with mood disorders have a 30 X greater risk of suicide than general population[535]
B. Population-based studies show that antidepressant prescriptions prevent suicide[1243]
C. Benefit of medication must outweigh risk
   1. All antidepressants carry a Black Box warning of risk of suicide when starting therapy
   2. Suicide risk is highest in the first 28 days of starting medication and 28 days after stopping[1244]
D. Adolescents – have an ↑ risk of suicide compared to adults over 25-years-old
   1. 55% of adolescents started some form of treatment prior to having suicidal behaviors[1245]
E. Over 70 years of age - highest rates
F. Women attempt suicide more than men, but men are more successful at completion[1246]
   1. For each completed suicide, 10-40 attempts are made
   2. Approximately 5% of adults have made a serious suicide attempt[1247]
G. Now the 10th leading cause of death in the US
H. 1 million people world-wide die by suicide each year[1246]
I. Suicide risks by disease state:
   1. Bipolar disorder – 10-19%; (25–56% attempt)[1248]
     i. Usually during mood transition or depressed phase
   2. Schizophrenia – 10-20% (1 out of 3 attempt)
   3. Depression – 15-20%

## II. POLYPHARMACY
A. Sometimes useful, sometimes harmful
B. Antipsychotics – use of multiple drugs is not justified in the medical literature[959,1072,1249,1250]
   1. American Psychiatric Association advises against it[452]
   2. Polypharmacy does not increase efficacy, only increases side effects
   3. Quetiapine and other antipsychotics should not be used as sleeping pills[452,1251]
   4. One meta-analysis found it may be superior under certain clinical situations[1252]
     i. Polypharmacy must start before any treatment failures can be determined
     ii. Use for > 10 weeks only in China on Chinese population
     iii. Clozapine + use of a Typical and Atypical antipsychotic
   5. Joint Commission requires reporting for inpatients discharged on >2 antipsychotics
     i. Hospital-based Inpatient Psychiatric Services (HBIPS-4 and HBIPS-5)
     ii. Appropriate justifications could be for cross-tapering of meds, clozapine augmentation, or at least 3 failed monotherapy trials[1253]
   6. A meta-analysis of clozapine augmentation showed weak benefits[1254]
   7. Estimates of polypharmacy for inpatients & outpatients is as high as 57.5%[1255]
   8. Caution if adding aripiprazole, because its DA agonist activity can worsen psychosis
C. Antidepressants – may be used if pt. has partial response once single agent maximized
   1. Use agents from different classes
   2. Some evidence supports initial polypharmacy to achieve higher remission rates[1256]
     i. Remission rate with mirtazapine + fluoxetine or venlafaxine or bupropion was superior to fluoxetine alone (52% vs. 58% vs. 46% vs. 25% respectively)
   3. CO-MED trial showed no differences between polypharmacy and monotherapy[1257]
     i. Escitalopram + placebo vs. bupropion + escitalopram vs. venlafaxine+ mirtazapine
   4. Other studies show similar results using a TCA + SSRI, antidepressant + L-methylfolate (Deplin®), and antidepressant + benzodiazepine receptor agonist, although some data conflicts with this[1258-1260]
D. Benzodiazepines (BZDs) and non-benzodiazepines for anxiety or sleep[1261]
   1. Common example: clonazepam for anxiety and temazepam for sleep
     i. Once tolerance develops to sedation, temazepam will no longer be effective for sleep
     ii. This includes non-benzodiazepines ("Z-drugs") for sleep
     iii. ALL of these medications work on exactly the same receptors
   2. Anxiolytics with antidepressants
     i. Can use BZDs prn (short-term) with antidepressants until they start to work
E. Mood stabilizers
   1. Studies show better results than single agent therapy
   2. Lithium, valproic acid, carbamazepine, lamotrigine with an atypical antipsychotic
   3. Can also use lower doses of each agent to reduce side effects

## III. BARIATRIC SURGERY[1262]
A. High pre-surgical risk of depression, anxiety, and eating disorders (over 60% of patients)
B. Post-surgery
   1. Decrease medication absorption
   2. Reduced GI surface area
   3. Reduced fat mass
   4. Effects on medication pharmacokinetics are drug-specific

5. Gastric emptying rate is increased
C. Bypassing duodenum reduces CYP3A4 and CYP3A5 enzymes
   1. Drugs metabolized by these enzymes may have higher blood levels
D. Changes in gastric pH can reduce medication bioavailability
E. *In vitro* analysis predicts ↓ dissolution of amitriptyline, fluoxetine, paroxetine, & sertraline in GI tract[1263]
   1. Bupropion dissolved to a greater extent
   2. Venlafaxine and citalopram were unchanged
F. Extended-release formulations should be avoided if possible

## IV. MEDICATION NON-ADHERENCE
A. Estimated at > 50% in 1 year[1264]
B. Similar or higher than those with other chronic conditions requiring medication (i.e., HTN/DM)
C. Dosing frequency <u>directly</u> correlates to non-adherence
D. Other factors contributing to non-adherence
   1. Polypharmacy
   2. Cost of medication / insurance co-pays
   3. Side effects
   4. Disbelief in being mentally ill

## V. MEDICAL COMORBIDITIES AND MENTAL ILLNESS[1265]
A. Bipolar & Schizophrenia patients are 2x more likely to have diabetes than general population
   1. Including increased risk of The Metabolic Syndrome: dyslipidemia, HTN, obesity
B. Pts >65 y.o. have a 19% greater 1 year risk for mortality with any mental disorder after an MI
C. Pts >65 y.o. have a 34% increased risk for mortality if they have schizophrenia[1266]
D. Some antipsychotics can increase risk of The Metabolic Syndrome, so monitoring of waist circumference, BMI, lipids, fasting glucose, HgA1C should be done periodically
E. Smoking cessation counseling can reduce mortality risks at any age

# 36. EATING DISORDERS

## I. FEEDING AND EATING DISORDERS (ED)
A. Includes: *Pica, Rumination Disorder, Avoidant/Restrictive Food Intake Disorder, Anorexia Nervosa* (Restrictive type or Binge-eating/purging type), *Bulimia Nervosa, Binge Eating Disorder,* and Other Specified or Unspecified Feeding or Eating Disorder
B. Prevalence > 6% of an ED among youths (ages 12-18 years) in the U.S.[1267]
C. Prevalence for males (14.3%) and females (19.7%) up to the age of 40 (peak at age 21)[1268]
D. Few randomized clinical trials (e.g., psychotherapy ± pharmacotherapy) in adolescents exist
E. Many antidepressants, naltrexone, anticonvulsants, and others have been tried with some success
F. May be from overactivity of neural transmission from the raphe nuclei to the hypothalamus[302]
G. Binge eating disorder (BED)
   1. Cognitive Behavioral Therapy is first-line
   2. Lisdexamfetamine (Vyvanse™) is the only FDA-approved medication (as of 10/2015)
      i. A prodrug, so it has to be metabolized to be active
         a. Has lower risk of abuse, because snorting the drug won't activate it
      ii. Topiramate and newer antidepressants are efficacious as well[1269]
H. Bulimia Nervosa
   1. Fluoxetine (Prozac®) is the only FDA-approved medication for the acute and maintenance treatment in adult patients
      i. Found to decrease the number of episodes of binging, as well the desire to vomit, in people with moderate to severe bulimia

## II. POTENTIAL FUTURE THERAPIES FOR EATING DISORDERS IN STUDY
A. **Dasotraline**[1270] by Sunovion Pharmaceuticals
   1. Submitted a New Drug Application for BED to the FDA in summer 2019
      i. Expected FDA response is the summer of 2020[1271]
   2. Balanced reuptake inhibitor of serotonin, norepinephrine and dopamine (SNDRI)
B. **D-Cycloserine**[357]
   1. Pediatric Feeding Disorders – in Phase I study
   2. Augments exposure therapy for food anxiety in patients with anorexia and bulimia nervosa

## I. BACKGROUND
  A. Thyroid dysfunction encompasses clinical, symptomatic, and asymptomatic factors
    1. Asymptomatic or symptomatic
    2. *Subclinical* hypothyroidism and hyperthyroidism
      i. Abnormal thyroid-stimulating hormone (TSH) levels but normal T4 and T3 levels
    3. Overt hypothyroidism and hyperthyroidism (i.e., abnormal TSH and T4 levels)
  B. Hypothalamus releases TRH (thyrotropin-releasing hormone) to tell the anterior pituitary gland to release TSH which tells the thyroid gland to release T3 (triiodothyronine) and T4 (thyroxine)
    1. Feedback mechanisms at each step help to regulate thyroid homeostasis
    2. Almost all thyroid hormone (>99.9%) is bound to plasma proteins
      i. Thyroxine-binding globulin, thyroid-binding pre-albumin, & albumin
    3. Only *free* unbound thyroid hormone is biologically active
    4. Most T3 (~80%) is formed by breaking down T4
      i. T3 is 5 X more biologically active than T4

## II. HYPOTHYROIDISM
  A. A syndrome characterized by the slowing down of all body processes due to deficiency of thyroid hormones
    1. Can occur in cats, dogs, and horses too
  B. Most common cause: *Hashimoto's disease*
    1. Antibodies attack the thyroid peroxidase enzyme
    2. TSH ↑ to between 5 and 10 IU/mL
  C. Other Causes
    1. Iodine deficiency or excess
      i. American Thyroid Assoc. recommends 150 µg/d
        a. 250 µg if pregnant/breastfeeding
    2. Genetic disorders (e.g., Down Syndrome)
  D. Primary hypothyroidism: Thyroid gland dysfunction (↓T4/T3 release)
    1. 7 X more likely to occur in women
    2. Overt hypothyroidism occurs in 0.3–0.4% of people[1275]
    3. Up to 8.5% of the population may have sub-clinical hypothyroidism
  E. Central (secondary) hypothyroidism: Pituitary dysfunction (↓ TSH release)
    1. Incidence: 1 in 1000
    2. May have other symptoms of generalized pituitary insufficiency
      i. Abnormal menses, decreased libido, galactorrhea
      ii. Symptoms of a pituitary adenoma (vision problems)
  F. *Myxedema coma* (rare complication of decompensated hypothyroidism)
      i. Symptoms: hypothermia and altered sensorium (delirium to coma)
      ii. Untreated disease has a high mortality rate
  G. Diagnosis
    1. Thyroid function tests: ↑ TSH, ↓ T4/T3 and clinical signs and symptoms[1276]
      i. Weakness, cold intolerance, headache, hoarseness, weight gain, galactorrhea, constipation
  H. Treatment
    1. Treat when TSH > 10 IU/mL or if symptomatic with TSH between 5 and 10 IU/mL
    2. Levothyroxine (L-thyroxine, T4) 1-1.5 mcg/kg/day IV/PO in a wide variety of doses
    3. Liothyronine (synthetic T3) - Not recommended today
      i. Can be used in treatment-resistant depression
      ii. Available in 5, 25, and 50 mcg tablets
    4. Desiccated thyroid extract (animal-based (usually pigs, cattle, or sheep) thyroid gland extract)
      i. 4.222 to 1 ratio of T4 to T3
      ii. 1 grain (equivalent to 60 mcg of T4)
      iii. Contains T1, T2, T3 and T4, as well as calcitonin (hormone released by the thyroid gland which regulates calcium levels)
    5. Liotrix (Thyrolar®)
      i. Synthetic T4 : T3 in 4 : 1 ratio
      ii. Available in 1/4, 1/2, 1, 2, and 3 tablet strengths (from 3.1/12.5 up to 37.5/150 mcg strengths)
    6. Drug interactions
      i. Drugs which impair levothyroxine absorption from the GI tract:
        a. Cholestyramine, calcium carbonate, sucralfate, aluminum hydroxide, ferrous sulfate, fiber supplements, H1 blockers, and proton pump inhibitors
      ii. Drugs which increase T4 clearance: Rifampin, carbamazepine, and possibly phenytoin
      iii. Amiodarone and selenium may block the conversion of T4 to T3
  I. Monitoring - TSH and T4 levels should both be checked every 6 weeks until euthyroid
  J. Guidelines
    1. U.S. Preventive Services Task Force (USPSTF)
      i. Mild, asymptomatic thyroid dysfunction should NOT be treated

**Signs and symptoms of**
**Hypothyroidism**

*Psychological*
- Poor memory and concentration
- Poor hearing

*Pharynx*
- Hoarseness

*Heart*
- Slow pulse rate
- Pericardial effusion

*Muscular*
- Delayed reflex relaxation

*Extremities*
- Coldness
- Carpal tunnel syndrome

*General*
- Fatigue
- Feeling cold
- Weight gain with poor appetite
- Hair loss

*Lungs*
- Shortness of breath
- Pleural effusion

*Skin*
- Paresthesia
- Myxedema

*Intestines*
- Constipation
- Ascites

*Reproductive system*
- Menorrhagia

Häggström, Mikael. "Medical gallery of Mikael Häggström 2014". Wikiversity Journal of Medicine 1(2). DOI:10.15347/wjm/2014.008. ISSN 20018762.

2. American Thyroid Association and American Association of Clinical Endocrinologists
  i. Screening for hypothyroidism should be considered in patients older than 60
  ii. Patients with overt asymptomatic thyroid dysfunction (TSH > 10 IU/ml) should be treated
K. Laboratory values

| Test | Lab Low | Optimal Range | Lab High |
|------|---------|---------------|----------|
| TSH | 0.5 µU/mL or IU/mL | 0.5-2 µU/mL or IU/mL | 5.0 µU/mL or IU/mL |
| Free T4 (thyroxine) | 0.8 ng/mL | 1.2-1.3 ng/mL | 2.7 ng/mL |
| Free T3 (triiodothyronine) | 60 ng/dL | 100-130 ng/dL | 181 ng/dL |

L. Thyroid disease's psychiatric effects
  1. Hypothyroidism ($\uparrow$ TSH, $\downarrow$ T4/T3)
    i. Slowing of mental processes/intellectual deterioration
    ii. Progressive loss of initiative and interest
    iii. Memory difficulties and lack of concentration
    iv. Depression with paranoid flavor
    v. Organic psychosis
    vi. Possible causative agents: Lithium, Amiodarone
  2. Hyperthyroidism ($\downarrow$ TSH, $\uparrow$ T4/T3)
    i. Marked anxiety and tension
    ii. Emotional lability
    iii. Irritability and impatience
    iv. Distractible over-activity
    v. Exaggerated sensitivity to noise
    vi. Fluctuating depression
    vii. Possible causative agent: Amiodarone (2-3% incidence)

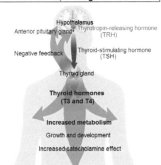

*Hypothalamic–Pituitary–Thyroid Axis*
http://upload.wikimedia.org/wikipedia/commons/c/cb/Thyroid_system.png

## III. HYPERTHYROIDISM / THYROTOXICOSIS
A. Excessive thyroid hormones cause increased metabolism of all body systems
  1. Occurs in 1.2% of the population[1277]
  2. Common in older domesticated cats (about 2%)
B. Most common cause: *Graves' disease* (autoimmune mediated)
  1. Affects ~0.1 per 100,000 children and 3 per 100,000 adolescents per year[388]
C. Many children get misdiagnosed with a mental illness instead (particularly ADHD at >68%)
  1. 1.7 times more likely to receive a mental health diagnosis and 5 times more likely to be suicidal
D. Diagnosis:
  1. Thyroid function tests (TFTs): ($\downarrow$ TSH, $\uparrow$ T4/T3)
  2. Clinical signs & symptoms: heat intolerance, weight loss, palpitation, pedal edema, amenorrhea, diarrhea, tremor, weakness, insomnia, thinning hair, proptosis, enlarged goiter, flushed moist skin
  3. Antibodies to thyroglobulin are further confirmation of autoimmune thyroid disease.
E. Treatment
  1. Surgery (thyroidectomy)
    i. Consider when malignancy is suspected, esophageal obstruction, or difficulty swallowing
  2. Radioactive Iodine (as Sodium Iodide 131)
  3. Potassium iodide (KI)
    i. **Lugol's Solution** (6.3 mg of iodide per drop) or
    ii. Saturated Solution of Potassium Iodide (SSKI) 38 mg iodide per drop
     a. D.O.C. in debilitated, cardiac, and older patients (poor surgery candidates)
     b. MOA: Inhibit thyroid hormone release
     c. Contraindicated in pregnancy
  4. Antithyroid Drugs
    i. MOA: Block effects of thyroid hormone production (no effect on actual disease) by inhibiting the peroxidase enzyme system of the thyroid gland, thus preventing oxidation of iodide
    ii. **PTU (Propylthiouracil)**: 100 mg – 150 mg q8h
     a. Also inhibits the peripheral conversion of T4 to T3
    iii. **Methimazole (Tapazole)**: 15 mg – 30 mg once daily or divided q8h
    iv. *Beta* Blockers
     a. Atenolol 50-100 mg PO daily
     b. Propranolol 20-40 mg PO TID
     c. Calcium channel blockers are also used

## IV. THYROID STORM
A. Described as an exaggerated form of thyrotoxicosis, characterized by diarrhea, tachycardia, high fever (>103°F), nausea, vomiting, arrhythmias, weakness, heart failure, confusion, disorientation
B. Treatment
  1. Hydrocortisone 300 mg initially, then 100 mg q8h
    i. MOA: Prevents peripheral conversion of T4 to T3
  2. Propanolol 60 mg – 80 mg PO q4h
  3. PTU 600mg-1000 mg PO then 200 mg-250 mg PO q4h
  4. Methimazole 20 mg PO q4h

I. **Drug selection criteria** in choosing a medication should involve a *process of elimination* based on these variables:

A. Non-pharmacologic alternatives
  1. Before even considering medication, can therapy or other alternatives be used?

B. Patient's specific symptoms and diagnosis
  1. Only consider evidence-based medications for the given diagnosis as first-line treatments

C. Possible medication and/or medical triggers that can induce or worsen psychiatric illness
  1. Is an untreated underlying condition the cause of the current psychiatric symptoms?
   i. Evaluate recent lab values, urinalysis, urine toxicology screens, EKG, and radiology reports
   ii. Removing an underlying drug cause of the illness may abrogate the need for treatment
   iii. Give strong consideration to recreational drug abuse, CNS depressants and CNS stimulants

D. Side effect profile of drug
  1. Can it be matched to patient's symptoms for better tolerability?

E. Prior-treatment history and previous medication trial(s)
  1. Consider previous doses, durations of treatment, and outcomes
  2. May choose a different class of medication or use similar ones
  3. If failed previous therapies, consider augmentation strategies or appropriate polypharmacy

F. Patient's medical co-morbidities
  1. A new medication should not worsen or exacerbate a pre-existing condition
  2. Might want to consider a therapy that can be used as both a medical and psychiatric treatment
   i. E.g., antihistamine or *beta*-blocker for anxiety or an SNRI for neuropathic pain

G. Patient's clinical severity / suicidality
  1. If an urgent response is needed, consider time delays for medication effectiveness
  2. Do not consider therapy that can be toxic in overdose to a patient who is potentially suicidal or has a history of suicide attempts (especially if by overdose)

H. Family psychiatric or medication history
  1. Did a relative have a good outcome with a specific medication?
  2. Can the medication possibly induce mania or psychosis in a genetically vulnerable individual?

I. Drug-drug interactions with prescribed, over-the-counter (OTC) and herbal medications
  1. Must also ask about vitamins and supplements
  2. Rule out medications that will have significant interactions with pre-existing therapy
  3. Should consider pharmacodynamic (e.g., agonist/antagonist combinations) and pharmacokinetic interactions

J. Patient's history of medication adherence
  1. If a history of poor adherence, consider longer half-life medications or long-acting injectables
  2. Reduce the frequency of dosing to once or twice a day if possible

K. Drug cost to patient
  1. Consider cash costs, deductibles, co-pays, and criteria for Patient Assistance Programs

II. Possible *pharmacotherapeutic interventions and recommendations* for existing pharmacotherapy

A. Reduce Polypharmacy:
  1. >2 Antidepressants of the same class (other than the addition of trazodone for sleep)
  2. >2 Antipsychotics (including Depots that are not the same as patient's p.o. antipsychotic)
  3. Using antipsychotic for sleep at low dose + another antipsychotic

B. Drug worsens side effects, which is then treated with another agent

C. Drug worsens one disease state when used to treat another

D. Dosing time of day (i.e., **A**ripiprazole should be dosed in **AM** because it may be stimulating)

E. Dosing frequency (TID or BID, when a drug could be given QD)

F. Drug used in a child, which is not approved, over one that is approved

G. Off-label use of drug that has no evidence-based efficacy (EBM)
  1. i.e., Some anticonvulsants being used for in Bipolar Disorder with no EBM support

H. Dose of Quetiapine too low to be therapeutic (i.e., 25-200 mg at HS being used for sleep)

I. QT-prolonging medications given to children/adolescents or elderly without ongoing EKG monitoring

J. Valproic acid proper monitoring (platelets, LFTs, blood levels)

K. Lithium proper monitoring (WBCs, SrCr, electrolytes, blood levels)

L. Dementia patients – Are they receiving BZDs or anticholinergics?

M. Other Key Drug Levels (*See page 18*)

# 39. DR. RAPPA'S TAKE HOME PSYCHOPHARMACY PEARLS

✓ Avoid bupropion or duloxetine if a patient is in ALCOHOL or BZD withdrawal or has a Substance Use Disorder
✓ Antipsychotic metabolic side effects are NOT dose-related
✓ Antipsychotic EPS side effects & QT-prolongation ARE dose-related
✓ Do not abruptly discontinue antipsychotics, which can cause a psychotic rebound
✓ Do not abruptly discontinue anticonvulsants, which can cause a seizure
✓ ALWAYS order thiamine for alcohol patients ASAP (+ folate & MVI) before giving them anything with glucose in it (to prevent causing Wernicke's Encephalopathy)
✓ Obtain an **EKG** for patients > 40 (or those with cardiovascular medications) when prescribing ANY arrhythmogenic drugs at baseline and again in 7 days
  ➤ e.g., TCAs, citalopram, ziprasidone, iloperidone, chlorpromazine, lithium, quetiapine, Bactrim, ciprofloxacin, levofloxacin, etc.
✓ Always check for a current **TSH** if a patient is on Levothyroxine
✓ Using 2 or more **proarrhythmic** drugs together is absolutely contraindicated
✓ For lamotrigine or clozapine please check adherence prior to re-starting at the most recent dose
  ➤ Per the Package Inserts - If a patient misses > **48 hours** then you should re-titrate from beginning doses to decrease the induction of life-threatening side effects
✓ Elderly patients on acetylcholinesterase inhibitors – avoid all anticholinergic drugs, which negate the benefits of increased acetylcholine in the brain
✓ Valproate with topiramate = increased risk of hyperammonemia
✓ Valproate with lamotrigine – must reduce the dose of lamotrigine by half
✓ Levels taken before steady state of Lithium (5 days) & Valproate (3 days) WILL NOT be accurate and cannot be forecast through extrapolation
✓ When considering a long-acting injectable antipsychotic (LAIA) for non-adherent patients, reduce their burden of taking other oral meds (especially Lithium or Valproate)
✓ Please check for affordability before starting an LAIA
  ➤ Includes formulary, co-pays, deductibles, Patient Assistance Programs, etc.
✓ Women on lamotrigine and **birth control pills** should skip the placebo week of pills
  ➤ Estrogen decreases lamotrigine levels.
    o On the placebo week, lamotrigine levels can spike, inducing a rash
✓ National average daily dose of haloperidol is approximately **2-5mg**.
  ➤ High doses can be neurotoxic
✓ Haloperidol decanoate dose = **20 times** the oral daily dose
✓ Invega Sustenna does NOT require an **oral** overlap
✓ Metabolic risks of antipsychotics increase *alphabetically* by **brand** name:
  ➤ Abilify / Geodon / Latuda < Risperdal/Invega < Seroquel < Zyprexa
✓ These medications SHOULD be taken with FOOD to increase absorption:
  ➤ Quetiapine XR, ziprasidone, lurasidone, & sertraline

## TAKEN FROM NATIONAL & INTERNATIONAL GUIDELINES

✓ Do not use quetiapine for sleep (Against APA's **Choosing Wisely** campaign)[452]
✓ Do not use antipsychotics for elderly behavioral problems (e.g., screaming, crying, sundowning)
  ➤ Treat with behavioral therapies & distractions
✓ Avoid using **antidepressants** in patients with Bipolar Disorder, including a current episode of Bipolar Depression
✓ If a patient is diabetic, obese, or has hyperlipidemia, use aripiprazole, brexpiprazole, cariprazine, lurasidone or ziprasidone
  ➤ Avoid quetiapine & olanzapine
✓ Consider trying clozapine if patient fails just 2 trials of other antipsychotics (> 6 weeks at full therapeutic doses)

## I. DEFINITIONS
  A. **SUBSTRATE** = a drug or medication (called a *"xenobiotic"*)
  B. **INHIBITOR** = a drug that slows a substrate's metabolism and ↑'s substrate blood levels
  C. INDUCER = a drug that accelerates a substrate's metabolism and ↓'s substrate blood levels
  D. **POLYMORPHISM**
   1. Genetic variation that results in an ↑ or ↓ in enzyme production
   2. People of different backgrounds can share some polymorphisms that can ↑ or ↓ a drug's metabolism
  E. PHARMACOGENOMICS
   1. An evolving field of psychopharmacology where a patient's genetic profile is used to make predictions about medication effectiveness or side effects
   2. DNA is analyzed for certain genotypes, alleles, or *single-nucleotide polymorphisms* (SNPs) involving specific cytochrome 450 enzymes of drug metabolism, polymorphic biomarkers for dopamine and/or serotonin receptor genes and human leukocyte antigens (HLA)[1299]
    i. Useful to predict or prevent certain side effects and tailor drug therapy to individual patients[1300]
    ii. Genetic testing is not routinely done because of cost, but it may actually be cost-saving[1301]
   3. Serotonin Transported Promoter Polymorphism (5HTTLPR)[1302-1305]
    i. Also called SL6 or SLC6A4
    ii. Serotonin Transporter (SRT) Gene has two allelic forms: one long ("l") and one short ("s")
    iii. Because we have one gene from each parent, there are 3 genetic possibilities
     a. 2 longs, 2 shorts, or a long and a short
    iv. Meta-analysis of 81 studies showed a significant association (p=0.0000009) with the short allele and an increased risk of depression and suicidality, but only when following any form of stress
     a. e.g., medical condition, childhood adversity or maltreatment, stressful life events
   4. Genetic tests for specific drugs
    i. Phenytoin / carbamazepine / lamotrigine
     a. HLA-A*3101, HLA-B*1502, and HLA-A*2402 polymorphisms increase the risk of serious rash and Stevens-Johnson Syndrome
    ii. Valproic acid
     a. Mutations in mitochondrial DNA polymerase γ (POLG) can cause acute liver failure
    iii. Clozapine
     a. "C" allele genotype in HLA-DQB1 (a major histocompatibility complex, class II, DQ *beta* 1) has been linked with agranulocytosis[1299]
    iv. More specific information can be found at:
     a. Cytochrome P450 database – http://bioinformatics.charite.de/supercyp/index.php?site=home
     b. **PharmGKB** – The National Institute of General Medical Sciences of the National Institutes of Health (NIH) - www.pharmgkb.org
     c. **CPIC** –Clinical Pharmacogenetics Implementation Consortium (CPIC) - www.cpicpgx.org
      1. A partnership between PharmGKB and Pharmacogenomics Research Network (PGRN)
   5. **FDA-cleared tests** for genotyping (just a few examples)[1306]
    i. eQ-PCR LC Warfarin Genotyping kit (TrimGen Corporation)
    ii. eSensor Warfarin Sensitivity Saliva Test (GenMark Diagnostics)
    iii. eSensor Warfarin Sensitivity Test and XT-8 Instrument (Osmetech Molecular Diagnostics)
    iv. Gentris Rapid Genotyping Assay - CYP2C9 & VKORCI (ParagonDx, LLC)
    v. INFINITI BioFilmChip® microarrays (AutoGenomics, Inc.)
    vi. Invader UGT1A1 Molecular Assay (Third Wave Technologies Inc.)
    vii. Roche AmpliChip® microarray (Roche Molecular Systems, Inc.)
    viii. Spartan RX (Spartan Bioscience, Inc.)
    ix. Verigene (Nanosphere, Inc.)
    x. xTAG (Luminex Molecular Diagnostics, Inc.)
## II. PHASE I STAGE OF DRUG METABOLISM[867,1082,1307-1311]
  A. To make lipophilic compounds more hydrophilic for excretion by the kidneys
   1. **Phase I** reactions include oxidation, reduction, hydrolysis, demethylation, cyclization, monoamine oxidase (MAO), xanthine oxidase, carboxylesterase, alcohol/aldehyde dehydrogenase, and more
  B. **CYTOCHROME P450 (CYP450):** A family of enzymes, common to all living organisms, that metabolize food, environmental substances & toxins, and medications
   1. Humans possess ~ 60 genes and 59 pseudogenes to make Cytochrome P450 enzymes
   2. Divided among **18 families** of cytochrome P450
   3. Discovered in 1958 - had a spectrophotometric peak at a wavelength of 450nm
   4. Cytochrome P450 enzymes are hemoproteins (i.e., contains a heme-iron center)
   5. Abbreviation CYP denotes cytochrome P450
    i. First # is the gene family number (i.e. CYP**1**), which share >40% amino acid sequences
    ii. First letter is the gene subfamily letter (i.e. CYP3**A**), which share >55% amino acid sequences
    iii. Last # is the gene number (i.e. CYP2D**6**), which share >97% amino acid sequences
   6. Not all human CYP enzymes are involved in drug metabolism
    i. Usually just CYP1, CYP2 & CYP3 families
   7. Six enzymes (CYP1A2, 2C9, 2C19, 2D6, 2E1, 3A4) metabolize >90% of xenobiotics in humans
    i. CYP1A2 (on Chromosome 15) comprises 10-15% of liver enzymes; metabolizes 5% of all drugs
    ii. CYP2A6 (on Chromosome 19) comprises 4% of liver enzymes; metabolizes 2% of all drugs

iii. CYP2B6 (on Chromosome 19) metabolizes 2-4% of all drugs
iv. CYP2C8 and CYP2C18 (on Chromosome 10) metabolizes 1% of all drugs
v. CYP2C9 (on Chromosome 10) comprises 12% of liver enzymes; metabolizes 10% of all drugs
vi. CYP2C19 (on Chromosome 10) comprises 6% of liver enzymes; metabolizes 5% of all drugs
vii. CYP2D6 (on Chromosome 22) comprises 2% of liver enzymes; metabolizes 30% of all drugs
   a. 50% of psychiatric drugs are metabolized by CYP2D6
   b. Also called *debrisoquine hydroxylase* or *sparteine hydroxylase*
viii. CYP2E1 (Chromosome 10) comprises 7% of liver enzymes; metabolizes 2-4% of all drugs
ix. CYP3A4 (on Chromosome 7) comprises 30% of liver enzymes; metabolizes 40-45% of all drugs
8. Various alleles are present in various populations that make cytochrome P450 enzymes
  i. Cytochrome P450 enzymes may vary among individuals based on their classification as a poor/slow, intermediate, normal/extensive, or rapid/ultra-rapid metabolizer[1312,1313]
  ii. Genetic testing for CYP2D6, CYP2C9, CYP2C19, and CYP1A2 are most common
C. **CYP ENZYME POLYMORPHISMS**
1. **Poor/slow metabolizers** lack functional enzyme activity due to defective, inactive or absent genes
  i. CYP1A2: 3-15% of Africans, 15-25% of Asians, 2-4% of Caucasians, 3.6-6% of Saudi Arabians
  ii. CYP2A6: 1% of African-Americans and Caucasians, 7-24% of Asians
  iii. CYP2B6: 16% of Africans
  iv. CYP2C9: 1-7% in Africans, 1.7-5% of Asians, 6-15% of Caucasians
  v. CYP2C19: 11-21% African-Americans, 12-36% of Asians, 7-22% of Caucasians, 18-23% of Japanese, 12-23% of native peoples
  vi. CYP2D6: 0-5% Africans, and 0-2% of Asians, 5-14% of Caucasians
  vii. CYP2E1: 1% of Asians
  viii. CYP3A4: up to 53% of Africans, 0-5% of Asians, 3-9% of Caucasians, up to 5% of Hispanics and Japanese - Have ↓ enzyme activity
  ix. CYP3A5: up to 81% of Africans, up to 74% of Asians, up to 96% of Caucasians - Have ↓ activity
  x. Consider using *half* the usual dose in poor metabolizers
  xi. Prone to more side effects from normal dosages
2. **Intermediate metabolizers** usually carry 1 functional and 1 defective allele, but may also carry 2 partially defective alleles
  i. Have underactive enzymes
  ii. CYP2C19: 30% of Caucasians and African Americans, 60% of Chinese
  iii. Consider using *usual* to *less than usual* doses of medications for intermediate metabolizers
3. **Normal/extensive metabolizers** carry 2 functional genes for enzyme production
  i. CYP1A2: 46-66% of Africans, 59-65% of Asians, 62-72% of Europeans, 75% of N & S Americans
  ii. CYP2D6: up to 37% of East Asians, 50% of Caucasians
  iii. CYP2C9: up to 60% of Caucasians
  iv. CYP2C19: up to 77% of Caucasians
  v. CYP3A4: 66-86% of Africans, 0% of Asians, 2-20% of Caucasians
  vi. Consider using *usual* doses of medications for normal/extensive metabolizers
4. **Rapid/ultra-rapid metabolizers** carry more than 2 active genes encoding a certain CYP enzyme
  i. Usually have overactive enzymes
  ii. CYP2D6: 29-37% of Africans, 4% of Caucasians, 18% of Ethiopians, 1.5-10% of Europeans, 1.3% of Japanese, 21% of Saudi Arabians
  iii. Consider using *higher than normal* doses of medications for rapid/ultra-rapid metabolizers
  iv. May have a poor drug response at normal dosages
III. **PHASE II STAGE OF DRUG METABOLISM**
A. *Conjugation* of Phase I metabolites that are not adequately hydrophilic enough for excretion
B. Metabolites are joined to highly polar ligands such as acetate, glutathione, glucuronate, glycine, methyl groups or sulfate
C. Enzymes involved include: aldo-keto reductase (**AKR**), thiopurine-S-methyltransferase (TPMT), glutathione S-transferase (**GST**), sulfotranserase (**SULT**), N-acetyltransferase (**NAT**), catachol-O-methyltransferase (**COMT**) and uridine diphospho [**UDP**] glucuronyl transferase (**UGT**)
1. In humans, most common are the **UGT1** and **UGT2** families
IV. **PHASE III STAGE OF DRUG METABOLISM**
A. Proteins responsible for *transport* (or *efflux*) of xenobiotics across cell membranes to be excreted
B. Most studied are adenosine triphosphate (ATP)-binding cassette (**ABC**) family of transporters
1. P-glycoprotein (**Pgp** or **P-gp**) is encoded by the ABCB1 gene[1307,1314]
  i. Also called the Multidrug Resistant 1 (**MDR1**), PGY1, and cluster of differentiation 243 (CD243)
  ii. Pgp inhibitors are of interest in Oncology to ↑ efficacy of chemotherapy drugs while ↓ toxicity
2. Multidrug Resistant Proteins 2 (**MRP2**/ABCC2) and 3 (**MDR3**/ABCB4)
3. Breast Cancer Resistance Protein (**BCRP**/ABCG2)
4. Solute Carrier Organic Anion Transporter (**OATP**1B1/SLCO1B1 and OATP1B3/SLCO1B3)
5. Organic Anion Transporter 1 & 3 (**OAT1**/SLC22A6 & **OAT3**/SLC22A8)
  i. Also known as Solute Carrier Family 22 Member 6
6. Multidrug and Toxin Extrusion Protein 1 & 2K (**MATE1**/SLC47A1 & MATE-2K/SLC47A2)
  i. Also known as Solute Carrier Family 47 Member 1
7. Organic Cation Transporter-2 (**OCT2**/SLC22A2) / Solute Carrier Family 22 Member 2
8. Bile Salt Export Protein (**BSEP**/ABCB11)

| ISO-ENZYME | SUBSTRATES | | INHIBITORS | | INDUCERS |
|---|---|---|---|---|---|
| 1A2 | acetaminophen agomelatine amitriptyline apremilast aprepitant asenapine bendamustine BZDs beta-blockers caffeine carbamazepine chlorpromazine cinacalcet clomipramine clopidogrel clozapine cyamemazine cyclobenzaprine desipramine deutrabenazine diphenhydramine disulfiram duloxetine estradiol febuxostat fluphenazine flutamide fluvoxamine | haloperidol heparin imipramine leflunomide loxapine maprotiline melatonin methadone metoclo- pramide mexiletine mianserin mirtazapine nabumetone naproxen nortriptyline olanzapine ondansetron perazine perphenazine phenacetin → APAP pimozide promazine propafenone propranolol ramelteon ranitidine rasagiline | riociguat [1A1] rotigotine [1A1&2] riluzole ropinirole ropivacaine (R)-warfarin stiripentol tacrine tasimelteon tetra- benazine theophylline thioridazine thiothixene tizanidine trifluo- perazine verapamil warfarin zileuton ziprasidone zolmitriptan zolpidem zotepine | acyclovir allopurinol amiodarone apiaceous vegetables: carrots, celery, parsnips, parsley artemisinin atazanavir cimetidine ciprofloxacin citalopram diltiazem duloxetine echinacea enoxacin ethanol [acute] ethinyl estradiol and oral contraceptives famotidine fluoro- quinolones fluoxetine fluvoxamine grapefruit juice hydromorphone interferon α2B | isoniazid Kava-Kava levofloxacin methoxsalen mexiletine mibefradil mirtazapine moxifloxacin nefazodone norfloxacin olanzapine omeprazole paroxetine peginterferon α2a perazine phenylpro- panolamine piperine propafenone propranolol sertraline stiripentol tacrine thiabendazole ticlopidine verapamil vemurafenib zafirlukast zileuton | barbiturates beta- naphthoflavone carbamazepine charbroiled foods cigarette smoking (polycyclic aromatic hydrocarbons) cruciferous vegetables: broccoli, cabbage, brussel sprouts deferasirox ethanol [chronic] fosphenytoin griseofulvin insulin lansoprazole marijuana methyl- cholanthrene modafinil nafcillin nevirapine phenytoin rifampin ritonavir St. John's Wort stiripentol teriflunomide |
| 2A6 | apremilast caffeine clomethiazole | disulfiram nicotine promazine | tolcapone valproate vortioxetine | isoniazid nicotine tranylcypromine | | phenobarbital secobarbital valproate |
| 2B6 | artemisinin bupropion cyclophos- phamide diazepam disulfiram efavirenz fluoxetine | ifosfamide ketamine levomethadone medazepam methadone nevirapine perampanel prasugrel | propofol selegiline sertraline tamoxifen temazepam valproate vortioxetine | citalopram clopidogrel cyclophos- phamide fluvoxamine orphenadrine paroxetine | quazepam sertraline stiripentol ticlopidine tenofovir venlafaxine voriconazole | barbiturates carbamazepine efavirenz esketamine fos-(phenytoin) lopinavir modafinil rifampin ritonavir stiripentol |
| 2C8 | amiodarone benzphetamine brivaracetam buprenorphine cabazitaxel carbamazepine chloroquine clonazepam clozapine cyamemazine dabrafenib diazepam diclofenac docetaxel enzalutamide febuxostat fluvastatin gemfibrozil | ibuprofen isotretinoin lapatinib levomilnacipran lomitapide loperamide loxapine mephobarbital methadone methobarbital montelukast morphine paclitaxel phenytoin pitavastatin ponatinib repaglinide | retinols sertraline simeprevir sitagliptin temazepam thiazole- dinediones tolbutamide torsemide treprostinil tretinoin valproate venlafaxine verapamil vortioxetine warfarin zolpidem zopiclone | abiraterone amiodarone atazanavir avandafil clopidogrel clozapine cotrimoxazole deferasirox fluvoxamine gemfibrozil ketoconazole lapatinib montelukast nefazodone nicardipine | nilotinib olanzapine paroxetine pazopanib quercetin sorafenib stiripentol telithromycin teriflun- omide thiazole- dinediones trimeth- oprim valproate vilazodone vismodegib | barbiturates carbamazepine dabrafenib fosphenytoin nilotinib phenytoin primidone rifabutin rifampin rifapentine |

*Italics = moderate*   Underlined & in italics = a drug class   **Bold = strong** (indicates that an inhibitor, inducer, or polymorphism will have significant impact on the drug's metabolism)

| ISO-ENZYME | SUBSTRATES | | | INHIBITORS | | INDUCERS |
|---|---|---|---|---|---|---|
| 2C9 | alosetron<br>amprenavir<br>azapropazone<br>azilsartan<br>bosentan<br>candesartan<br>carbamazepine<br>carvedilol<br>celecoxib<br>chlorpropamide<br>clopidogrel<br>clozapine<br>cotrimoxazole<br>desogestrel<br>diclofenac<br>**dronabinol**<br>etravirine<br>febuxostat<br>flurbiprofen | fluvastatin<br>fluvoxamine<br>glimepiride<br>glipizide<br>glyburide<br>ibuprofen<br>irbesartan<br>ketamine<br>losartan<br>**marijuana**<br>**(THC)**<br>mefenamic<br>acid<br>melatonin<br>meloxicam<br>methadone<br>montelukast<br>naproxen<br>nateglinide<br>pitavastin | pioglitazone<br>piroxicam<br>ramelteon<br>rosiglitazone<br>rosuvastatin<br>sildenafil<br>sulfamethox-<br>azole<br>sulfonylureas<br>(S)-warfarin<br>tamoxifen<br>torsemide<br>valdecoxib<br>valsartan<br>vardenafil<br>zafirlukast<br>zileuton<br>zolpidem | **amiodarone**<br>**azapropazone**<br>**berberine**<br>**bosentan**<br>**capecitabine**<br>cimetidine<br>clozapine<br>**cotrimoxazole**<br>cranberries<br>diosmin<br>disulfiram<br>**doxifluridine**<br>**ethanol [acute]**<br>**felbamate**<br>**fluconazole**<br>**fluorouracil**<br>*fluvastatin*<br>fluvoxamine<br>gemfibrozil<br>ginkgo<br>milk thistle<br>hydromorphone<br>**imatinib**<br>**indomethacin**<br>ketoconazole<br>**leflunomide**<br>lovastatin<br>luliconazole<br>marijuana (THC) | metronidazole<br>miconazole<br>**nafcillin**<br>nefazodone<br>nilotinib<br>norethindrone<br>oxandrolone<br>phenobarbital<br>phenylbutazone<br>phenytoin<br>**piperine**<br>pomegranate<br>propoxyphene<br>ritonavir<br>secobarbital<br>sertraline<br>**sulfamethizole**<br>**sulfamethoxazole**<br>sulfaphenazole<br>**sulfinpyrazone**<br>**tamoxifen**<br>tolbutamide<br>toremifene<br>valproate<br>vemurafenib<br>vismodegib<br>voriconazole<br>*zafirlukast* | aminoglu-<br>tethimide<br>**aprepitant**<br>dabrafenib<br>elvitegravir<br>**enzalutamide**<br>**griseofulvin**<br>nilotinib<br>**rifampin**<br>**rifapentine**<br>**ritonavir**<br>St. John's<br>Wort<br>vigabatrin |
| 2C19 | agomelatine<br>**aprepitant**<br>**atomoxetine**<br>axitinib<br>bortezomib<br>brivaracetam<br>**bromazepam**<br>bupropion<br>**cannabidiol**<br>carisoprodol →<br>meprobamate<br>chlorphenir-<br>amine<br>cilostazol<br>**citalopram**<br>**clobazam**<br>**clomipramine**<br>clopidogrel<br>clorazepate<br>**clozapine**[24%]<br>cyclophos-<br>phamide<br>desvenlafaxine<br>dexlansoprazole | desipramine<br>diazepam +<br>desmethyl-<br>diazepam<br>**dothiepin**<br>**escitalopram**<br>esomeprazole<br>etravirine<br>flunitrazepam<br>flurazepam<br>**imipramine**<br>lacosamide<br>lansoprazole<br>lapatinib<br>letrozole<br>levomilnacipran<br>lomitapide<br>loxapine<br>**medazepam**<br>methadone<br>**moclobemide**<br>nelfinavir<br>nilutamide<br>**norclobazam** | nordazepam<br>omeprazole<br>pantoprazole<br>pentamidine<br>perphenazine<br>**prazepam**<br>primidone<br>progesterone<br>proguanil→<br>cycloguanil<br>promazine<br>propranolol<br>rabeprazole<br>(R)-warfarin<br>→ 8-OH<br>**rotigotine**<br>simeprevir<br>suvorexant<br>temazepam<br>teniposide<br>thalidomide<br>thioridazine<br>tofacitinib<br>vilazodone | arformoterol<br>armodafinil<br>avanafil<br>bortezomib<br>carbamazepine<br>**chloramphetacol**<br>**cimetidine**<br>citalopram<br>diazepam<br>disulfiram<br>eslicarbazepine<br>**esomeprazole**<br>ethinyl estradiol<br>felbamate (weak)<br>**fluconazole**<br>**fluoxetine &<br>norfluoxetine**<br>**fluvoxamine**<br>indomethacin | hydromorphone<br>lansoprazole<br>letrozole<br>**moclobemide**<br>nicardipine<br>**omeprazole**<br>oxcarbazepine<br>pantoprazole<br>rabeprazole<br>rotigotine<br>stiripentol<br>telmisartan<br>**ticlopidine**<br>topiramate<br>tranylcypromine<br>vilazodone<br>vismodegib<br>voriconazole | **artemisinin**<br>dabrafenib<br>**efavirenz**<br>**enzalutamide**<br>ginkgo biloba<br>norethindrone<br>**phenytoin**<br>prednisone<br>**rifampin**<br>**ritonavir**<br>tipranavir<br>vilazodone |
| Both<br>2C9 &<br>2C19 | **amitriptyline**<br>*barbiturates*<br>celecoxib<br>cyamemazine<br>diclofenac<br>diphenhydramine<br>divalproex sodium<br>**doxepin**<br>**fluoxetine**<br>formoterol<br>fosphenytoin<br>imipramine<br>indomethacin<br>mefenamic acid<br>mephenytoin<br>mirtazapine<br>ospemifene | perazine<br>phenytoin<br>piroxicam<br>prasugrel<br>quetiapine<br>(S)-naproxen →<br>norsuprofen<br>**sertraline**<br>TCA demethylation<br>tetrahydrocannabinol<br>tolbutamide<br>trimipramine<br>valproate<br>**venlafaxine**<br>voriconazole<br>vortioxetine<br>zonisamide | | **clopidogrel**<br>**delavirdine**<br>**efavirenz**<br>**etravirine**<br>fenofibrate<br>**fluconazole**<br>**fluoxetine**<br>**fluvoxamine**<br>fosphenytoin<br>**isoniazid** | Kava-Kava<br>ketoconazole<br>**modafinil**<br>olanzapine<br>paroxetine<br>probenecid<br>valproate<br>**voriconazole** | *barbiturates*<br>**carbam-**<br>**azepine**<br>cigarette<br>smoking<br>enzalutamide<br>ethanol<br>[chronic]<br>nevirapine<br>**phenytoin**<br>**primidone**<br>**rifampin**<br>**ritonavir** |
| 2C18 | clozapine | THC - tetrahydrocannabinol | | | | carbamazepine |

*Italics = moderate*     <u>*Underlined & in italics = a drug class*</u>     **Bold = strong (indicates that an inhibitor,**
**inducer, or polymorphism will have significant impact on the drug's metabolism) )**

149

| ISO-ENZYME | SUBSTRATES | | | INHIBITORS | | INDUCERS |
|---|---|---|---|---|---|---|
| 2D6 | alogliptin<br>alprenolol<br>amitriptyline →<br>nortriptyline<br>amphetamines<br>[most]<br>amoxapine<br>arformoterol<br>aripiprazole<br>asenapine<br>atomoxetine<br>benztropine<br>bisoprolol<br>brexpiprazole<br>brofaromine<br>bufuralol<br>cariprazine<br>carvedilol<br>cevimeline<br>chloroquine<br>chlorpheniramine<br>chorprothixene<br>chlorpromazine<br>ciclesonide &<br>des-ciclesonide<br>cinacalcet<br>citalopram &<br>n-desmethyl-<br>citalopram<br>clomipramine<br>clonidine<br>clozapine<br>cobicistat<br>codeine →<br>morphine<br>cyclobenzaprine<br>dapoxetine<br>darifenacin<br>debrisoquine<br>sulfate<br>desipramine<br>deutetrabenazine<br>dexfenfluramine<br>dextro-<br>amfetamine<br>dextro-<br>methorphan<br>dihydrocodeine<br>diphen-<br>hydramine<br>dolasetron<br>donepezil | dothiepin<br>doxepin<br>duloxetine<br>ecstasy<br>[MDMA]<br>encainide<br>escitalopram<br>fesoterodine<br>fingolimod<br>flecainide<br>flunarizine<br>fluoxetine &<br>norfluoxetine<br>flupenthixol<br>fluphenazine<br>fluvoxamine<br>formoterol<br>galantamine<br>guanoxan<br>haloperidol<br>hydrocodone<br>ibrutinib<br>iloperidone<br>imipramine →<br>desipramine<br>indoramin<br>levomilnacipran<br>lidocaine<br>lisdex-<br>amfetamine<br>lisuride<br>lovastatin<br>loxapine<br>maprotiline<br>meperidine<br>methadone<br>methylphenidate<br>metoclopramide<br>metoprolol<br>mexiletine<br>mianserin<br>miconazole<br>minaprine HCl<br>mirabegron<br>mirtazapine<br>moclobemide<br>moricizine<br>morphine<br>nebivolol<br>nefazodone<br>nortriptyline<br>olanzapine | ondansetron<br>opipramol<br>oxycodone<br>paliperidone<br>palonsetron<br>paroxetine<br>perhexiline<br>perphenazine<br>phenacetin [combo]<br>phenformin [combo]<br>pimozide<br>pomegranate<br>ponatinib<br>prajmaline<br>promethazine<br>propafenone<br>propranolol<br>protriptyline<br>quetiapine<br>ranolazine<br>remoxipride<br>risperidone→9-<br>OH (paliperidone)<br>ritonavir<br>rotigotine<br>selegiline<br>sertindole<br>sertraline<br>(S) metoprolol<br>(S) mexiletine<br>sparteine sulfate<br>tacrolimus<br>tamoxifen<br>(prodrug)<br>tetrabenazine<br>thioridazine<br>timolol<br>tolterodine<br>tramadol<br>trazodone &<br>mCPP metabolite<br>treprostinil<br>trimipramine<br>valbenazine<br>venlafaxine<br>verapamil<br>vilazodone<br>vortioxetine<br>yohimbine<br>zolpidem<br>zotepine<br>zuclopenthixol | abiraterone<br>amiodarone<br>asenapine<br>avanafil<br>berberine<br>bupropion<br>celecoxib<br>chloramphenicol<br>chloroquine<br>chlor-<br>pheniramine<br>chlorpromazine<br>cimetidine<br>cinacalcet<br>citalopram<br>clemastine<br>clobazam<br>cobicistat<br>clomipramine<br>clozapine<br>cobicistat<br>cocaine<br>codeine<br>darifenacin<br>darunavir<br>desipramine<br>desvenlafaxine<br>diltiazem<br>diphen-<br>hydramine<br>doxepin<br>doxorubicin<br>dronedarone<br>duloxetine<br>escitalopram<br>ethanol [acute]<br>everolimus<br>flecainide<br>fluoxetine &<br>nor-fluoxetine<br>fluphenazine<br>fluvoxamine<br>goldenseal<br>halofantrine<br>haloperidol<br>hydromorphone<br>hydroxy-<br>chloroquine<br>hydroxyzine<br>iloperidone | imatinib<br>Kava-Kava<br>labetalol<br>levo-<br>mepromazine<br>lorcaserin<br>lumefantrine<br>melperone<br>methadone<br>metoclopramide<br>mibefradil<br>mirabegron<br>moclobemide<br>modafinil<br>nefazodone<br>nicardipine<br>nilotinib<br>olanzapine<br>paroxetine<br>pazopanib<br>perphenazine<br>pomegranates<br>promethazine<br>propranolol<br>quinacrine<br>quinidine<br>quinine<br>ranitidine<br>ranolazine<br>risperidone<br>rotigotine<br>sertraline<br>terbinafine<br>thioridazine<br>thiothixene<br>ticlopidine<br>trazodone<br>tripelennamine<br>valproate<br>vemurafenib<br>venlafaxine<br>vilazodone<br>vincristine<br>ziprasidone | barbiturates<br>dexa-<br>methasone<br>ethanol<br>[chronic]<br>phenytoin<br>rifampin |
| 2E1 | acetaminophen<br>acetone<br>aniline<br>benzene<br>chloral hydrate<br>chlorzoxazone<br>clozapine<br>disulfiram | enflurane<br>ethanol<br>felbamate<br>halothane<br>isoflurane<br>isoniazid<br>n,n-dimethyl-<br>formamide | methoxyflurane<br>pyrazone<br>pyridine<br>sevoflurane<br>theophylline<br>toxins&<br>carcinogens<br>valproate | clomethiazole<br>disulfiram<br>ethanol [acute]<br>rufinamide (weak)<br>theophylline | | cigarette<br>smoking<br>ethanol<br>[chronic]<br>isoniazid |

Italics = moderate    Underlined & in italics = a drug class    Bold = strong (indicates that an inhibitor, inducer, or polymorphism will have significant impact on the drug's metabolism) )

| ISO-ENZYME | SUBSTRATES | | | | |
|---|---|---|---|---|---|
| 3A4/5/7 | abiraterone | citalopram | felodipine | nefazodone | sertraline |
| | acetaminophen | clarithromycin | fentanyl | nevirapine | sibutramine |
| | ado-trastuzumab | clindamycin | fesoterodine | nicardipine | sildenafil |
| |   emtansine | clomethiazole | fexofenadine | nifedipine | silodosin |
| | agomelatine | clomipramine | finasteride | nilotinib | simeprevir |
| | alfentanil | clopidogrel | fingolimod | nimodipine | simvastatin |
| | alfuzosin | clozapine | fluoxetine | nisoldipine | sirolimus |
| | aliskiren | cobicistat | fluspirilene | nitrendipine | sitagliptin |
| | alitretinoin | cocaine | flutamide | nortriptyline | solifenacin |
| | almotriptan | codeine-n- | fluticasone | olanzapine | sorafenib |
| | alogliptin |   demethylation | fluvoxamine | omeprazole | stiripentol |
| | amiodarone | colchicine | frovatriptan | ondansetron | sufentanil |
| | amitriptyline | conivaptan | fulvestrant | *oral contraceptives* | sunitinib |
| | amlodipine | corticosteroids | galantamine | ospemifene | suvorexant |
| | amprenavir | crizotinib | glyburide | oxybutynin | tacrolimus |
| | apixaban | cyamemazine | granisetron | oxycodone | tadalafil |
| | apremilast | cyclobenzaprine | guanfacine | paclitaxel | tamoxifen |
| | aprepitant | cyclophosphamide | halofantrine | paliperidone | tasimelteon |
| | **aripiprazole** | cyclosporine | **haloperidol** | pantoprazole | telaprevir |
| | armodafinil | dabrafenib | hydrocortisone | paricalcitol | telithromycin |
| | artemether | dapsone | ifosfamide | paroxetine | temsirolimus |
| | asenapine | darifenacin | iloperidone | pasireotide | teniposide |
| | astemizole | dasatinib | imatinib | pazopanib | terfenadine |
| | atorvastatin | delavirdine | imipramine | **perampanel** | testosterone |
| | avanafil | desvenlafaxine | indacaterol | perazine | theophylline |
| | axitinib | deutetrabenazine | irinotecan | pergolide | thioridazine |
| | azelastine | dexamethasone | isradipine | perphenazine | tiagabine |
| | azithromycin | dexlansoprazole | itraconazole | phentermine | ticagrelor |
| | bazedoxifene | dextromethorphan | ivabradine | **pimozide** | tinidazole |
| | beclomethasone | **dihydroergotamine** | ivacaftor | pioglitazone | tofacitinib |
| | bedaquiline | diltiazem | ixabepilone | pomalidomide | tolcapone |
| | *benzodiazepines* | disopyramide | ketoconazole | ponatinib | tolterodine |
| | benzphetamine | disulfiram | lansoprazole | prasugrel | tolvaptan |
| | bepridil | docetaxel | lapatinib | praziquantel | topotecan |
| | bexarotene | dofetilide | lercanidipine | prednisone | toremifene |
| | boceprevir | dolasetron | letrozole | progesterone | tramadol |
| | bortezomib | dolutegravir | **levomepromazine** | propafenone | **trazodone** |
| | bosentan | domperidone | **levomethadone** | promazine | triamcinolone |
| | bosutinib | donepezil | **levomilnacipran** | propranolol | trifluoperazine |
| | brentuximab | doxorubicin | levonorgestrel | *protease inhibitors* | trimipramine |
| | **brexpiprazole** | **dronabinol** | lidocaine | quazepam | ulipristal |
| | **bromocriptine** | dronedarone | linagliptin | **quetiapine** | valbenazine |
| | **bromperidol** | droperidol | lisuride | quinacrine | vandetanib |
| | **brotizolam** | dutasteride | lomitapide | quinidine (not 3A5) | vardenafil |
| | budesonide | ebastine | loperamide | quinine | vemurafenib |
| | bupivacaine | efavirenz | loratadine | (R)-warfarin | venlafaxine |
| | **buprenorphine** | eletriptan | losartan | rabeprazole | verapamil |
| | **buspirone** | elvitegravir | lovastatin | ramelteon | vesnarinone |
| | cabazitaxel | enzalutamide | loxapine | ranolazine | **vilazodone** |
| | cabozantinib | eplerenone | lumefantrine | reboxetine | vinblastine |
| | caffeine [also by | ergotamines | lurasidone | regorafenib | vincristine |
| |   aldehyde oxidase] | erlotinib | macitentan | repaglinide | vinorelbine |
| | canagliflozin | ethosuximide | maraviroc | rifabutin | vismodegib |
| | *cannabinoids* | erythromycin (not | mefloquine | rilpivirine | vorapaxar |
| | **carbamazepine** |   3A5) | methadone | riociguat | voriconazole |
| | **cariprazine** | escitalopram | mianserin | risperidone | vortioxetine |
| | cerivastatin | esomeprazole | milnacipran | rivaroxaban | **zaleplon** [also by |
| | chloroquine | eszopiclone | mifepristone | roflumilast |   aldehyde oxidase] |
| | chlorpheniramine | ethosuximide | mirabegron | romidepsin | zileuton |
| | chlorpromazine | etoposide | mirtazapine | ropinirole | ziprasidone [also by |
| | chlorprothixene | etravirine | modafinil | rotigotine |   aldehyde oxidase] |
| | ciclesonide & | everolimus | mometasone | ruxolitinib | **zolpidem** |
| |   des-ciclesonide | exemestane | montelukast | salmeterol | zonisamide |
| | cilostazol | felbamate | morphine | saxagliptin | **zopiclone** |
| | cinacalcet | | nateglinide | sertindole | **zotepine** |

*Italics = moderate*    <u>*Underlined & in italics = a drug class*</u>    **Bold = strong (indicates that an inhibitor, inducer, or polymorphism will have significant impact on the drug's metabolism) )**

| 3A4/5/7 INHIBITORS | | | | 3A4/5/7 INDUCERS | |
|---|---|---|---|---|---|
| **amiodarone** | **dasatinib** | **indinavir** | omeprazole | **amino-glutethimide** | garlic supplements |
| **amprenavir** | deferasirox | interleukin-10 | **paritaprevir** | amprenavir | _glucocorticoids_ |
| _aprepitant_ | **delavirdine** | _isavuconazole_ | paroxetine | **apalutamide** | **griseofulvin** |
| **atazanavir** | diazepam | **isoniazid** | pazopanib | aprepitant | _lorlatinib_ |
| avanafil | diethyldithio- | istradefylline | phenytoin | **armodafinil** | **mitotane** |
| _**barbiturates**_ | carbamate | **itraconazole** | pomegranate | **artemether** | _modafinil_ |
| basiliximab | _diltiazem_ | ivacaftor | **posaconazole** | _**barbiturates**_ | nafcillin |
| **berberine** | **dronedarone** | **ketoconazole** | quinidine/quinine | _bexarotene_ | **nevirapine** |
| bicalutamide | _duvelisib_ | **lapatinib** | **quinupristin** | _bosentan_ | **oxcarbazepine** |
| **boceprevir** | echinacea | _lefamulin_ | ranitidine | **carbamazepine** | **oxybutynin** |
| brentuximab | **efavirenz** | _letermovir_ | ranolazine | cigarette | perampanel |
| carfilzomib | **elvitegravir** | linagliptin | _ribociclib_ | smoking | phenylbutazone |
| _ceritinib_ | ethanol [acute] | lomitapide | **ritonavir** | clobazam | **phenytoin** |
| **chloramphenicol** | **ethinyl estradiol** | **lopinavir** | **saquinavir** | _dabrafenib_ | _rifabutin_ |
| chlorzoxazone | _everolimus_ | lovastatin | _schisandra_ | deferasirox | **rifampin** |
| cilostazol | _fedratinib_ | luliconazole | sertraline | **dexamethasone** | _rifapentine_ |
| **cimetidine** | _fluconazole_ | _**macrolides**_ | stiripentol | echinacea | rifaximin |
| **ciprofloxacin** | fluoxetine & norfl. | marijuana | synercid | _efavirenz_ | ritonavir (hi dose) |
| **clotrimazole** | **fluvoxamine** | mibefradil | tacrolimus | _etravirine_ | rofecoxib |
| **cobicistat** | **fosamprenavir** | **miconazole** | **tamoxifen** | **enzalutamide** | rufinamide (weak) |
| _conivaptan_ | **fosaprepitant** | **mifepristone** | **telaprevir** | esketamine | _St. John's Wort_ |
| _crizotinib_ | _gestodene [combo]_ | mirabegron | ticagrelor | _eslicarbazepine_ | stiripentol |
| crofelemer | ginkgo | **nefazodone** | **tipranavir** | ethanol [chronic] | topiramate |
| _cyclosporine_ | _goldenseal_ | **nelfinavir** | **tofisopam** | flutamide | troglitazone |
| **dalfopristin** | _grapefruit juice_ | nicardipine | valproate | **fosphenytoin** | **vemurafenib** |
| **danazol** | _haloperidol_ | nifedipine | _verapamil_ | | |
| **danoprevir** | **idelalisib** | nilotinib | **voriconazole** | | |
| **darunavir** | _imatinib_ | netupitant | **zafirlukast** | | |
| **dasabuvir** | interferon _gamma_ | **ombitasvir** | zileuton | | |

_Italics = moderate_    Underlined & in italics = a drug class    **Bold = strong (indicates that an inhibitor, inducer, or polymorphism will have significant impact on the drug's metabolism) )**

## VI. PHASE II SUBSTRATES AND INDUCERS[1315,1316]

| ENZYME | SUBSTRATES | | | INDUCERS |
|---|---|---|---|---|
| **AKR1C** (aldo-keto reductase) | haloperidol<br>naloxone | **naltrexone**<br>**(AKR1C4)** | oxcarbazepine<br>(AKR1C1-1C4) | |
| **UGT** (uridine diphospho-glucuronyl transferase) | desvenlafaxine<br>guanfacine<br>haloperidol<br>heroin | nalmefene<br>paliperidone<br>retigabine | rotigotine<br>tolcapone<br>topiramate | |
| - **UGT1A1** | ezetimibe<br>clozapine<br>desmethyl-clozapine | _beta_-estradiol<br>etoposide<br>nicotine | perampanel<br>_R_-carvedilol<br>sertraline | |
| - **UGT1A2** | nicotine | | | |
| - **UGT1A3** | amitriptyline<br>buprenorphine | ezetimibe<br>telmisartan | valproate | |
| - **UGT1A4** | amitriptyline<br>asenapine<br>clozapine<br>desmethyl-clozapine | diphenhydramine<br>imipramine<br>**lamotrigine**<br>midazolam | **olanzapine**<br>perampanel<br>phenobarbital<br>trifluoperazine | _barbiturates_<br>carbamazepine<br>_cigarette smoking_<br>estrogen-containing<br>  oral contraceptives<br>lamotrigine<br>_protease inhibitors_<br>phenytoin<br>rifampin |
| - **UGT1A6** | acetaminophen | deferiprone | valproate | |
| - **UGT1A7** | cannabidiol | dronabinol (1A7 to A10) | | |
| - **UGT1A9** | acetaminophen<br>cannabidiol (_also inhibits_) | entacapone<br>indomethacin<br>mycophenolic acid | propofol _R_-<br>oxazepam<br>valproate | |
| - **UGT2B4** | codeine | | | |
| - **UGT2B7** | buprenorphine<br>cannabidiol (_also inhibits_)<br>carbamazepine<br>**codeine**<br>diazepam<br>diclofenac | epirubicin<br>flurbiprofen<br>**lamotrigine**<br>lorazepam<br>**morphine**<br>naloxone<br>naproxen | oxazepam<br>S-carvedilol<br>temazepam<br>valproate (_also inhibits_)<br>zidovudine | |
| - **UGT2B10** | amitriptyline<br>clomipramine<br>**diphenhydramine** | imipramine<br>nicotine | olanzapine<br>trimipramine | |
| - **UGT2B15** | lorazepam<br>oxazepam | oxcarbazepine<br>phenytoin | | |
| - **UGT3B7** | lamotrigine | | | |
| **SULT** (sulfotransferase) | rotigotine (SULT1A1, SULT1A2, SULT1A3, SULT1B1, SULT1C4, and SULT1E1) | | | |

**Bold** = highly dependent on this enzyme / inhibitors or inducers will have significant effects on levels

| TRANSPORTER (GENE) | SUBSTRATES | | INHIBITORS | | |
|---|---|---|---|---|---|
| P-gp (ABCB1) | 2-amino-1-methyl-6-phenylimidazo[4,5-b]pyridine (PhIP) amitriptyline amprenavir aripiprazole atomoxetine bromocriptine cabergoline carbamazepine chlorpromazine cimetidine citalopram clozapine dabigatran diazepam digoxin diphenhydramine donepezil duloxetine escitalopram fexofenadine fluoxetine fluvoxamine haloperidol lamotrigine | levetiracetam levomilnacipran levosulpiride loperamide methadone milnacipran nortriptyline olanzapine oxcarbazepine paliperidone paroxetine pitavastatin prazosin quetiapine quinidine rifampin risperidone sertraline sulpiride talinolol topiramate venlafaxine vilazodone vinblastine vortioxetine | *(Most P-gp inhibitors also inhibit CYP3A4)* actinomycin D amiodarone annamycin **aripiprazole** atorvastatin biricodar (VX-710) carvedilol chlorpromazine citrus fruit (diosmin) clarithromycin colchicine cyclosporine diltiazem doxorubicin dronedarone elacridar (GF120918) erythromycin esomeprazole felodipine fenofibrate fluphenazine gallopamil | garlic ginseng green tea (quercetin) gomisin A itraconazole ketoconazole lamellarin lansoprazole lapatinib lopinavir mitotane (NSC-38721) MS-209 nifedipine omeprazole pantoprazole paroxetine polyethylene glycol progesterone propafenone quinidine ranolazine reserpine | reversin 121&125 ritonavir saquinavir sertraline silymarin St. John's Wort stiripentol tacrolimus tamoxifen tariquidar (XR9576) telaprevir tipranavir toremifene trifluoperazine valspodar verapamil vinblastine vincristine yohimbine zosuquidar (LY335979) zonisamide (weak) |

| **P-GP INDUCERS:** | artemisinin carbamazepine dexamethasone | doxorubicin nefazodone phenobarbital | phenytoin prazosin rifampin | risperidone St. John's Wort tenofovir | tipranavir trazodone vinblastine |
|---|---|---|---|---|---|

| TRANSPORTER (GENE) | SUBSTRATES | | | INHIBITORS | |
|---|---|---|---|---|---|
| BCRP (ABCG2) (Breast Cancer Resistance Protein) | 2-amino-1-methyl-6-phenylimidazo[4,5-b]pyridine (PhIP) carbamazepine coumestrol daidzein dantrolene | estrone-3-sulfate genistein glyburide lamotrigine methotrexate [also by aldehyde oxidase] | paliperidone pitavastatin prazosin risperidone rosuvastatin sulfasalazine | curcumin cyclosporine A elacridar (GF120918) estradiol-17β-glucuronide estrone-3-sulfate | eltrombopag fumitremorgin c ko134 ko143 novobiocin stiripentol sulfasalazine |
| OATP1B1 (SLCO1B1) (Solute Carrier Organic Anion Transporter) OATP1B3 (SLCO1B3) | asunaprevir benzylpenicillin bosentan cerivastatin cholecystokinin (cck-8) octapeptide (1B3) danoprevir digoxin | docetaxel (1B3) estradiol-17β-glucuronide fexofenadine estrone-3-sulfate (1B1) glyburide methotrexate | _HMG CoA reductase inhibitors_ nateglinide paclitaxel repaglinide telmisartan (1B3) | atazanavir clarithromycin cyclosporine erythromycin estradiol-17β-glucuronide estrone-3-sulfate gemfibrozil | lopinavir probenecid rifampin (single dose) rifamycin ritonavir simeprevir tacrolimus |
| OAT1 (SLC22A6) (Organic Anion Transporter 1) | adefovir cefaclor ceftizoxime cidofovir furosemide | ganciclovir methotrexate p-aminohippuric acid (PAH) tenofovir | | benzylpenicillin p-aminohippuric acid (PAH) probenecid teriflunomide | |
| OAT3 (SLC22A8) | benzylpenicillin estrone-3-sulfate famotidin | methotrexate oseltamivir carboxylate | penicillin G pravastatin rosuvastatin | cimetidine | |
| MATE1 (SLC47A1) MATE-2K (SLC47A2) | 1-methyl-4-phenylpyridinium (MPP+) dofetilide metformin tetraethylammonium (TEA) | | | cimetidine pyrimethamine | |
| OCT2 (SLC22A2) (Organic Cation Transporter-2) | 1-methyl-4-phenylpyridinium (MPP+) dofetilide metformin tetraethylammonium (TEA) | | | cimetidine dolutegravir isavuconazole quinidine | ranolazine trimethoprim vandetanib verapamil |

157

# 42. REFERENCES

1. Adderall mixed amphetamine salts [package insert]. Teva Select Brands, Horsham, PA. 12/2016.
2. Adderall XR® mixed amphetamine salts [package insert]. Shire US Inc., Lexington, MA.; 8/2019.
3. Evekeo®™ amphetamine sulfate. [package insert]. Arbor Pharmaceuticals, LLC. Atlanta, GA. 9/2016.
4. Strattera™ atomoxetine [package insert]. Indianapolis, IN: Ely Lily & Co.; 5/2017.
5. Catapres® clonidine [package insert]. Boehringer Ingelheim, Ridgefield, CT, 1998.
6. Kapvay® clonidine [package insert]. Shionogi Pharma, Inc., Atlanta, GA, 8/2016.
7. Focalin®/Focalin XR® dexmethylphenidate. [package insert]. Novartis Pharmaceuticals Corp. East Hanover, NJ. 1/2019.
8. Dextroamphetamine [package insert]. Research Triangle Park, NC: GlaxoSmithKline; 2007 November.
9. Dexedrine Spansules (dextroamphetamine) [package insert]. Catalent Pharma Solutions, Winchester, KY, 10/2013.
10. Dextroamphetamine sulfate [package insert]. Lupin Pharmaceuticals, Inc., Baltimore, MD, 4/2017
11 Dextrostat (dextroamphetamine) [package insert]. Shire Richwood, Florence, KY, 6/2006.
12. ProCentra® dextroamphetamine [package insert]. Independence Pharmaceuticals, LLC. Newport, KY. Feb 2017.
13. Zenzedi® (dextroamphetamine) [package insert]. Arbor Pharmaceuticals, LLC, Atlanta, GA, 2/2017
14. Intuniv™ guanfacine [package insert]. Shire US Inc., Wayne, PA, 7/2016.
15. Vyvanse® lisdexamfetamine [package insert]. Shire US Inc., Wayne, PA. 1/2018.
16. Desoxyn® methamphetamine [package insert]. AbbVie LTD, Barceloneta, PR. 10/2013.
17. Methylphenidate ER [package insert]. Amneal Pharmaceuticals of NY LLC, Brookhaven, NY, 6/2017.
18. Adhansia XR™ methylphenidate [package insert]. Purdue Pharmaceuticals LP, Wilson, NC, Feb. 2019.
19. Aptensio XR™ methylphenidate [package insert]. Patheon Manufacturing Services LLC, Greenville, NC. 10/2016.
20. Concerta® methylphenidate [package insert]. Janssen Pharmaceuticals, Inc. Titusville, NJ. 1/2017
21. Cotempla XR-ODT® (methylphenidate) [package insert]. Neos Therapeutics Brands, LLC, Grand Prairie, TX 6/2017.
22. Daytrana® methylphenidate patch [package insert]. Noven Pharmaceuticals, Inc., Miami, FL. 11/2017
23. Quillichew ER® methylphenidate [package insert]. Tris Pharma, Inc., Monmouth Junction, NJ, 8/2018.
24. Jornay PM™. methylphenidate [package insert]. Ironshore Pharmaceuticals, Inc., Cherry Hill, NJ, 4/2019.
25. Quillivant XR® methylphenidate [package insert]. Tris Pharma, Inc., Monmouth Junction, NJ, 8/2018.
26. Relexxii™ methylphenidate [package insert]. Vertical Pharmaceuticals, LLC, Bridgewater, NJ, 2/2019.
27 Metadate CD/ER methylphenidate [package insert]. UCB, Inc. Smyrna, GA, 1/2014.
28. Methylin® and Methylin ER. methylphenidate [package insert]. Mallinckrodt Inc. Hazelwood, MO. 10/2013.
29. Methylin® Chewable and Methylin Oral Soln. methylphenidate [package insert]. Mallinckrodt Inc. Hazelwood, MO. 9/2016.
30. Ritalin® / Ritalin SR methylphenidate [package insert]. Novartis Pharmaceuticals, East Hanover, NJ, 1-2019.
31. Adzenys ER® (dextroamphetamine) [package insert]. Neos Therapeutics, Inc., Grand Prairie, TX, 9/2017.
32. Adzenys XR-ODT® (dextroamphetamine) [package insert]. Neos Therapeutics, Inc., Grand Prairie, TX, 12/2017.
33. Dyanavel® XR amphetamine sulfate. [package insert]. Tris Pharma Inc., Monmouth Junction, NJ, 2/2019.
34. Evekeo ODT™ amphetamine sulfate. [package insert]. Arbor Pharmaceuticals, LLC. Atlanta, GA. 3/2019.
35. Mydayis® (amphetamine sulfate) [package insert]. Shire US Inc., 300 Shire Way, Lexington, MA, 6/2017.
36. Xanax®, alprazolam [package insert]. Pharmacia & Upjohn Company, Kalamazoo, MI, 12/2016.
37. Librium®, chlordiazepoxide [package insert]. Roche Laboratories, Nutley, NJ, 1995.
38. Klonopin® clonazepam [package insert]. Roche Laboratories, Inc., Nutley, NJ, 10/2017.
39. Tranxene T-TAB (clorazepate) [package insert]. AbbVie LTD, Barceloneta, PR. 9/2016.
40. Valium®, diazepam. [package insert]. Roche Pharmaceuticals. Nutley, New Jersey, 7/2017.
41. Diastat® (diazepam rectal gel) [package insert]. DPT Laboratories, LTD., San Antonio, Texas, Sept 2005.
42. Valtoco (diazepam nasal spray) [package insert]. Neurelis, Inc. San Diego, CA 1/2020.
43. Prosom® estazolam [package insert]. Abbott Laboratories, North Chicago, IL, 12/2018.
44. Flurazepam (Dalmane) [package insert]. Mylan Pharmaceuticals Inc. Morgantown, WV 12/2018.
45. Ativan®, lorazepam [package insert]. Wyeth pharmaceuticals Inc. Philadelphia, Pennsylvania, 9/2016.
46. Serax®, oxazepam [package insert]. Faulding and Wyeth-Ayerst Laboratories, Philadelphia, PA, 2000.
47. Doral (quazepam) [package insert]. Meda Pharmaceuticals, Inc. Somerset, NJ, 10/2016.
48. Restoril®, temazepam [package insert]. Mallinckrodt. St. Louis, Missouri, 9/2017.
49. Halcion®, triazolam. [package insert]. Pharmacia & Upjohn Company. Kalamazoo, Michigan, 2002.
50. BuSpar®, buspirone [package insert]. Bristol-Myers Squibb Company, Princeton, NJ, 12/2016.
51. Inderal®, propranolol [package insert]. Wyeth Pharmaceuticals, Inc, Philadelphia, PA, 11/2010.
52. Armodafinil - Nuvigil® [package insert]. Teva Pharmaceuticals, Inc., North Wales, PA; 2015 April.
53. Benadryl® diphenhydramine [package insert]. Parke-Davis, Morris Plains, NJ, 6/2018.
54. Doxepin [package insert]. New York, NY: Pfizer, Inc.; 6/2015.
55. Silenor® doxepin [package insert]. Somaxon Pharmaceuticals, Inc, San Diego, CA. March 2010.
56. Lunesta® (eszopiclone) [package insert]. Sunovion Pharmaceuticals Inc., Marlborough, MA, 8/2019.
57. Hydroxyzine [package insert]. AA Pharma Inc. Vaughan, ON, Canada, July 2018.
58. Atarax® (hydroxyzine HCl) [package insert]. ERFA Canada 2012 Inc. Montréal, QC, Jan 2015.
59. Ucerax (hydroxyzine hydrochloride) 25 mg film-coated tablets. Summary of product characteristics. (PDF). Irish Medicines Board. 2013.
   http://www.imb.ie/images/ uploaded/swedocuments/LicenseSPC_PA0891-005-001_16082013162208.pdf Retrieved 9/3/19.
60. Vistaril® hydroxyzine pamoate [package insert]. Pfizer Inc, New York, NY, 9/2019.
61. Meprobamate Miltown® [package insert]. Wallace Laboratories, Cranbury, NJ, 1/2016.
62. Modafinil - Provigil® [package insert]. Frazer, PA: Cephalon, Inc.; 11/2018.
63. Wakix® (pitolisant) [package insert]. Harmony Biosciences, LLC, Plymouth Meeting, PA. 8/2019.
64. Rozerem® ramelteon [package insert]. Takeda Pharmaceuticals America, Inc., Deerfield, IL, 12/2018.
65. Sunosi™ (solriamfetol) [package insert]. Jazz Pharmaceuticals, Inc., Palo Alto, CA. 6/2019.
66. Belsomra® suvorexant [package insert]. Merck and Co, Inc. Whitehouse Station, NJ 7/2018.
67. Xyrem (sodium oxybate) oral solution [package insert]. Jazz Pharmaceuticals, Inc., Palo Alto, CA. 10/2018.
68. Hetlioz® tasimelteon [package insert]. Vanda Pharmaceuticals Inc., Washington, D.C. Dec. 2014.
69. Trazodone [package insert]. Pomona, NY: Barr Laboratories, Inc.; 6/2017.
70. Sonata® zaleplon [package insert]. King Pharmaceuticals, Inc., New York, NY, 8/2019.
71. Ambien® zolpidem [package insert]. Sanofi-Aventis US,LLC, Bridgewater, NJ, 8/2019.
72. INTERMEZZO (zolpidem tartrate) sublingual tablets. [package insert]. Purdue Pharma L.P. Stamford, CT 8/2019.
73. ZOLPIMIST (zolpidem tartrate) Oral Spray [package insert]. Aytu BioScience, Inc. Englewood, CO 8/2019.
74. Edluar (zolpidem tartrate) sublingual tablets [package insert]. Meda Pharmaceuticals Inc. Somerset, NJ 8/2019
75. Osmolex ER™ (amantadine) [package insert]. Vertical Pharmaceuticals, LLC, Bridgewater, NJ, 2/2018.
76. Gocovri™ (amantadine) [package insert]. Adamas Pharma LLC. Emeryville, CA. 8/2017.
77. Apokyn (apomorphine hydrochloride injection) [package insert]. US WorldMeds, LLC, Louisville, KY, 5/2019.
78. Cycloset (bromocriptine mesylate) [package insert]. VeroScience, LLC, Tiverton, RI 2/2017.
79. Parlodel® (bromocriptine mesylate) [package insert]. Novartis Pharmaceuticals Corporation East Hanover, NJ, 1/2012.
80. Dostinex® (Cabergoline) [package insert]. Pharmacia & Upjohn, NY, NY 7/2011.
81. Lodosyn® (carbidopa) [package insert]. Valeant Pharmaceuticals, Bridgewater, NJ 2/2017
82. Sinemet® / Sinemet CR® (carbidopa/levodopa) [package insert]. Mylan Pharmaceuticals, Morgantown WV, 4/2018.
83. Parcopa® (carbidopa/levodopa) [package insert]. CIMA LABS INC. Eden Prairie, MN 2/2006.
84. Rytary® (extended-release carbidopa/levodopa) [package insert]. Impax Pharmaceuticals, Hayward, CA, 1/2015.
85. Duopa® (carbidopa/levodopa enteral suspension). [package insert]. AbbVie Inc North Chicago, IL 9/2016.
86. Stalevo® (carbidopa, levodopa and entacapone) [package insert]. Novartis Pharmaceuticals Corporation, East Hanover, NJ 2/2016.
87. Aricept® (donepezil) [package insert]. Woodcliff Lake, NJ: Eisai Inc. 12/2018.
88. Comtan (entacapone) [package insert]. Novartis Pharmaceuticals Corporation East Hanover, NJ, 6/2018.
89. Razadyne® (galantamine) [package insert]. Titusville, NJ: Janssen Pharmaceuticals, Inc. 5/2018.
90. Nourianz (istradefylline) [package insert]. Kyowa Kirin, Inc., Bedminster, NJ 8/2019.
91. Inbrija™ (levodopa inhalation powder) [package insert]. Acorda Therapeutics, Inc. Ardsley, NY, 12/2018.
92. Namenda XR® memantine [package insert]. St. Louis, MO, Forest Pharmaceuticals, Inc. 10/2016.
93. Namzaric™ (memantine + donepezil) [package insert]. Forest Pharmaceuticals, Dublin, Ireland. 1/2019.
94. Permax (pergolide mesylate) [package insert]. Eli Lilly and Company, Indianapolis, IN 3/2007.

95. Mirapex® and Mirapex ER® (pramipexole) [package insert]. Boehringer Ingelheim Pharmaceuticals, Inc. Ridgefield, CT 5/2018.
96. Azilect (rasagiline) [package insert]. Teva Pharmaceuticals USA, Inc., North Wales, PA, 12/2018.
97. Exelon (rivastigmine) [package insert]. East Hanover, NJ: Novartis Pharmaceuticals Corporation. 12/2018.
98. Requip (ropinirole) and Requip XL (extended-release) [package insert]. GlaxoSmithKline, Research Triangle Park, NC 2/2018.
99. Neupro (rotigotine transdermal system) [package insert]. UCB, Inc., Smyrna, GA 1/2019.
100. Xadago (safinamide) [package insert]. US WorldMeds, LLC, Louisville, KY, 5/2017.
101. Eldepryl (selegiline) [package insert]. Somerset Pharmaceuticals, Inc., Morgantown, WV, 6/2012.
102. Zelapar (selegiline) [package insert]. Valeant Pharmaceuticals North America LLC, Bridgewater, NJ 8/2016.
103. Emsam (selegiline) [package insert]. Somerset Pharmaceuticals, Inc., Morgantown, WV 7/2017.
104. Tasmar (tolcapone) [package insert]. Valeant Pharmaceuticals North America LLC, Bridgewater, NJ, 12/2018.
105. Cogentin injection (benztropine) [package insert]. Hospira, Inc., McPherson, KS, 9/2016.
106. Benztropine 2 mg tablets, Prescribing Information, Pendopharm, Division of Pharmascience Inc. Control number 179633. 2/2015.
107. Artane® (trihexyphenidyl) [package insert] Wyeth-Ayerst Laboratories, Pearl River, NY, 10/2003.
108. Amantadine [package insert].Actavis Pharma Inc. Parsippany, NJ 1/2017.
109. Symmetrel® (amantadine) [package insert]. Endo Pharmaceuticals Inc., Chadds Ford, PA, 1/2009
110. Austedo® (deutetrabenazine) [package insert]. Teva Pharmaceuticals USA, Inc., North Wales, PA 8/2017.
111. Ingrezza® (valbenazine) [package insert]. Neurocrine Biosciences, Inc., San Diego, CA, 12/2018.
112. Xenazine® (tetrabenazine) [package insert]. Lundbeck, Deerfield, IL 9/2018.
113. Carbatrol® (carbamazepine extended-release) [package insert]. Shire US Inc., Wayne, PA. 9/2018.
114. Epitol® (carbamazepine) [package insert]. TEVA Pharmaceuticals, Sellersville, PA. 12/2018.
115. Equetro® (carbamazepine extended-release) [package insert]. Validus Pharmaceuticals LLC, Parsippany, NJ, 10/2016.
116. Tegretol® (carbamazepine) [package insert]. Novartis Pharmaceuticals, East Hanover, 3/2018.
117. Lamictal® (lamotrigine) [package insert]. GlaxoSmithKline, Research Triangle Park, NC, 9/2018.
118. LAMICTAL XR (lamotrigine) [package insert]. GlaxoSmithKline, Research Triangle Park, NC, 9/2019.
119. Eskalith® Lithium [package insert]. GlaxoSmithKline, Research Triangle Park, NC, 9/2003.
120. Lithobid® (lithium) [package insert]. GlaxoSmithKline ANI Pharmaceuticals, Inc., Baudette, MN 11/2018
121. Symbyax®, Olanzapine + Fluoxetine [package insert]. Eli Lilly and Company, Indianapolis, IN, 3/2018.
122. Depakote®, Depakene® valproic Acid [package insert]. AbbVie Inc., North Chicago, IL, 2/2019.
123. Brivaracetam (Briviact®) [package insert]. UCB, Inc., Smyrna, GA 5/2018.
124. Cannabidiol (Epidiolex®) [package insert]. Greenwich Biosciences, Inc., Carlsbad, CA 12/2018.
125. Onfi® (clobazam) [package insert]. Lundbeck , Deerfield, IL. 6/2018.
126. APTIOM® (eslicarbazepine acetate) [package insert]. Sunovion Pharmaceuticals Inc., Marlborough, MA, 3/2019.
127. Ethotoin (Peganone®) [package insert]. UPM Pharmaceuticals, Bristol, TN 7/2016.
128. Zarontin® ethosuximide capsules [package insert]. Parke-Davis Div of Pfizer, New York, NY, 7/2018.
129. FELBATOL® (felbamate) [package insert]. Meda Pharmaceuticals, Somerset, NJ, 2/2018.
130. CEREBYX® (fosphenytoin) [package insert] Pfizer Inc., New York, NY, 6/2015.
131. Neurontin® gabapentin [package insert]. Pfizer Inc., New York, NY, 10/2017.
132. Gralise™ gabapentin [package insert]. Depomed, Inc., Menlo Park, CA, 9/2015.
133. HORIZANT® (gabapentin enacarbil) [package insert]. XenoPort, Inc., Santa Clara, CA, 10/2016.
134. VIMPAT® (lacosamide) [package insert]. UCB, Inc., Smyrna, GA, 6/2019.
135. KEPPRA / KEPPRA XR (levetiracetam) [package insert]. UCB, Inc., Smyrna, GA, 10/2017.
136. Elepsia™ (levetiracetam) [package insert]. Sun Pharmaceutical Industries, Inc., Cranbury, NJ, March 2015.
137. ROWEEPRA (levetiracetam) [package insert]. OWP Pharmaceuticals, Inc. West Chicago, IL 11/2016.
138. SPRITAM (levetiracetam) [package insert]. Aprecia Pharmaceuticals, LLC, Blue Ash, OH 9/2018.
139. FDA approves levetiracetam as first 3D printed drug product. Spritam-Aprecia Pharmaceuticals Co.
http://www.aphadruginfoline.com/supplemental-approvals/fda-approves-levetiracetam-first-3d-printed-drug-product Accessed on 8/4/15.
140. Methsuximide (Celontin) [package insert]. Pfizer, New York, NY 8/2013.
141. Midazolam Nayzilam [package insert]. UCB, Inc., Smyrna, GA 5/2019.
142. Trileptal®, oxcarbazepine [package insert]. Novartis, East Hanover, NJ, 1/2019.
143. OXTELLAR XR™ (oxcarbazepine) [package insert]. Supernus Pharmaceuticals, Inc., Rockville, MD, 12/2018.
144. FYCOMPA® (perampanel) [package insert]. Eisai Inc., Woodcliff Lake, NJ, 5/2019.
145. Phenobarbital oral solution [package insert]. manufacturer e5 Pharma, LLC, Boca Raton, FL. 10/2017.
146. Phenytoin sodium [package insert]. Upsher-Smith Laboratories, Inc., Maple Grove, MN. 9/2018.
147. Phenytek® (phenytoin) [package insert] Mylan Pharmaceuticals, Inc., Morgantown, WV, 2/2018.
148. LYRICA (pregabalin) ) [package insert]. Parke-Davis, New York, NY, 6/2019.
149. Lyrica CR (pregabalin controlled-release) [package insert]. Parke-Davis, New York, NY, 6/2019
150. Mysoline® (primidone). Valeant Pharmaceuticals N.A., Aliso Viejo, CA, Mar 2009.
151. BANZEL® (rufinamide) [package insert]. Eisai Inc., Woodcliff Lake, NJ, June 2015.
152. Diacomit (stiripentol) [package insert]. BIOCODEX, 60000 BEAUVAIS – France 8/2018.
153. Gabitril® (tiagabine) [package insert]. Cephalon, Inc., Frazer, PA, 5/2018.
154. Topamax® topiramate [package insert]. Janssen Pharmaceuticals, Inc., Titusville, NJ, 5/2019.
155. Trokendi XR™ (topiramate) [package insert]. Supernus Pharmaceuticals, Inc., Rockville, MD, 2/2019.
156. QUDEXY® XR (topiramate) [package insert]. Upsher-Smith Laboratories, Inc., Maple Grove, MN, 2/2019.
157. Tridione (trimethadione) [package insert]. AbbVie Inc. North Chicago, IL 4/2013.
158. Sabril® (vigabatrin) [package insert]. Lundbeck, Deerfield, IL, 7/2018.
159. Vigadrone (vigabatrin) [package insert]. UPSHER-SMITH LABORATORIES, LLC, Maple Grove, MN 10/2018.
160. ZONEGRAN® (zonisamide) [package insert]. Eisai Inc., Teaneck, NJ, 6/2017.
161. Elavil® amitriptyline [package insert]. West Point, PA: Zeneca Pharmaceuticals; 5/2016.
162. Tofranil® (imipramine) [package insert]. Hazelwood, MO: Mallinckrodt Inc.; 2007 September.
163. Surmontil® (trimipramine) [package insert].Research Triangle Park, NC: GlaxoSmithKline; 5/2014.
164. Nortriptyline [package insert]. Corona CA: Watson Laboratories, Inc.; 2007 August.
165. Pamelor® (nortriptyline) [package insert]. Patheon Inc., Whitby, Ontario, Canada. 4/2019.
166. Desipramine [package insert]. Bridgewater, NJ: Sanofi-Aventis; 2007 July.
167. Protriptyline [package insert]. West Point, PA; Merck&Co., Inc.; 5/2014.
168. Amoxapine [package insert]. Corona, CA: Watson Laboratories; 7/2010.
169. Maprotiline (Ludiomil®) [package insert].Summit, NJ: Ciba-Geigy Co.; 2/2008.
170. Nardil® phenelzine [package insert]. NY, NY: Park David, 6/2018.
171. Parnate® tranylcypromine [package insert]. Research Triangle Park, NC: GlaxoSmithKline, 1/2018.
172. Marplan® isocarboxazid [package insert]. Parsippany, NJ: Validus Pharmaceuticals, 4/2019.
173. Fluoxetine [package insert]. Pomona, NY: Barr Laboratories, Inc.; 3/2017.
174. Sertraline [package insert]. Morgantown, WV: Mylan Pharmaceuticals, Inc.; 12/2016.
175. Paroxetine [package insert]. Sellersville, PA: Teva Pharmaceuticals; 6/2014.
176. Pexeva (paroxetine mesylate) [package insert]. Norwich Pharmaceuticals, Inc., Norwich, NY. 2/2018.
177. Brisdelle (paroxetine) [package insert]. Noven Therapeutics, LLC, Miami, FL, 3/2018.
178. Fluvoxamine [package insert]. Sellersville, PA: Teva Pharmaceuticals; 2008 February.
179. Celexa® Citalopram [package insert]. Bonita Springs, FL: Forest Pharmaceuticals; 1/2019.
180. Lexapro® Escitalopram [package insert]. St. Louis, MO: Forrest Laboratories, Inc.; 1/2017.
181. Nefazodone [package insert]. Sellersville, PA: Teva Pharmaceuticals; 6/2014.
182. Oleptro™ trazodone [package insert]. Labopharm Europe Limited, Dublin, Ireland, 7/2014.
183. Trintellix® vortioxetine [package insert]. Lundbeck, Deerfield, IL, 7/2016.
184. Venlafaxine [package insert]. Sellersville, PA: Teva Pharmaceuticals, 12/2018.
185. Pristiq™ Desvenlafaxine [package insert]. Philadelphia, PA: Wyeth Pharmaceuticals, Inc.; 11/2018.
186. Cymbalta® Duloxetine [package insert]. Indianapolis, IN: Eli Lilly & Co.; 12/2017.
187. Irenka™ (Duloxetine) [package insert]. Lupin Pharmaceuticals Baltimore, MD 6/2015.
188. Drizalma Sprinkle™ (duloxetine delayed-release) [package insert]. Sun Pharmaceutical Industries, Inc. Cranbury, NJ 7/2019.
189. Pristiq™ Desvenlafaxine [package insert]. Philadelphia, PA: Wyeth Pharmaceuticals, Inc.; 11/2018.
190. Remeron® Mirtazapine [package insert]. Organon Inc., West Orange, NJ. 9/2019.
191. Wellbutrin® bupropion [package insert]. Research Triangle Park, NC: GlaxoSmithKline; 8/2017.

192. Viibryd™ vilazodone [package insert]. Trovis Pharmaceuticals, LLC. 5/2018
193. Spravato™ esketamine [package insert]. Janssen Pharmaceutical Companies, Inc., Titusville, NJ, 2019.
194. Zulresso™ (brexanolone) [package insert]. Sage Therapeutics,Inc., Cambridge, MA 6/2019.
195. Deplin® L-methylfolate calcium [package insert]. PAMLAB, L.L.C. Covington, LA. February 2010.
196. Thorazine®, Chlorpromazine [package insert]. Sandoz Inc, Broomfield, CO, 6/20111.
197. Prolixin®, Fluphenazine [package insert]. Ben Venue Inc, Bedford, OH, 8/2018.
198. Fluphenazine Decanoate [package insert]. Bedford Laboratories™, Bedford, OH, 8/2018
199. Haldol®, haloperidol [package insert]. Apotex Inc, Toronto, Canada, 12/2018.
200. Haloperidol Decanoate [package insert]. Bedford Laboratories™, Bedford, OH 5/2017.
201. Loxitane® [package insert]. Watson Pharma Inc, Corona, CA, 9/2010.
202. Adasuve (loxapine) [package insert]. Teva Pharmaceuticals, Inc. Horsham, PA, 8/2017.
203. Moban®, Molindone [package insert]. Endo Pharmaceuticals Inc, Chadds Ford, PA, 10/2018.
204. Trilafon®, perphenazine [package insert]. Schering Corporation, Kenilworth, NJ, 5/2017.
205. Mellaril®, Thioridazine [package insert]. Novartis Pharmaceuticals Corporation, East Hanover, NJ. 11/2016.
206. Navane®, thiothixene [package insert]. Pfizer Inc, NY, NY, 1/2010.
207. Stelazine®, trifluoperazine [package insert]. GlaxoSmithKline, Research Triangle Park, NC, 9/2010.
208. Abilify® aripiprazole [package insert]. Otsuka Pharmaceutical Co. Ltd., Tokyo, Japan, 8/2019.
209. Abilify Maintena™ [package insert]. Otsuka Pharmaceutical Co. Ltd., Tokyo, Japan, 2/2019.
210. Aristada (aripiprazole lauroxil) [package insert]. Alkermes, Inc. Waltham, MA 11/2018.
211. Aristada Initio (aripiprazole lauroxil) [package insert]. Alkermes, Inc. Waltham, MA 6/2018.
212. Saphris® (asenapine) [package insert]. Merck & Co., Inc., Whitehouse Station, NJ, 2/2017.
213. Secuado® (asenapine transdermal system) [package insert]. Noven Therapeutics, LLC, Miami, FL 10/2019.
214. Rexulti® (brexpiprazole) [package insert]. Otsuka America Pharmaceutical, Inc., Rockville, MD. 2/2018.
215. Cariprazine (Vraylar™) [package insert]. Actavis Pharma, Inc., Parsippany, NJ. May 2019.
216. Clozaril® clozapine [package insert]. Novartis Pharmaceuticals Corporation, East Hanover, NJ, 2/2017.
217. Fazaclo® clozapine [package insert]. Azur Pharma, Inc, Philadelphia, PA 2010. 2/2017.
218. Versacloz™ (clozapine) [package insert]. Jazz Pharmaceuticals Inc. Palo Alto, CA. 1/2018.
219. Fanapt® iloperidone [package insert]. Vanda Pharmaceuticals, Inc., Washington, D.C., 2/2017.
220. Latuda® lurasidone [package insert]. Sunovion Pharmaceuticals, Marlborough, MA 3/2018.
221. Zyprexa® olanzapine [package insert]. Eli Lilly and Company, Indianapolis, IN 1/2018.
222. Zyprexa® Relprevv™ [package insert]. Eli Lilly and Company, Indianapolis, IN 1/2018.
223. Invega® paliperidone [package insert]. ALZA Corporation, Mountain View, CA, 1/2019.
224. Invega® Sustenna® [package insert]. Janssen Pharmaceuticals, Inc., Titusville, NJ, 1/2019.
225. Invega Trinza™ [package insert]. Janssen Pharmaceuticals, Inc., Titusville, NJ, 1/2019.
226. Nuplazid™ (pimavanserin) [package insert]. ACADIA Pharmaceuticals Inc. San Diego, CA, 5/2019.
227. Seroquel® XR Quetiapine [package insert]. AstraZeneca Pharmaceuticals, Wilmington, DE, 11/2018.
228. Risperdal® risperidone [package insert]. Ortho-McNeil-Janssen Pharmaceuticals Inc, Gurabo, Puerto Rico, 1/2019.
229. Risperdal® Consta® [package insert]. Janssen Pharmaceuticals, Inc., Titusville, NJ, 1/2019.
230. Perseris™ (risperidone) subcutaneous injection. Indivior Inc., North Chesterfield, VA, 7/2018.
231. Geodon® ziprasidone [package insert]. Pfizer Inc, NY, NY, 11/2018.
232. Guallar E. Coffee gets a clean bill of health. BMJ. 2017;359(November):j5356. doi:10.1136/bmj.j5356
233. Saleh N. 6 surprising benefits of caffeine. MDLinx 11/19/19. https://www.mdlinx.com/internal-medicine/article/5160 Accessed on 12/16/19.
234. Poole R, Kennedy OJ, Roderick P, Fallowfield JA, Hayes PC, Parkes J. Coffee consumption and health: umbrella review of meta-analyses of multiple health outcomes. BMJ. 2017;359:j5024. doi:10.1136/bmj.j5024
235. Cohen TF. The Power of Drug Color. The Atlantic website. http://www.theatlantic.com/health/archive/2014/10/the-power-of-drug-color/381156/ Accessed on 4/8/15.
236. Tuttle AH, Tohyama S, Ramsay T, et al. Increasing placebo responses over time in U.S. clinical trials of neuropathic pain. Pain. 2015;156(12):2616-2626. doi:10.1097/j.pain.0000000000000333
237. Leibowitz KA, Hardebeck EJ, Goyer JP, Crum AJ. Physician Assurance Reduces Patient Symptoms in US Adults: an Experimental Study. J Gen Intern Med. 2018;33(12):2051-2052. doi:10.1007/s11606-018-4627-z
238. Chesney E, Goodwin GM, Fazel S. Risks of all-cause and suicide mortality in mental disorders: a meta-review. World Psychiatry. 2014;13:153-160. doi: 10.1002/wps.20128.
239. Sheehan R, Hassiotis A, Walters K, et al. Mental illness, challenging behaviour, and psychotropic drug prescribing in people with intellectual disability: UK population based cohort study. BMJ 2015(Sep 1);351:h4326. http://dx.doi.org/10.1136/bmj.h4326.
240. Matone M, Zlotnik S, Miller D, Kreider A, Rubin D, & Noonan K. (2015). Psychotropic Medication Use by Pennsylvania Children in Foster Care and Enrolled in Medicaid: An Analysis of Children Ages 3-18 Years. Philadelphia: PolicyLab at The Children's Hospital of Philadelphia.
241. Scudder L, Matone M, and Noonan K. Antipsychotic Drugs in Kids. Editorial. Medscape Pediatrics. http://www.medscape.com/viewarticle/849949_print Accessed on 9/1/15.
242. US Office of Inspector General. SGA Use Among Medicaid-Enrolled Children: Quality-of-Care Concerns (OEI-07-12-00320). http://oig.hhs.gov/oei/reports/oei-07-12-00320.pdf Accessed on 9/5/15.
243. dosReis S, Yoon Y, Rubin DM, et al. Antipsychotic Treatment Among Youth in Foster Care. Pediatrics. 2011 Dec; 128(6): e1459–e1466. doi: 10.1542/peds.2010-2970. PMCID: PMC3387900.
244. American Psychiatric Association. Diagnostic and Statistical Manual of Mental Disorders, 4th ed. text revised (DSM-IV-TR). Washington DC. American Psychiatric Association. 2000.
245. American Psychiatric Association. Diagnostic and Statistical Manual of Mental Disorders (Fifth ed.). Arlington, VA: American Psychiatric Publishing. ISBN 978-0-89042-555-8. 2013.
246. Sher Y and Lolak S. Ethical Issues: The Patient's Capacity to Make Medical Decisions. http://www.psychiatrictimes.com/special-reports/ethical-issues-patients-capacity-make-medical-decisions?GUID=631E98CE-0053-4441-9560-14CD338CC37E&rememberme=1&ts=30122014#sthash.OM7REOWp.dpuf. Accessed on 12/30/14.
247. New Psychotropic Drug Classification System Unveiled. Medscape. 11/3/14. http://www.medscape.com/viewarticle/834238 Accessed on 12/5/14.
248. Goodier R. Ten Drugs Cause Majority of ER Visits in Adults for Adverse Psych Med Effects. Medscape 7/14/14.
249. Weiss AJ (Truven Health Analytics), Barrett ML (M.L. Barrett, Inc.), Heslin KC (AHRQ), Stocks C (AHRQ). Trends in Emergency Department Visits Involving Mental and Substance Use Disorders, 2006–2013.HCUP Statistical Brief #216. December 2016. Agency for Healthcare Research and Quality, Rockville, MD. http://www.hcup-us.ahrq.gov/reports/statbriefs/sb216-Mental-Substance-Use-Disorder-ED-Visit-Trends.pdf.
250. Hampton LM, Daubresse M, Chang HY, et al. Emergency department visits by adults for psychiatric medication adverse events. JAMA Psychiatry. 2014 Sep;71(9):1006-14. doi: 10.1001/jamapsychiatry.2014.436
251. Williams LJ, Pasco JA, Stuart AL, et al. Psychiatric Disorders, Psychotropic Medication Use and Falls Among Women: An Observational Study. BMC Psychiatry. 2015;15(75).
252. Access to Health Services – Healthy People 2020. https://www.healthypeople.gov/2020/topics-objectives/topic/Access-to-Health-Services. Accessed on 9/20/19.
253. Sultan RS, Correll CU, Schoenbaum M, King M, Walkup JT, Olfson M. National Patterns of Commonly Prescribed Psychotropic Medications to Young People. J Child Adolesc Psychopharmacol. 2018;28(3):158–165. doi:10.1089/cap.2017.0077
254. Rubin R. Use of Illicit Drugs Continues to Rise. JAMA 2019 (Oct.22/29);322(16):1543.
255. The Silent Shortage: How Immigration Can Help Address the Large and Growing Psychiatrist Shortage in the United States. October 23, 2019. http://www.newamericaneconomy.org/wp-content/uploads/2017/10/NAE_PsychiatristShortage_V6-1.pdf Accessed on 10/11/19.
256. Substance Abuse and Mental Health Services Administration. (2019). Key substance use and mental health indicators in the United States: Results from the 2018 National Survey on Drug Use and Health(HHS Publication No. PEP19-5068, NSDUH Series H-54). Rockville, MD: Center for Behavioral Health Statistics and Quality, Substance Abuse and Mental Health Services Administration. Retrieved from https://www.samhsa.gov/data/
257. Mental Health in America - Access to Care Data. Access to Care Ranking 2020. https://www.mhanational.org/issues/mental-health-america-access-care-data. Accessed 9/30/19.
258. The State of Mental Health in America 2019. Mental Health America Inc. Alexandria, VA. https://www.mentalhealthamerica.net/sites/default/files/2019%20MH%20in%20America%20Final.pdf Accessed on 8/3/19.
259. Moore TJ. Adult Utilization of Psychiatric Drugs and Differences by Sex, Age, and Race. JAMA Internal Medicine 2017;177(2):274-5.
260. Substance Abuse and Mental Health Services Administration. (2018). Key substance use and mental health indicators in the United States: Results from the 2017 National Survey on Drug Use and Health(HHS Publication No. SMA 18-5068, NSDUH Series H-53). Rockville, MD: Center for Behavioral Health Statistics and Quality, Substance Abuse and Mental Health Services Administration. Retrieved from https://www.samhsa.gov/data/

261. di Giacomo E, Krausz M, Colmegna F, Aspesi F, Clerici M. Estimating the risk of attempted suicide among sexual minority youths. JAMA Pediatr. 2018:1-8. doi:10.1001/jamapediatrics.2018.2731

262. Sara R. Collins, Herman K. Bhupal, and Michelle M. Doty, Health Insurance Coverage Eight Years After the ACA: Fewer Uninsured Americans and Shorter Coverage Gaps, But More Underinsured (Commonwealth Fund, Feb. 2019). https://doi.org/10.26099/penv-q932

263. Burstein B, Agostino H, Greenfield B. Suicidal Attempts and Ideation among Children and Adolescents in US Emergency Departments, 2007-2015. JAMA Pediatr. 2019;173(6):598-600. doi:10.1001/jamapediatrics.2019.0464

264. Anglin D, Link B, Phelan J. Racial differences in stigmatizing attitudes toward people with mental illness. Psychiatr Serv 2006;57(6):857-862.

265. Strakowski SM. Racial Disparity in Mental Illness: Advice for Clinicians. Medscape. 7/2/15. http://www.medscape.com/viewarticle/847096_print Accessed on 7/7/15.

266. Diaz FJ and DeLeon J. Excessive antipsychotic dosing in 2 U.S. State hospitals. J Clin Psychiatry 63(11):998-1003, 2002 Nov.

267. Bakare MO. Effective therapeutic dosage of antipsychotic medications in patients with psychotic symptoms: Is there a racial difference?. BMC Research Notes. 1:25, 2008.

268. Masimirembwa CM, Hasler JA: Genetic polymorphism of drug metabolizing enzymes in African populations: implications for the use of neuroleptics and antidepressants. Brain Res Bull 1997, 44(5):561-571.

269. Gara MA, Vega WA, Arndt S, et al. Influence of Patient Race and Ethnicity on Clinical Assessment in Patients with Affective Disorders. Arch Gen Psychiatry. 2012;69(6):593-600. doi:10.1001/archgenpsychiatry.2011.2040.

270. Chow EA, HF, Foster Gonzalez VG, et al. The Disparate Impact of Diabetes on Racial/Ethnic Minority Populations. Clinical Diabetes July 2012 vol. 30 no. 3 130-133. doi: 10.2337/diaclin.30.3.130.

271. Cockcroft DW, Gault MH. Prediction of creatinine clearance from serum creatinine. Nephron 1976;16(1):31-41.

272. Wiesner R, Edwards E, Freeman R, et al. Model for end-stage liver disease (MELD) and allocation of donor livers. Gastroenterology. 2003;124:91-6.

273. Huhn M, Tardy M, Spineli LM, et al. Efficacy of pharmacotherapy and psychotherapy for adult psychiatric disorders: a systematic overview of meta-analyses. JAMA Psychiatry. 2014;71(6):706-15.

274. King V, Robinson S, Bianco T, et al. Choosing antidepressants for adults: clinicians guide. Agency for Healthcare Research and Quality Advancing Excellence in Health Care. AHRQ Publication No. 07-EHC007-3. August 2007. http://www.effectivehealthcare.ahrq.gov

275. Solomon DA, Keller MB, Leon AC, et al. Multiple Recurrences of Major Depressive Disorder. Am Journal Psychiatry 2000;157(2):229-233.

276. Weilburg JB, O'Leary KM, Meigs JB, et al. Evaluation of the adequacy of outpatient antidepressant treatment. Psychiatr Serv 2003;54:1233-9.

277. Ruhe HG MD, Huyser J MD, Swinkels JA, et al. Dose escalation for insufficient response to standard-dose maximal first-step serotonin reuptake inhibitors in major depressive disorder: Systematic review. British Journal of Psychiatry 189(4):309-316, October 2006.

278. Watanabe N, Omori IM, Nakagawa A, et al. Mirtazapine versus other antidepressants in the acute-phase treatment of adults with major depression: systematic review and meta-analysis. Journal of Clinical Psychiatry 69(9):1404-15, 2008 Sep.

279. Miyamoto S, Duncan G, Marx C, et al. Treatments for schizophrenia: a critical review of pharmacology and mechanisms of action of antipsychotic drugs. Molecular Psychiatry. 10(1):79-104, January 2005.

280. Webber M, Marder S. Better pharmacotherapy for schizophrenia: What does the future hold? Current Psychiatry Reports 2008;10(4):352-8.

281. Gardner D, Baldessarini R, Waraich P. Modern antipsychotic drugs: a critical overview. CMAJ Canadian Medical Association Journal. 172(13):1703-1711, June 21, 2005.

282. Katzman M. Current Considerations in the Treatment of Generalized Anxiety Disorder. CNS Drugs. 23(2):103-120, January 2009.

283. Sramek J, Zarotsky V, Cutler Neal. Generalized Anxiety Disorder: Treatment Options. Drugs. 62(11):1635-1648, January 2002.

284. Thase ME. Maintenance therapy for bipolar disorder. Journal of Clinical Psychiatry. 69(11):e32, 2008 Nov.

285. Smith LA, Cornelius V, Warnock A, et al. Effectiveness of mood stabilizers and antipsychotics in the maintenance phase of bipolar disorder: a systematic review of randomized controlled trials. Bipolar Disorders. 9(4):394-412, June 2007.

286. Gelenberg AJ MD, Pies R MD. Matching the Bipolar Patient and Mood Stabilizer. Ann Clin Psychiatry. 15(3-4):203-216, Sept/Dec 2003.

287. Zyvox® linezolid [package insert]. Pfizer, Pharmacia & Upjohn Co. New York, NY, 7/2018.

288. Ionso A, Rodríguez LA, Logroscino G, Hernán MA. Use of antidepressants and the risk of Parkinson's disease: a prospective study. J Neurol Neurosurg Psychiatry. 2009;80(6):671–674. doi:10.1136/jnnp.2008.152983.

289. Sidney H, Kennedy, Henning F, et al. Efficacy of escitalopram in the treatment of major depressive disorder compared with conventional selective serotonin reuptake inhibitors and venlafaxine XR: a meta-analysis. J Psychiatry Neurosci 2004;31(2):122-31.

290. S. Svensson and P.R. Mansfield. Escitalopram: superior to citalopram or a chiral chimera? Psychother Psychosom 2004;73(1):10-6.

291. S. K. Teo et al. Clinical pharmacokinetics of thalidomide. Clin Pharmacokinet. 2004;43(5):311-27.

292. PL Detail Document, "Ghost" Tablets. Pharmacist's Letter/Prescriber's Letter. March 2013.

293. Tungaraza TE, Talapan-Manikoth P, and Jenkins R. Curse of the ghost pills: the role of oral controlled-release formulations in the passage of empty intact shells in faeces. Two case reports and a literature review relevant to psychiatry. Ther Adv Drug Saf. 2013 Apr; 4(2): 63–71. doi: 10.1177/2042098612474681.

294. Pigott TA. Gender differences in the epidemiology and treatment of anxiety disorders. J Clin Psychiatry 1999;60 Suppl.8:4-15.

295. Bandelow B, Michaelis S, and Wedekind D. State of the Art Treatment of anxiety disorders. Dialogues Clin Neurosci. 2017;19:93-106.

296. Facts & Statistics. Anxiety & Depression Assoc. of America (ADAA). https://adaa.org/about-adaa/press-room/facts-statistics Accessed on 9/5/19.

297. Hilimire MR, DeVylder JE, and Forestell CA. Fermented foods, neuroticism, and social anxiety: An interaction model. Psychiatry Research 2015(August 15);228(2):203–208.

298. Velotis C, Wodarski S. Highlights From Current Research on Anxiety Disorders: The Most Common Psychiatric Illnesses Affecting Children and Adults. PsycCRITIQUES. 50(42), October 2005.

299. Jongsma A, Nichols K. Comprehensive Treatment of Anxiety Disorders. PsycCRITIQUES. 49(Sup11), Dec. 2004.

300. Bystritsky A. Treatment-resistant anxiety disorders. Molecular Psychiatry. 11(9):805-814, September 2006.

301. Spett M. Treating Anxiety Disorders: Drugs, Psychotherapy, or Both? PsycCRITIQUES. 49 (Supplement 4), October 2004.

302. Fasipe OJ. The emergence of new antidepressants for clinical use: Agomelatine paradox versus other novel agents. IBRO Reports. 2019;6(July 2018):95-110. doi:10.1016/j.ibror.2019.01.001

303. Frick A, Åhs F, Engman J, et al. Serotonin Synthesis and Reuptake in Social Anxiety Disorder: A Positron Emission Tomography Study. JAMA Psychiatry. Published online June 17, 2015. doi:10.1001/jamapsychiatry.2015.0125

304. Batelaan NM, Bosman RC, Muntingh A, Scholten WD, Huijbregts KM, van Balkom AJLM. Risk of relapse after antidepressant discontinuation in anxiety disorders, obsessive-compulsive disorder, and post-traumatic stress disorder: systematic review and meta-analysis of relapse prevention trials. BMJ. 2017;358:j3927. doi:10.1136/bmj.j3927

305. Hussain FS, Dobson ET, Strawn JR. Pharmacologic Treatment of Pediatric Anxiety Disorders. Curr Treat Options Psychiatry. 2016;3(2):151-160. doi:10.1007/s40501-016-0076-7

306. Lader M, Scotto JC. A multicentre double-blind comparison of hydroxyzine, buspirone and placebo in patients with generalized anxiety disorder. Psychopharmacology (Berl). 1998;139(4):402-406. doi:10.1007/s002130050731

307. Pecknold, J. C., Matas, M., Howarth, B. G., Ross, C., Swinson, R., Vezeau, C., & Ungar, W. (1989). Evaluation of Buspirone as an Antianxiety Agent: Buspirone and Diazepam versus Placebo*. The Canadian Journal of Psychiatry, 34(8), 766–771. https://doi.org/10.1177/070674378903400804

308. Mitte K, Noack P, Steil R, Hautzinger M. A meta-analytic review of the efficacy of drug treatment in generalized anxiety disorder. *J Clin Psychopharmacol.* 2005;25(2):141-150. doi:10.1097/01.jcp.0000155821.74832.f9

309. Olajide D, Lader M. A comparison of buspirone, diazepam, and placebo in patients with chronic anxiety states. J Clin Psychopharmacol. 1987 Jun;7(3) 148-152. PMID: 2885344.

310. Kubo N, Shirakawa O, Kuno T, And Tanak C. Antimuscarinic Effects of Antihistamines: Quantitative Evaluation by Receptor-Binding Assay. The Japanese Journal of Pharmacology Vol. 43 (1987) No. 3 P 277-282. http://dx.doi.org/10.1254/jjp.43.277

311. Ferreri M, Hantouche EG. Recent clinical trials of hydroxyzine in generalized anxiety disorder. Acta Psychiatr Scand Suppl. 1998;393:102-8.

312. PRAC recommends new measures to minimize known heart risks of hydroxyzine-containing medicines. European Medicines Agency website. http://www.ema.europa.eu/ema/index.jsp?curl=pages/news_and_events/news/2015/02/news_detail_002255.jsp&mid=WC0b01ac058004d5c1. Accessed on 4/8/2015.

313. Meeting highlights from the Pharmacovigilance Risk Assessment Committee (PRAC) 9-12 February 2015. http://www.ema.europa.eu/ema/index.jsp?curl=pages/news_and_events/news/2015/02/news_detail_002264.jsp&mid=WC0b01ac058004d5c1. Accessed on 8/22/15.

314. Llorca PM, Spadone C, Sol O, et al. Efficacy and Safety of Hydroxyzine in the Treatment of Generalized Anxiety Disorder: A 3-Month Double-Blind Study. J Clin Psychiatry 2002;63:1020–1027.

315. Tyrer P. Anxiolytics not acting at the benzodiazepine receptor: beta blockers. Prog Neuropsychopharmacol Biol Psychiatry. 1992 Jan;16(1):17-26.

316. A Head, M J Kendall, R Ferner, and C Eagles. Acute effects of beta blockade and exercise on mood and anxiety. Br J Sports Med. 1996 Sep; 30(3): 238–242. doi: 10.1136/bjsm.30.3.238

317. Peet M. The treatment of anxiety with beta-blocking drugs. Postgrad Med J 1988;64(Suppl 2):45-9.

318. Turner P. Therapeutic uses of beta-adrenocepter blocking drugs in the central nervous system in man. Postgrad Med J. 1989;65(759):1-6. doi:10.1136/pgmj.65.759.1
319. Steenen SA, Van Wijk AJ, Van Der Heijden GJ MG, Van Westrhenen R, De Lange J, De Jongh A. Propranolol for the treatment of anxiety disorders: Systematic review and meta-analysis. J Psychopharmacol. 2016;30(2):128-139. doi:10.1177/0269881115612236
320. Khadke VV, Khadke VS, and Khare A. Oral propranolol- Efficacy and comparison of two doses for peri-operative anxiolysis. Journal of the Indian Medical Association June 2012;110(7):457-60.
321. Ye L, Lippmann S. Reduction of anxiety after treatment with transdermal clonidine. Am J Heal Pharm. 2018;75(11):1-2. doi:10.2146/ajhp180064
322. Hoehn-Saric R, Merchant AF, Keyser ML, Smith VK. Effects of Clonidine on Anxiety Disorders. Arch Gen Psychiatry. 1981;38:1278-1282.
323. Strawn JR, Compton SN, Robertson B, Albano AM, Hamdani M, Rynn MA. Extended Release Guanfacine in Pediatric Anxiety Disorders: A Pilot, Randomized, Placebo-Controlled Trial. J Child Adolesc Psychopharmacol. 2017;27(1):29-37. doi:10.1089/cap.2016.0132
324. Baldwin DS, den Boer JA, Lyndon G, Emir B, Schweizer E, Haswell H. Efficacy and safety of pregabalin in generalised anxiety disorder: a critical review of the literature. J Psychopharmacol. 2015;29(10):1047-1060.
325. Generoso MB, Trevizol AP, Kasper S, Cho HJ, Cordeiro Q, Shiozawa P. Pregabalin for generalized anxiety disorder: An updated systematic review and meta-analysis. Int Clin Psychopharmacol. 2017;32(1):49-55. doi:10.1097/YIC.0000000000000147
326. Schjerning O, Damkier P, Lykkegaard SE, Jakobsen KD, Nielsen J. Pregabalin for anxiety in patients with schizophrenia — A randomized, double-blind placebo-controlled study. Schizophr Res. 2018;195:260-266. doi:10.1016/j.schres.2017.09.014
327. Bach DR, Korn CW, Vunder J, Bantel A. Effect of valproate and pregabalin on human anxiety-like behaviour in a randomised controlled trial. Transl Psychiatry. 2018;8(1). doi:10.1038/s41398-018-0206-7
328. el-Guebaly N, Sareen J, Stein MB. Are there guidelines for the responsible prescription of benzodiazepines? Can J Psychiatry. 2010;55(11):709-714. doi:10.1177/070674371005501104
329. Ott CA. Treatment of anxiety disorders in patients with comorbid bipolar disorder. Ment Health Clin [Internet]. 2018;8(6):256-63. DOI: 10.9740/mhc.2018.11.256.
330. Schmitz A. Benzodiazepine use, misuse, and abuse: A review. Ment Heal Clin. 2016;6(3):120-126. doi:10.9740/mhc.2016.05.120
331. Wongsamitkul N, Maldifassi MC, Simeone X, Baur R, Ernst M, Sigel E. α subunits in GABAA receptors are dispensable for GABA and diazepam action. Sci Rep. 2017;7(1):1-11. doi:10.1038/s41598-017-15628-7
332. Zhu S, Noviello CM, Teng J, Walsh RM, Kim JJ, Hibbs RE. Structure of a human synaptic GABAA receptor. Nature. 2018;559(7712):67-88. doi:10.1038/s41586-018-0255-3
333. Sieghart W. Pharmacology of benzodiazepine receptors: An update. J Psychiatry Neurosci. 1994;19(1):24-29.
334. Santhakumar V, Wallner M, Otis TS. Ethanol acts directly on extrasynaptic subtypes of GABAA Receptors To Increase Tonic Inhibition. October. 2007;41(3):211-221.
335. Jones CM, Mack KA, Paulozzi LJ. Pharmaceutical overdose deaths, United States, 2010. JAMA. 2013;309(7):657-9. DOI:10.1001/jama.2013.272. PubMed PMID: 23423407.
336. Vinkers CH, Olivier B. Mechanisms underlying tolerance after long-term benzodiazepine use: a future for subtype-selective GABA(A) receptor modulators? Advances in Pharmacological Sciences 2012;2012:416864. [PUBMED:22536226]
337. Taipale H, Koponen M, Tanskanen A, et al. Long-term use of benzodiazepines and related drugs among community-dwelling individuals with and without Alzheimer's disease. Int Clin Psychopharmacol. 2015 Jul;30(4):202-8. doi: 10.1097/YIC.0000000000000080.
338. Billioti de Gage S, Begaud B, Bazin F, et al. Benzodiazepine use and risk of dementia: prospective population based study. BMJ 2012;345(27):e6231.
339. Gallacher J, Elwood P, Pickering J, Bayer A, Fish M, Ben-Shlomo Y. Benzodiazepine use and risk of dementia: evidence from the Caerphilly Prospective Study (CaPS). Journal of Epidemiology and Community Health 2012;66(10):869–73
340. Wu CS, Wang SC, Chang IS, Lin KM. The association between dementia and long-term use of benzodiazepine in the elderly: nested case-control study using claims data. American Journal of Geriatric Psychiatry 2009;17(7):614–20.
341. Imfeld P, Bodmer M, Jick SS, et al. Benzodiazepine Use and Risk of Developing Alzheimer's Disease or Vascular Dementia: A Case-Control Analysis. Drug Saf. 2015 Jun 30. [Epub ahead of print]
342. Canadian Agency for Drugs and Technologies in Health. Discontinuation Strategies for Patients with Long-term Benzodiazepine Use: A Review of Clinical Evidence and Guidelines. Rapid Response Rep Summ with Crit Apprais. 2015;1(July):1-28. doi:10.1017/CBO9781107415324.004
343. Vicens C, Fiol F, Llobera J, et al. Withdrawal from long-term benzodiazepine use: Randomised trial in family practice. Br J Gen Pract. 2006;56(533):958-963.
344. Brett J, Murnion B. Management of benzodiazepine misuse and dependence. Aust Prescr. 2015;38(5):152-155.
345. Baandrup L, Ebdrup BH, Rasmussen JO, Lindschou J, Gluud C, Glenthøj BY. Pharmacological interventions for benzodiazepine discontinuation in chronic benzodiazepine users. Cochrane Database Syst Rev. 2018;2018(3). doi:10.1002/14651858.CD011481.pub2
346. Kaylee Caniff, Emily Telega, Jolene R. Bostwick, Kristen N. Gardner, Pregabalin as adjunctive therapy in benzodiazepine discontinuation, American Journal of Health-System Pharmacy, Volume 75, Issue 2, 15 January 2018, Pages 67–71, https://doi.org/10.2146/ajhp160712
347. Liebrenz M, Gehring MT, Buadze A, Caflisch C. High-dose benzodiazepine dependence: a qualitative study of patients' perception on cessation and withdrawal. BMC Psychiatry. 2015;15(1):1-12. doi:10.1186/s12888-015-0493-y
348. Bandelow B, Sher L, Bunevicius R, et al. Guidelines for the pharmacological treatment of anxiety disorders, obsessive-compulsive disorder and posttraumatic stress disorder in primary care. Int J Psychiatry Clin Pract. 2012;16(2):77-84. doi:10.3109/13651501.2012.667114
349. Strawn JR, Geracioti L, Rajdev N, et al. Pharmacotherapy for Generalized Anxiety Disorder in Adults and Pediatric Patients: An Evidence-Based Treatment Review. Expert Opin Pharmacother. 2018 July; 19(10):1057–1070. doi:10.1080/14656566.2018.1491966.
350. Baldwin DS, Anderson IM, Nutt DJ, et al. Evidence-based pharmacological treatment of anxiety disorders, post-traumatic stress disorder and obsessive-compulsive disorder: a revision of the 2005 guidelines from the British Association for Psychopharmacology. J Psychopharmacol. 2014; 28(5):403–439.
351. Greenblatt HK, Greenblatt DJ. Gabapentin and Pregabalin for the Treatment of Anxiety Disorders. Clin Pharmacol Drug Dev. 2018;7(3):228-232. doi:10.1002/cpdd.446
352. Clarke H, Kirkham KR, Orser BA, et al. Gabapentin reduces preoperative anxiety and pain catastrophizing in highly anxious patients prior to major surgery: A blinded randomized placebo-controlled trial. Can J Anesth. 2013;60(5):432-443. doi:10.1007/s12630-013-9890-1
353. Srour H, Pandya K, Flannery A, Hatton K. Enteral Guanfacine to Treat Severe Anxiety and Agitation Complicating Critical Care After Cardiac Surgery. Semin Cardiothorac Vasc Anesth. 2018;22(4):403-406. doi:10.1177/1089253218768537
354. Pande AC, Davidson JRT, Jefferson JW, et al. Treatment of Social Phobia with Gabapentin: A Placebo-Controlled Study Journal of Clinical Psychopharmacology 1999;19(4):341-348.
355. Lavigne JE, Mustian K, Mathews JL, et al. A Randomized, Controlled, Double-Blinded Clinical Trial of Gabapentin 300 mg versus 900 mg versus Placebo for Anxiety Symptoms in Breast Cancer Survivors. Breast Cancer Res Treat. 2012 Nov;136(2):479–486. doi:10.1007/s10549-012-2251-x.
356. Stein MB, Sareen J, Hami S, Chao J. Pindolol potentiation of paroxetine for generalized social phobia. A double-blind, placebo-controlled, cross-over study. Am J Psychiatry 2001;158:1725–1727.
357. Schade S, Paulus W. D-Cycloserine in Neuropsychiatric Diseases: A Systematic Review. Int J Neuropsychopharmacol. 2016;19(4):1-7. doi:10.1093/ijnp/pyv102
358. Qureshi NA, Mohammed A, Al-Bedah. Mood disorders and complementary and alternative medicine: A literature review. Neuropsychiatr Dis Treat. 2013;9:639-658. doi:10.2147/NDT.S43419
359. Anheyer, D., Haller, H., Klose, P. et al. Phytotherapy in Psychiatric Disorders Nervenarzt (2018) 89:1009. https://doi.org/10.1007/s00115-018-0539-8 (Translated to English from German)
360. Muszyńska B, Łojewski M, Rojowski J, Opoka W, Sułkowska-Ziaja K. Natural products of relevance in the prevention and treatment of depression. Psychiatr Pol. 2015;49(3):435-453. doi:10.12740/pp/29367
361. Szafrański T. Herbal remedies in depression – state of the art. Psychiatr Pol 2014;48(1):59-73.
362. Sarris J, Panossian A, Schweitzer I, Stough C, Scholey A. Herbal medicine for depression, anxiety and insomnia: A review of psychopharmacology and clinical evidence. Eur Neuropsychopharmacol. 2011;21(12):841-860. doi:10.1016/j.euroneuro.2011.04.002
363. Dwyer A V, Whitten DL, Hons B, Hawrelak JA, Hons B. Herbal Medicines, other than St. John's Wort, in the Treatment of Depression: A Systematic Review. Altern Med Rev. 2010;16(1):40-49.
364. Möller HJ, Volz HP, Dienel A, Schläfke S, Kasper S. Efficacy of Silexan in subthreshold anxiety: meta-analysis of randomised, placebo-controlled trials. Eur Arch Psychiatry Clin Neurosci. 2019;269(2):183-193. doi:10.1007/s00406-017-0852-44
365. Donelli D, Antonelli M, Bellinazzi C, Gensini GF, Firenzuoli F. Effects of lavender on anxiety: A systematic review and meta-analysis. Phytomedicine. 2019;65(September):153099. doi:10.1016/j.phymed.2019.153099
366. 2017 Medicines in Development for Mental Illness. https://www.phrma.org/-/media/Project/PhRMA/PhRMA-Org/PhRMA-Org/PDF/MID_Mental-Illness-2017-Drug-List_Final.pdf Accessed 9/22/19.
367. New Anxiety Medications. https://mentalhealthdaily.com/2018/02/17/new-anxiety-medications-2018-drugs-in-clinical-trials/ Accessed 8/2/19.

162

368. Valdoxan (agomelatine) Summary of product characteristics and package leaflet. European Medicine Agency. Les Laboratoires Servier, Suresnes cedex, France. April 2019. http://www.ema.europa.eu/docs/en_GB/document_library/EPAR_-_Product_Information/human/000915/WC500046227.pdf

369. Morris G, Anderson G, Berk M, Maes M. Coenzyme Q10 Depletion in Medical and Neuropsychiatric Disorders: Potential Repercussions and Therapeutic Implications. Mol Neurobiol. 2013;48(3):883-903. doi:10.1007/s12035-013-8477-8

370. Travivo™ for Major Depression. Available at: https://www.fabrekramer.com/products/tgfk07ad/tgfk07ad-2/ Accessed on 8/8/19.

371. A Safety and Efficacy Study of JNJ-42165279 in Participants With Social Anxiety Disorder (Clinical Research Trial Listing) (Claustrophobia) (NCT02432703)". www.centerwatch.com. Retrieved 2019-03-02.

372. Gold Standard, Inc. Benzodiazepines. Clinical Pharmacology [online]. http://www.clinicalpharmacology.com Accessed: 2/2/12.

373. Radley DC, Finkelstein SN, Stafford RS. Off-label prescribing among office based physicians. Arch Intern Med. 2006;166:1021-26.

374. Bridge JA, Birmaher B, Iyenger S, et al. Placebo response in randomized controlled trials of antidepressants for pediatric major depressive disorder. American Journal of Psychiatry. 166(1):42-9, 2009 Jan.

375. Ackermann RT, Williams JW Jr. Rational treatment choices for non-major depressions in primary care: an evidence-based review. Journal of General Internal Medicine. 17(4):293-301, 2002 Apr.

376. Tsapakis EM, Soldani F, Tondo L, et al. Efficacy of antidepressants in juvenile depression: meta-analysis. Brit J Psych 2008;193(1):10-7.

377. Dubicka B, MRCPsych; Hadley S, Roberts C. Suicidal behavior in youths with depression treated with new-generation antidepressants: Meta-analysis. British Journal of Psychiatry. 189(5):393-398, November 2006.

378. Hall WD, Lucke J. How have the selected serotonin reuptake inhibitor antidepressants affected suicide mortality?. Australian & New Zealand Journal of Psychiatry 40(11-12): 941-950, November/December 2006.

379. Cheung AH, Emslie GJ, Mayes TL. The use of antidepressants to treat depression in children & adolescents. CMAJ 2006;174(2):193-200.

380. Southammakosane C and Schmitz K. Pediatric Psychopharmacology for Treatment of ADHD, Depression, and Anxiety. Pediatrics 2015. peds.2014-1581; Published online July 6, 2015 (10.1542/peds.2014-1581).

381. Merikangas KR, He JP, Burstein M, et al. Lifetime prevalence of mental disorders in U.S. adolescents: results from the National Comorbidity Survey Replication - Adolescent Supplement (NCS-A). J Am Acad Child Adolesc Psychiatry. 2010;49(10):980–989.

382. American Academy of Pediatrics. Policy Statement. Off-Label Use of Drugs in Children. Committee on Drugs. Pediatrics 2014(Mar 1);133(3): 563-567. (doi: 10.1542/peds.2013-4060).

383. The National Institute of Mental Health (NIMH) website on Attention Deficit Hyperactivity Disorder (ADHD). Accessed on 2/6/2012 at http://www.nimh.nih.gov/health/topics/attention-deficit-hyperactivity-disorder-adhd/index.shtml

384. Jefferson B Prince , Peter S. Jensen, Amy Vierhile. Piecing together the ADHD Puzzle: Treatment Strategies for attention deficit Hyperactivity Disorder (ADHD) From Childhood to Adolescence and through the Transition years. Found at http://cme.medscape.com/viewprogram/6043. Accessed on 3/23/09.

385. Stephen V. Faraone, Norra MacReady, Highlights of the 2008 U.S. Psychiatric and Mental Health Congress. New Research on Pharmacological Therapy in ADHD. Found at http://cme.medscape.com/viewprogram/17840_pnt. Accessed on 3/1/09.

386. Scott H. Kollins, Laurie E. Scudder, Elizabeth Samander. ADHD in Childhood and Adolescence: New Evidence in Diagnosis and Treatment. Found at http://cme.medscape.com/viewprogram/18705_pnt. Accessed on 3/23/09.

387. Liew Z, Ritz B, Rebordosa C, Lee PC, Olsen J. Acetaminophen use during pregnancy, behavioral problems, and hyperkinetic disorders. JAMA Pediatr. 2014;168(4):313-20.

388. Zader SJ, Williams E, Buryk MA. Mental Health Conditions and Hyperthyroidism. Pediatrics. 2019;144(5): e20182874

389. Visser SN, Bitsko RH, Danielson ML, et al. Treatment of Attention Deficit/Hyperactivity Disorder among Children with Special Health Care Needs. J Pediatr 2015 (ahead of print). http://dx.doi.org/10.1016/j.jpeds.2015.02.018.

390. Reinblatt SP, Mahone EM, Tanofsky-Kraff M, et al. Pediatric loss of control eating syndrome: association with attention-deficit/hyperactivity disorder and impulsivity. Int J Eat Disord. 2015 Apr 9. [Epub ahead of print].

391. Dalsgaard S, Leckman JF, Mortensen PB, et al. Effect of drugs on the risk of injuries in children with attention deficit hyperactivity disorder: a prospective cohort study. The Lancet Psychiatry. Published Online: 21 July 2015. DOI: http://dx.doi.org/10.1016/S2215-0366(15)00271-0.

392. Florida Psychotherapeutic Medication Guidelines for Children and Adolescents 2015 (January). http://medicaidmentalhealth.org. Accessed on 8/15/15.

393. Häggkvist J and Franck J. Biological Research on Addiction: Comprehensive Addictive Behaviors and Disorders, Volume 2. Book Chapter 7 - Animal Models of Addiction other than Alcohol: Amphetamines. 2013, pgs 61-68. ISBN: 978-0-12-398335-0. DOI: https://doi.org/10.1016/C2011-0-07782-7. Academic Press. Elsevier Inc. Karolinska Institutet, Stockholm, Sweden.

394. King GR and Ellinwood EH. Amphetamines and other stimulants. Substance Abuse: A Comprehensive Textbook, 3rd edition. 1997; 207-22. Williams & Wilkins, Baltimore, MD.

395. Baldessarini RJ. Drugs and the treatment of psychiatric disorders: Psychosis and anxiety / Depression and Mania. Goodman and Gilman's The Pharmacological Basis of Therapeutics, 9th edition. 1996;400-6,432. McGraw-Hill, New York, NY.

396. Musto DF. Historical Perspectives. Substance Abuse: A Comprehensive Textbook 3rd Ed. 1997;1-9. Williams & Wilkinson, Baltimore, MD.

397. Heal DJ, Smith SL, Gosden J, et al. Amphetamine, past and present – a pharmacological and clinical perspective. J Psychopharmacol. 2013 Jun;27(6):479–496. doi: 10.1177/0269881113482532 PMCID: PMC3666194.

398. Myerson A. The effect of benzedrine sulphate on mood and fatigue in normal and neurotic persons. Arch Neur Psychiatry 1936; 36:816–22.

399. Guttmann E and Sargant W. Observations on Benzedrine. The British Medical Journal 1937 (May 15):1013-1015.

400. Bett WR. Benzedrine Sulphate in Clinical Medicine. Post-Graduate Medical Journal 1946 (August):205-218.

401. Haelle T. About one in four youths prescribed stimulants also use the drugs nonmedically. 6/25/19. https://www.mdedge.com /familymedicine/article/203549/ mental-health/about-one-four-youths-prescribed-stimulants-also-use Accessed 6/26/19.

402. Habel LA, Cooper WO, Sox CM, et al. ADHD medications and risk of serious cardiovascular events in young and middle-aged adults. JAMA 2011 Dec 28;306(24):2673-83.

403. Cooper WO, Habel LA, Sox CM, et al. ADHD drugs & serious cardiovascular events in children & young adults. NEJM 2011;365:1896-904.

404. MacKenzie LE, Abidi S, Fisher HL, et al. Stimulant Medication and Psychotic Symptoms in Offspring of Parents With Mental Illness. Pediatrics. 2016;137(1):e20152486. doi:10.1542/peds.2015-2486

405. Vitiello B, Elliott GR, Swanson JM, et al. Blood Pressure and Heart Rate Over 10 Years in the Multimodal Treatment Study of Children with ADHD. Am J Psychiatry 2012;169:167-177.

406. Biederman J, DiSalvo M, Fried R, Woodworth KY, Biederman I, Faraone S V. Quantifying the Protective Effects of Stimulants on Functional Outcomes in Attention-Deficit/Hyperactivity Disorder: A Focus on Number Needed to Treat Statistic and Sex Effects. J Adolesc Heal. 2019:1-6. doi:10.1016/j.jadohealth.2019.05.015

407. Steingard R, Taskiran S, Connor DF, Markowitz JS, Stein MA. New Formulations of Stimulants: An Update for Clinicians. J Child Adolesc Psychopharmacol. 2019;29(5):1-16. doi:10.1089/cap.2019.0043

408. van Wyk GW, Hazell PL, Kohn MR, et al. How oppositionality, inattention, and hyperactivity affect response to atomoxetine versus methylphenidate: a pooled meta-analysis. J Atten Disord 2012;16(4):314-324.

409. Childress Ann C, Brams Matthew, Cutler Andrew J., et al. Journal of Child and Adolescent Psychopharmacology. June 2015, 25(5): 402-414. doi:10.1089/cap.2014.0176.

410. FDA Drug Safety Communication: FDA reporting permanent skin color changes associated with use of Daytrana patch (methylphenidate transdermal system) for treating ADHD. 6/24/15. http://www.fda.gov/Drugs/DrugSafety/ucm452244.htm

411. Ghasri P, Gattu S, Saedi N, Ganesan AK. Chemical leukoderma after the application of a transdermal methylphenidate patch. J Am Acad Dermatol. 2012 Jun;66(6):e237-8.

412. Monarch® eTNS® System for Pediatric ADHD. https://www.monarch-etns.com/ Accessed on 9/24/19.

413. Hirota T, Schwartz S, Correll CU. Alpha-2 agonists for attention-deficit/hyperactivity disorder in youth: A systematic review and meta-analysis of monotherapy and add-on trials to stimulant therapy. J Am Acad Child Adolesc Psychiatry. 2014;53(2):153-173. doi:10.1016/j.jaac.2013.11.009

414. Medications used in the Treatment of ADHD. In: Managing Medication for Children and Adolescents with ADHD. National Resource Center on ADHD Children. A Program of CHADD. May 2011. http://www4adhd.org/documents/WWWK3.pdf

415. A.D.D Warehouse. Medication chart to treat attention deficit hyperactivity disorder. http://www.addwarehouse.com/shopsite_sc/store/html/42/article13.htm. Accessed 2/9/12.

416. The official 2010 TCPR ADHD medication comparison chart. The Carlat Psychiatry Report. October 2010. http://thecarlatreport.com/article/official-2010-tpcr-adhd-medication-comparison-chart

417. Gold Standard, Inc. Amphetamines. Clinical Pharmacology [database online]. http://www.clinicalpharmacology.com. Accessed: June 16, 2012.

418. Bostwick JR, Demehri A. Pills to powder: A clinician's reference for crushable psychotropic medications. Curr Psychiatr. 2014;13(5):e1-e4.

419. Jafarinia M, Mohammadi M-R, Modabbernia A, et al. Bupropion versus methylphenidate in the treatment of children with attention-deficit/hyperactivity disorder: randomized double-blind study. Hum. Psychopharmacol Clin Exp2012;27:411–418. DOI: 10.1002/hup.2242.

420. Harrison P. Dementia Drug May Help Improve ADHD Symptoms. Medscape Medical News. Presented at the 12th World Congress of Biological Psychiatry on June 15, 2015. Accessed on 6/20/15. http://www.medscape.com/viewarticle/846627?nlid=83065_2051&src=wnl_edit_medn_psyc&uac=39316CJ&spon=12

421. Bolea-Alamañac B, Nutt DJ, Adamou M, et al. Evidence-based guidelines for the pharmacological management of attention deficit hyperactivity

disorder: Update on recommendations from the British Association for Psychopharmacology. J Psychopharmacol, March 2014; vol. 28, 3: pp. 179-203, first published on February 12, 2014.

422. Anheyer D, Lauche R, Schumann D et al (2017) Herbal medicines in children with attention deficit hyperactivity disorder (ADHD): a systematic review. Complement Ther Med 30:14–23 3. Apaydin EA, Maher AR, Shanman R et al (2016) A systematic review of St. John's wort for major depressive disorder. Syst Rev 5:148 4.

423. Koopman-Verhoeff ME, van den Dries MA, van Seters JJ, Luijk MPCM, Tiemeier H, Luik AI. Association of Sleep Problems and Melatonin Use in School-aged Children. JAMA Pediatr. 2019;173(9):883–885. doi:https://doi.org/10.1001/jamapediatrics.2019.2084

424. Mental Health Daily. http://mentalhealthdaily.com/2015/09/14/new-adhd-medications-in-the-pipeline-2015/. Accessed 4/28/16.

425. LeClerc S and Easley D. Pharmacologic Therapies for Autism Spectrum Disorder: A Review. P&T 2015;40(6):389-397.

426. Singh K, Connors SL, Macklin EA, et al. Sulforaphane treatment of autism spectrum disorder (ASD). Proc Natl Acad Sci USA. 2014;111(43):15550-5.

427. Chemical derived from broccoli sprouts shows promise in treating autism. Eureka Alert website. http://www.eurekalert.org/pub_releases/2014-10/ihm-cdf100814.php. Accessed April 10, 2015.

428. Investor Update. https://www.roche.com/investors/updates/inv-update-2018-01-29.htm Accessed 10/30/19.

429. Lemonnier E, Degrez C, Phelep M, et al. A randomized controlled trial of bumetanide in the treatment of autism in children. Trans Psychiatry 2012;2:e202. doi 10.1038/tp.2012.124.

430. Science behind NBTX-001. http://www.nobilistx.com/science-behind-nbtx-001/ Accessed on 8/18/19.

431. NIMH – Major Depression. https://www.nimh.nih.gov/health/statistics/major-depression.shtml Accessed 12/11/19.

432. Patton GC et al. The prognosis of common mental disorders in adolescents: A 14-year prospective cohort study. Lancet 2014 Jan 16; [e-pub ahead of print]. (http://dx.doi.org/10.1016/S0140-6736(13)62116-9)

433. Boers E, Afzali MH, Newton N, Conrod P. Association of Screen Time and Depression in Adolescence. JAMA Pediatr. 2019. doi:10.1001/jamapediatrics.2019.1759

434. Bowes L, Johnson C, Wolke D, et al. Peer victimization during adolescence and its impact on depression in early adulthood: prospective cohort study in the United Kingdom. BMJ 2015;350:h2469. doi:10.1136/bmj.h2469.

435. Miron O, Yu K-H, Wilf-Miron R, Kohane IS. Suicide Rates Among Adolescents and Young Adults in the United States, 2000-2017. JAMA. 2019;321(23):2362-2364. doi:10.1001/jama.2019.5054

436. Curtin SC, Heron M. Death rates due to suicide and homicide among persons aged 10-24: United States, 2000-2017 key findings data from the National Vital Statistics System. 2019;(352):1-8. https://www.cdc.gov/nchs/data/databriefs/db352-h.pdf

437. Food and Drug Administration. Relationship between psychotropic drugs and pediatric suicidality. August 16, 2004. http://www.fda.gov/ohrms/dockets/ac/04/briefing/2004-4065b1-10-TAB08-Hammads-Review.pdf Accessed May 7, 2015.

438. Cooper WO, Callahan ST, Shintani A, et al. Antidepressants and suicide attempts in children. Pediatrics 2014;133(2):204-10.

439. Rahn KA, Cao Y-J, Hendrix CW,and Kaplin AI. The role of 5HT1A receptors in mediating acute negative effects of antidepressants: implications in pediatric depression. Transl Psychiatry (2015)5, e563; doi:10.1038/tp.2015.57.

440. Miller M, Swanson SA, Azrael D, Pate V, Sturmer T. Antidepressant dose, age, and the risk of deliberate self-harm. JAMA Intern Med 2014;174:899–909.

441. Phased SSRI Dosages Could Mitigate Suicide Risks in Youngsters. US Pharmacist WeeklyNewsUpdate. May 20, 2015. http://www.uspharmacist.com/weekly_news_update/nl/54820.

442. Locher C, Koechlin H, Zion SR, et al. Efficacy and safety of selective serotonin reuptake inhibitors, serotonin-norepinephrine reuptake inhibitors, and placebo for common psychiatric disorders among children and adolescents: A systematic review and meta-analysis. JAMA Psychiatry. 2017;74(10):1011-1020. doi:10.1001/jamapsychiatry.2017.2432

443. Shamseddeen W, Clarke G, Keller MB, et al. Adjunctive sleep medications and depression outcome in the treatment of serotonin-selective reuptake inhibitor resistant depression in adolescents study. J Child Adolesc Psychopharmacol. 2012;22(1):29-36.

444. Cipriani A, Zhou X, Del Giovane C, et al. Comparative efficacy and tolerability of antidepressants for major depressive disorder in children and adolescents: a network meta-analysis. Lancet. 2016;388(10047):881-890. doi:10.1016/S0140-6736(16)30385-3

445. Le Noury J, Nardo JM, Healy D, et al. Restoring Study 329: efficacy and harms of paroxetine and imipramine in treatment of major depression in adolescence. BMJ 2015;351:h4320 doi: http://dx.doi.org/10.1136/bmj.h4320 (Published 16 September 2015).

446. Wagner KD. Anxiety Disorders in Children and Adolescents: New Findings. Psychiatric Times 2019(2):8.

447. Correll CU and Blader JC. Antipsychotic use in youth without psychosis: A double-edged sword. Editorial. JAMA Psychiatry. Published online July 1, 2015. E1-E2.

448. Gotay N. Neurobiology and Clinical Management of Childhood Onset Schizophrenia. Psychiatric Times 2019(4):11-13.

449. Hee Han, D. Autoimmunity May Play a Role in Pediatric Psychosis. MPR website. http://www.empr.com/autoimmunity-may-play-a-role-in-pediatric-psychosis/article/406434/ Accessed April 8, 2015.

450. Margari L, Matera E, Petruzzelli mg et al. Prolactin variations during risperidone therapy in a sample of drug-naïve children and adolescents. Int Clin Psychopharmacology 2014 (Dec. 15). Doi:10.1097/YIC.0000000000000063.

451. Olfson M, King M, and Schoenbaum M. Treatment of Young People With Antipsychotic Medications in the United States. JAMA Psychiatry. doi:10.1001/jamapsychiatry.2015.0500. Published online July 1, 2015.

452. American Psychiatric Association. Choosing Wisely: Five Things Physicians and Patients Should Question. Released September 20, 2013; recommendation #3 updated August 21, 2014; recommendation #4 updated April 22, 2015. http://www.choosingisely.org/wp-content/uploads/2015/02/APA-Choosing-Wisely-List.pdf Accessed on 6/28/2019.

453. Galling B, Roldán A, Nielsen RE, et al. Type 2 diabetes mellitus in youth exposed to antipsychotics: A systematic review and meta-analysis. JAMA Psychiatry. 2016;73(3):247-259. doi:10.1001/jamapsychiatry.2015.2923

454. Phelps J. Before Bipolar: Is there a prodrome? Psychiatric Times. July 3, 2015. http://www.psychiatrictimes.com/bipolar-disorder/bipolar-there-prodrome Accessed on 7/7/15.

455. Steven Marwaha, Catherine Winsper, Paul Bebbington, Daniel Smith. Cannabis Use and Hypomania in Young People: A Prospective Analysis. Schizophrenia Bulletin, 2017; DOI: 10.1093/schbul/sbx158

456. Peruzzolo TL, Tramontina S, Rohde LA, et al. Pharmacotherapy of bipolar disorder in children and adolescents: an update. Revista Brasileira de Psiquatria. 2013;35:393–405.

457. Vitiello B. How effective are the current treatments for children diagnosed with manic/mixed bipolar disorder? CNS Drugs 2013;27(5):331-3.

458. Amerio A, Ossola P, Scagnelli F, et al. Safety and efficacy of lithium in children and adolescents: A systematic review in bipolar illness. Eur Psychiatry. 2018;54:85-97. doi:10.1016/j.eurpsy.2018.07.012

459. Findling RL, McNamara JK, Youngstrom EA, Stansbrey R, Gracious BL, Reed MD, et al. Double-blind 18-month trial of lithium vs. divalproex maintenance treatment in pediatric bipolar disorder. J Am Acad Child Adolesc Psychiatry 2005;44:409-17.

460. Chang K, Saxena K, and Howe M. An Open-label study of lamotrigine adjunct or monotherapy for the treatment of adolescents with bipolar depression. J Am Acad Child Adolesc Psychiatry 2006;45(3):298-304.

461. Wagner KD. Treatment of Bipolar Depression in Children and Adolescents. Psychiatric Times 201(8):8.

462. University of Utah. Uridine Adolescent Bipolar De-pression Randomized Controlled Trial. https:clinicaltrials.gov/ct2/sho w/stud y/NCT01805440. Accessed July 9, 2018.

463. Nierenberg AA. Effective agents in treating bipolar depression. J Clin Psy Oct 2008;69(10):e29.

464. Bond DJ, Noronha MM, Kauer-Sant'Anna, et al. Antidepressant-associated mood elevations in bipolar II disorder compared with bipolar I disorder and major depressive disorder a systematic review and meta-analysis. Journal of Clinical Psychiatry. 69(10):1589-601, 2008 Oct.

465. Goldberg JF, Ghaemi S, Nassir. Benefits and limitations of antidepressants and traditional mood stabilizers for treatment of bipolar depression. Bipolar Disorders Supplement. 7 (Supplement 5):3-12, December 2005.

466. Taylor MJ, Goodwin GM. Long-term prophylaxis in bipolar disorder. CNS Drugs 2006;20(4):303-10.

467. Barnes C, Mitchell P. Considerations in the management of bipolar disorder in women. Aust N Z J Psychiatry. 2005 Aug;39(8):662-7.

468. Bourin M, Prica C. The role of mood stabilisers in the treatment of the depressive facet of bipolar disorders. Neurosci Biobehav Rev 2007;31(6):963-75

469. Nolen WA. Anticonvulsants, Antidepressants and Traditional Mood Stabilisers: Review of the Latest Data. Bipolar Disorders. 10 (Supplement 1): 16, February 2008.

470. Davis JM, Janicak PG, Hogan DM. Mood stabilizers in the prevention of recurrent affective disorders: a meta-analysis. Acta Psychiatrica Scandinavia. 100(6):406-417, December 1999.

471. Merikangas KR, Jin R, He JP, et al., Prevalence and Correlates of Bipolar Spectrum Disorder in the World Mental Health Survey Initiative. Arch Gen Psychiatry. 2011 Mar; 68(3): 241–251. doi: 10.1001/archgenpsychiatry.2011.12

472. Rowland TA, Marwaha S. Epidemiology and risk factors for bipolar disorder. Ther Adv Psychopharmacol. 2018;8(9):251-269. doi:10.1177/2045125318769235

473. Miller JJ. Major Depressive Episode : Is It Bipolar I or Unipolar Depression? Psychiatric Times 2018;(July):17-18.

474. Phelps J. Borderline or Bipolar: Objective Data Support a Difference. Psychiatr Times. 2016:4-5.

475. Vöhringer PA, Barroilhet SA, Alvear K, et al. The International Mood Network (IMN) Nosology Project: differentiating borderline personality from bipolar illness. Acta Psychiatr Scand. 2016;134:504-510.

476. Miller S, Dell'Osso B, and Ketter, TA. The prevalence and burden of bipolar depression. Journal of Affective Disorders 2014(Dec);169(suppl.1):S3-S11.
477. Pallaskorpi S, Suominen K, Ketoki vi M, et al. Incidence and predictors of suicide attempts in bipolar I and II disorders: A 5-year follow-up study. Bipolar Disord. 2017;19(1):13-22. doi:10.1111/bdi.12464
478. Patel R, Reiss P, Shetty H, et al. Do antidepressants increase the risk of mania and bipolar disorder in people with depression? A retrospective electronic case register cohort study. BMJ Open. 2015;5(12). doi:10.1136/bmjopen-2015-008341
479. Viktorin A, Lichtenstein P, Thase ME, et al. The Risk of Switch to Mania in Patients with Bipolar Disorder During Treatment With an Antidepressant Alone and in Combination with a Mood Stabilizer. Am J Psychiatry 2014;171:1067-73.
480. Pacchiarotti I, Bond DJ, Baldessarini RJ, et al. The International Society for Bipolar Disorders (ISBD) Task Force Report on Antidepressant Use in Bipolar Disorders. The American Journal of Psychiatry 2013;170(11):1249–1262. http://dx.doi.org/10.1176/appi.ajp.2013.13020185
481. Sachs GS, Nierenberg AA, Calabrese JR, et al. Effectiveness of adjunctive antidepressant treatment for bipolar depression. N Engl J Med 2007;356(17):1711–1722.
482. Ghaemi SN, Ostacher MM, El-Mallakh RS, et al. Antidepressant Discontinuation in Bipolar Depression: A Systematic Treatment Enhancement Program for Bipolar Disorder (STEP-BD) Randomized Clinical Trial of Long-Term Effectiveness and Safety. J Clin Psychiatry 2010;71(4):372-380. 10.4088/JCP.08m04909gre.
483. McInerney SJ and Kennedy SH. Review of Evidence for Use of Antidepressants in Bipolar Depression. Prim Care Companion CNS Disord 2014;16(5):doi:10.4088/PCC.14r01653.
484. El-Mallakh RS. Adjunctive antidepressant treatment for bipolar depression. N. Engl. J. Med.357(6), 615 (2007).
485. Baldessarini RJ, Faedda GL, Offidani E, et al. Psychiatric Times. November 08, 2013. "Switching" of Mood from Depression to Mania with Antidepressants. http://www.psychiatrictimes.com/bipolar-disorder/switching-mood-depression-mania-antidepressants. Accessed on June 18, 2015.
486. Soreff S. Bipolar Affective Disorder: Practice Essentials, Background, Pathophysiology. Updated: Mar 16, 2015. http://emedicine.medscape.com/article/286342-overview. Accessed on June 18, 2015.
487. Canetta SE, Bao Y, Co MD, et al. Serological documentation of maternal influenza exposure and bipolar disorder in adult offspring. Am J Psychiatry. 2014;171(5):557-63.
488. Kessing LV et al. Starting Lithium prophylaxis early v. late in bipolar disorder. BR J Psychiatry 2014 Jul 10; http://dx.doi.org/10.1192/bjp.bp.113.142802.
489. Nivoli AMA, Murru A, Goikolea JM, et al. New treatment guidelines for acute bipolar mania: A critical review. Journal of Affective Disorders 2012 (Oct);140(2):125-141.
490. Calabrese JR, Keck PE, Starace A, et al. Efficacy and Safety of Low- and High-Dose Cariprazine in Acute and Mixed Mania Associated With Bipolar I Disorder: A Double-Blind, Placebo-Controlled Study. J Clin Psychiatry 2015;76(3):284–292.
491. Sachs GS, Greenberg WM, Starace A, et al. Cariprazine in the treatment of acute mania in bipolar I disorder: A double-blind, placebo-controlled, Phase III trial. Journal of Affective Disorders March 15, 2015;174:296–302.
492. Bose A, Starace A, Wang Q, et al. Cariprazine in the treatment of acute mania in bipolar disorder: a double-blind, placebo-controlled, phase III trial. Eur Neuropsychopharm. 2012;22(suppl 2):S285. doi:10.1016/s0924-977x(12)70432-7.
493. Durgam S, Starace A, Li D, et al. The efficacy and tolerability of cariprazine in acute mania associated with bipolar I disorder: a phase II trial. Bipolar Disorders 2015 (Feb);17(1):63–75.
494. Berk M and Malhi GS. Should antipsychotics take pole position in mania treatment? The Lancet Oct. 8, 2011;378:1279-81.
495. Fuerst ML. Antidepressants Not Safer for Either Bipolar Depression Subtype. Psychiatric Times 9/10/15. http://www.psychiatrictimes.com/bipolar-disorder/antidepressants-not-safer-either-bipolar-depression-subtype Accessed on 8/21/17.
496. University of Wisconsin-Madison News. Research explains lithium's dual anti-manic/ anti-depressive effect. July 1, 1998. http://www.news.wisc.edu/3353 Accessed on June 18, 2015.
497. Rybakowski JK. Factors associated with lithium efficacy in bipolar disorder. Harv Rev Psychiatry.2014 Nov-Dec;22(6):353-7. doi: 10.1097/HRP.0000000000000006.
498. Stern S, Santos R, Marchetto MC, et al. Neurons derived from patients with bipolar disorder divide into intrinsically different sub-populations of neurons, predicting the patients' responsiveness to lithium. Mol Psychiatry. 2018;23(6):1453-1465. doi:10.1038/mp.2016.260
499. Phelps J. Mitochondrial clues to Bipolar Disorder. Psychiatric Times May 11, 2017. http://www.psychiatrictimes.com/bipolar-disorder/mitochondrial-clues-bipolar-disorder Accessed 5/17/17.
500. Terao T, Okuno K, Okuno T, et al. A simpler and more accurate equation to predict daily lithium dose. J Clin Psychopharmacol. 1999 Aug;19(4):336-40.
501. Zetin M, Garber G, De Antonio M et al. Prediction of lithium dose: a mathematical alternative to the test dose method. J Clin Psychiatry 1983;44:144-145.
502. Epstein RA, Moore KM, and Bobo WV. Treatment of bipolar disorders during pregnancy: maternal and fetal safety and challenges. Drug, Healthcare and Patient Safety 2015;7:7–29.
503. Murru A, Popovic D, Pacchiarotti I, Hidalgo D, León-Caballero J, Vieta E. Management of Adverse Effects of Mood Stabilizers. Curr Psychiatry Rep. 2015;17(8). doi:10.1007/s11920-015-0603-z
504. Malik K, Chand PK, Marimuthu P, Suman LN. Efficacy of Transcranial Direct Current Stimulation in the Treatment: Resistant Patients who Suffer from Severe Obsessive-compulsive Disorder. Indian J Psychol Med. 2017;39(5):611-618. doi:10.4103/IJPSYM.IJPSYM
505. Kirov G, Tredget J, John R, Owen MJ, et al. A cross-sectional and a prospective study of thyroid disorders in lithium-treated patients. J Affect Disord. 2005 Aug;87(2-3):313-7.
506. Charnow, JA, ed. Renal tumor risk higher in lithium-treated patients. Renal and Urology News August 2014 ed.
507. McKnight RF, Adida M, Budge K, et al. Lithium toxicity profile: a systematic review and meta-analysis. The Lancet, Early Online Publication, 20 January 2012. doi:10.1016/S0140-6736(11)61516-X. Accessed on 1/20/2012 at www.thelancet.com.
508. Singh LK, Nizame SH, Akhtar S, Praharal SK. Improving tolerability of lithium with a once-daily dosing schedule. Am J Ther. 2011;18(4):288–291.
509. Mitchell PB and Hadzi-Pavlovic D. Lithium treatment for bipolar disorder. Bulletin of the World Health Organization 2000,78(4):515-517.
510. Schrauzer GN, Shrestha KP. Lithium in drinking water and the incidence of crimes, suicides and arrests related to drug addictions.Biol Trace Elem Res 1990;25: 105–13.
511. Dawson EB, Moore TD, McGanity WJ. Relationship of lithium metabolism to mental hospital admissions and homicide. Dis Nerv Syst 1972;33:546–56.
512. Gonzalez R, Bernstein I, Suppes T. An investigation of water lithium concentrations and rates of violent acts in 11 Texas counties: Can an association be easily shown? Clin Psych 2008;69: 325-26. Letter.
513. Kendall T, Burbeck R, Bateman A. Lithium in drinking water. British Journal of Psychiatry 2011;199:159-60.
514. Ohgami H, Terao T, Shiotsuki I, et al. Lithium levels in drinking water and risk of suicide. Br J Psychiatry 2009;194: 464-5.
515. Young AH. Invited commentary on…lithium levels in drinking water and levels of suicide. Br J Psychiatry 2009;194: 466.
516. Kabacs N, Memon A, Obinwa T, et al. Lithium in drinking water and suicide rates across the East of England. Brit J Psychiatry 2011;198: 406-7.
517. Kapusta ND, Mossaheb N, Etzersdorfer E, et al. Lithium in drinking water and suicide mortality. British J Psychiatry 2011;198:346-50.
518. Corcoran AC, Taylor RD, Page IH. Lithium poisoning from the use of salt substitutes. JAMA 1949;139:685–688.
519. Shorter E. The history of lithium therapy. Bipolar Disord 2009:11(Suppl. 2):4–9.
520. Huthwaite MA, Stanley J. Lithium in drinking water. Br J Psychiatry. 2010 Feb;196(2):159; author reply 160. doi: 10.1192/bjp.196.2.159.
521. Hoosier State Chronicals. The Daily Banner, Greencastle, Putnam County, 19 February 1949. Page 1. https://newspapers.library.in.gov/cgi-bin/indiana?a=d&d=TDB19490219-01.1.1&txq=lithium+AND+%22salt+substitutes%22 Accessed 10/30/19
522. Cade JF. Lithium Salts in the Treatment of Psychotic Excitement. The Medical Journal of Australia 1949;2(10):349-51.
523. Vita A, De Peri L, and Sacchetti E. Lithium in drinking water and suicide prevention: a review of the evidence. International Clinical Psychopharmacology 2015 (Jan);30(1):1-58.
524. Phelps J. Low-Dose Lithium: A Different, Important Tool. Psychiatric Times 9/13/16. https://www.psychiatrictimes.com/bipolar-disorder/low-dose-lithium-different-important-tool/page/0/1 Accessed 9/14/16
525. Llewellyn A, Stowe ZN, Strader JR. The use of lithium and management of women with bipolar disorder during pregnancy and lactation. J Clin Psychiatry 1998;59 Suppl 6:57-64; discussion 65.
526. Ward S, Wisner KL. Collaborative management of women with bipolar disorder during pregnancy and postpartum: Pharmacological considerations. J Midwifery Womens Health 2007 Jan-Feb;52(1):3-13.
527. Iqbal MM, Sohhan T, Mahmud SZ. The effects of lithium, valproic acid, and carbamazepine during pregnancy and lactation. J Toxicol Clin Toxicol 2001;39(4):381-92.
528. Goodnick PJ, Chaudry T, Artadi J, Arcey S. Women's issues in mood disorders. Expert Opin Pharmacother 2000 Jul;1(5):903-16.
529. Sharma V. Management of bipolar II disorder during pregnancy and the postpartum period—Motherisk Update 2008. Can J Clin Pharmacology/Journal Canadian de Pharmacologic Clinique 2009;16(1):e33-41.
530. Gentile S. Prophylactic treatment of bipolar disorder in pregnancy and breastfeeding: focus on emerging mood stabilizers. Bipolar Disorders. 8(3):207-220, June 2006.

531. Mood stabilisers 'safe' to use while breastfeeding. Inpharma Weekly. (1232);5, April 8, 2000.
532. Baldessarini RJ, Tondo L, and Hennen J. Treating the suicidal patient with bipolar disorder. Reducing suicide risk with lithium. Ann N Y Acad Sci. 2001 Apr;932:24-38; discussion 39-43.
533. Lewitzka. What role does (should) Lithium play in suicide treatment/prevention? Psychiatric Times. http://www.psychiatrictimes.com/special-reports/what-role-does-should-lithium-play-in-suicide-treatment-prevention?GUID=631E98CE-0053-4441-9560-14CD338CC37E&rememberme=1&ts=20012015 Accessed on 12/31/14.
534. The BALANCE investigators and collaborators. Lithium plus valproate combination therapy versus monotherapy for relapse prevention in bipolar I disorder (BALANCE): a randomized open-label trial. Lancet 2010(Jan 30);375:385-95.
535. Cipriani A, Kawton K, Stockton S, Geddes JR. Lithium in the prevention of suicide in mood disorders: updated systematic review and meta-analysis. BMJ 2013;346:f3646 doi: 10.1136/bmj.f3646 and Appendices 1-5.
536. Reed RC, Dutta S. Does it really matter when a blood sample for valproic acid concentration is taken following once-daily administration of divalproex-ER? Ther Drug Moni. 2006;28(3):413-8.
537. Meador KJ, Baker GA, Browning N, et al. Cognitive Function at 3 Years of Age after Fetal Exposure to Antiepileptic Drugs. N Engl J Med 2009; 360:1597-1605. April 16, 2009.
538. Bromley RL, Mawer R, Clayton-Smith J, et al. Autism spectrum disorders following in utero exposure to antiepileptic drugs. Neurology December 2, 2008;71(23):1923-1924. doi: 10.1212/01.wnl.0000339399.64213.1a
539. Gunes A, Bilir E, Zengil H, et al. Inhibitory effect of valproic acid on cytochrome P450 2C9 activity in epilepsy patients. Basic Clin Pharmacol Toxicol. 2007 Jun;100(6):383-6.
540. Allen MH, Hirschfeld RM, Wozniak PJ, et al. Linear Relationship of Valproate Serum Concentration to Response and Optimal Serum Levels for Acute Mania. Am J Psychiatry 2006;163:272-275.
541. Shi YW, Min FL, Zhou D et al. HLA-A*24:02 as a common risk factor for antiepileptic drug-induced cutaneous adverse reactions. Neurology. 2017;88(23):2183. Epub 2017 May 5.
542. Cambell R, Beall J. Pharmacogenomics of Lamotrigine: a possible link to serious cutaneous adverse reactions. Mental Health Clin (Internet). 2015;5(2):78-81. DOI: 10.9740/mhc.2015.03.078.
543. Harden CL, Herzog AG, Nikolov BG, et al. Hormone replacement therapy in women with epilepsy: a randomized, double-blind, placebo-controlled study. Epilepsia 2006;47(9):1447-1451.
544. Sandlin EKL, Gao Y, & El-Mallakh RS. Pharmacotherapy of bipolar disorder: current status and emerging options. Clin Pract 2014;11(1):39-48.
545. Thigpen J, Miller S, Pond BB. Behavioral side effects of antiepileptic drugs. US Pharmacist. 2013;38(11):HS15-HS20.
546. Wagner KD, Kowatch RA, Emslie GJ, et al. A double-blind, randomized, placebo-controlled trial of oxcarbazepine in the treatment of bipolar disorder in children and adolescents. Am J Psychiatry 2006 Jul;163(7):1179-86.
547. MacMillan CM, Korndorfer SR, Rao S, et al. A comparison of divalproex and oxcarbazepine in aggressive youth with bipolar disorder. Journal of Psychiatric Practice. 2006 Jul;12(4):214–222.
548. Calabrese JR, Keck PE Jr., McElroy S. A pilot study of topiramate as monotherapy in the treatment of acute mania. J Clin Psychopharmacol 2001;21:340-342.
549. Chengappa KNR, Gerson S, and Levine J. The evolving role of topiramate among other mood stabilizers in the management of bipolar disorder. Bipolar Disord 2001;3:215-232.
550. Gurnze HC, Normann C, Langosch J, et al. Antimanic efficacy of topiramate in 11 patients in an open clinical trial with an off-on design. J Clin Psychiatr 2001;62:464-468.
551. Knaba S, Yagi G, Kamijima K, et al. The first open study of Zonisamide, a novel anticonvulsant, shows efficacy in mania. Prog Neuropsychopharmacol Biol Psychiatr 1994;18:707-715.
552. Gurnze H, Erfurth A, Marcuse A, et al. Tiagabine appears not to be efficacious in the treatment of acute mania. J Clin Psychiatr 1999;60:759-762.
553. Pande AC, Crockatt JG, Janney CA, et al. Gabapentin in bipolar disorder: A placebo controlled trial of adjunctive therapy. Bipolar Disord 2000;2(3):249-255.
554. Schaffer LC, Schaffer CB, Miller AR, et al. An open trial of pregabalin as an acute and maintenance adjunctive treatment for outpatients with treatment resistant bipolar disorder. J Affect Disord. 2013 May;147(1-3):407-10. doi: 10.1016/j.jad.2012.09.005. Epub 2012 Oct 4.
555. Nath K, Bhattacharya A, Praharaj SK. Eslicarbazepine acetate in the management of refractory bipolar disorder. Clin Neuropharmacol. 2012 Nov-Dec;35(6):295. doi: 10.1097/WNF. 0b013e318271220b.
556. Norris ER, Karen Burke, Correll JR, et al. A double-blind, randomized, placebo-controlled trial of adjunctive ramelteon for the treatment of insomnia and mood stability in patients with euthymic bipolar disorder. J Affect Disord. 2013;144(1-2):141-147. doi:10.1016/j.jad.2012.06.023
557. Zarate Jr. CA, Quiroz JA, Singh JB, et al. An open-label trial of the glutamate-modulating agent riluzole in combination with lithium for the treatment of bipolar depression. Biol Psychiatry 2005;57(4):430–432.
558. Dubovsky SL, Franks RD, Allen S, et al. Calcium antagonists in mania: A double-blind study of verapamil. Psychiatr Res 1986;18:309-320.
559. Garza-Trevino ES, Overall JE, and Hollister LE Verapamil versus lithium in acute mania. Am J Psychiatr 1992;149:121-122.
560. Giannini AJ, Houser WL Jr, Loiselle RH, et al. Antimanic effects of verapamil. Am J Psychiatry 1984; 141:1602-1603.
561. Höschl C and Kozeny J. Verapamil in affective disorders: a double-blind, controlled study. Biol Psychiatr 1989;25:128-140.
562. Brunet G, Cerlich B, Robert P et al. Open trial of a calcium antagonist, nimodipine, in acute mania. Clin Neuropharmacol 1990;13:224-228.
563. DeBeaurepaire R. Treatment of neuroleptic-resistant mania and schizoaffective disorder. Am J Psychiatr 1992;149:1614-1615.
564. Chaudhry HR, Arshad N, Niaz S et al. Efficacy of nimodipine as a combination therapy in the treatment of bipolar disorder.Bipolar Disorders 2008;10(Suppl 1):41-42.
565. Murphy BL, Stoll AL, Harris PQ, et al. Omega-3 fatty acid treatment, with or without cytidine, fails to show therapeutic properties in bipolar disorder: a double-blind, randomized add-on clinical trial. J Clin Psychopharmacol. 2012(Oct.);(5):699-703.
566. Turnbull T, Cullen-Drill M, Smaldone A. Efficacy of omega-3 fatty acid supplementation on improvement of bipolar symptoms: a systematic review. [Review] Archives of Psychiatric Nursing 2008 Oct.22;(5):305-11.
567. Montgomery P, Richardson AJ. Omega-3 fatty acids for bipolar disorder. Cochrane Database of Systematic Reviews 2008,Issue 2. Art. No.: CD005169. DOI: 10.1002/14651858.CD005169.pub2.
568. Aiken C. What's New in Bipolar Depression? Psychiatric Times 5/10/17. http://www.psychiatrictimes.com/bipolar-disorder/whats-new-bipolar-depression Accessed on 6/17/17.
569. Henriksen TE, Skrede S, Fasmer OB, et al. Blue-blocking glasses as additive treatment for mania: A randomized placebo-controlled trial. Bipolar Disord. 2016;18(3):221-232. doi:10.1111/bdi.12390
570. Aiken C. A Hopeful Contender for Bipolar Depression. Psychiatric Times. https://www.psychiatrictimes.com/bipolar-disorder/hopeful-contender-bipolar-depression Accessed on 6/17/17.
571. McIntyre RS, Subramaniapillai M, Lee Y, et al. Efficacy of Adjunctive Infliximab vs Placebo in the Treatment of Adults With Bipolar I/II Depression: A Randomized Clinical Trial. JAMA Psychiatry 76(8):783-790. Published online 5/8/19. doi:10.1001/jamapsychiatry.2019.0779
572. Loebel A, Cucchiaro C, Silva R, et al. Lurasidone Monotherapy in the treatment of Bipolar I Depression: A randomized, double-blind, Placebo-controlled study. Am J Psychiatry 2014;171:160-168.
573. Yatham, LN, Kennedy, SH, Parikh, SV, et al. Canadian Network for Mood and Anxiety Treatments (CANMAT) and International Society for Bipolar Disorders (ISBD) 2018 guidelines for the management of patients with bipolar disorder. Bipolar Disord. 2018; 20: 97– 170. https://doi.org/10.1111/bdi.12609
574. Stamm TJ, Lewitzka U, Sauer C, et al. Supraphysiologic doses of levothyroxine as adjunctive therapy in bipolar depression: A randomized, double-blind, placebo-controlled study. J Clin Psychiatry. 2014;75(2):162-168. doi:10.4088/JCP.12m08305
575. Walshaw PD, Gyulai L, Bauer M, et al. Adjunctive thyroid hormone treatment in rapid cycling bipolar disorder: A double-blind placebo-controlled trial of levothyroxine (L-T 4 ) and triiodothyronine (T 3 ). Bipolar Disord. 2018;20(7):594-603. doi:10.1111/bdi.12657
576. Ketter TA, Miller S, Dell'Osso B, et al. Balancing benefits and harms of treatments for acute bipolar depression. Journal of Affective Disorders 2014;169(S1):S24–S33.
577. Selle V, Schalkwijk S, Vázquez GH, et al. Treatments for Acute Bipolar Depression: Meta-analyses of Placebo-controlled, Monotherapy Trials of Anticonvulsants, Lithium and Antipsychotics. Pharmacopsychiatry 2014 (Feb); 47: 43–52.
578. Vázquez GH, Holtzman JN, Tondo L, et al. Efficacy & tolerability of treatments for bipolar depression. J Affect Disord 2015(9-1);183:258-62.
579. Fountoulakis KN. A Critical Consideration of the Most Recent Guidelines for Bipolar Depression. Psychiatric Times. http://www.psychiatrictimes.com/special-reports/critical-consideration-most-recent-guidelines-bipolar-depression/page/0/2?GUID=631E98CE-0053-4441-9560-14CD338CC37E&rememberme=1&ts=12082014#sthash.dKzhUJPc.dpuf Accessed on Aug 19, 2014.
580. Stoner SC, Worrel JA, Vlach D, et al. Retrospective analysis of serum valproate levels and need for an antidepressant drug. Pharmacotherapy 2001;21:850-854.
581. Alkermes Announces Positive Topline Results from Complete Six-Month Phase II Clinical Trial of ALKS 3831 in Schizophrenia. http://phx.corporate-ir.net/phoenix.zhtml?c=92211&p=irol-newsArticle&ID=2032249 Accessed on 6/28/15.
582. Nunez N, Singh B, Romo-Nava F, et al. Efficacy and tolerability of adjunctive modafinil /armodafinil in bipolar depression: a meta-analysis of randomized controlled trials. Bipolar Disord. 2019;0(ja). doi:10.1111/bdi.12859
583. Aiken C. A Common Antioxidant Shows Promise in Bipolar Depression. http://www.psychiatrictimes.com/bipolar-disorder/common-antioxidant-shows-promise-bipolar-depression Oct 31, 2018. Accessed on 11/3/18.

584. NRX-100/NRX-101. http://www.neurorxpharma.com/nrx-100nrx-101-overview.html Accessed on 8/3/19.
585. Kantrowitz JT, Halberstam B, and Gangwisch J. Single-Dose Ketamine Followed by Daily d-Cycloserine in Treatment-Resistant Bipolar Depression. J Clin Psychiatry 2015;76(6):737–738 (doi:10.4088/JCP.14l09527).
586. Lumateperone. https://www.intracellulartherapies.com/products-and-technology/lumateperone/ Accessed on 8/2/19.
587. Tundo A, de Filippis R, De Crescenzo F. Pramipexole in the treatment of unipolar and bipolar depression. A systematic review and meta-analysis. Acta Psychiatr Scand. 2019;140(2):116-125. doi:10.1111/acps.13055
588. Palacios, J., Yildiz, A., Young, A. H., & Taylor, M. J. (2019). Tamoxifen for bipolar disorder: Systematic review and meta-analysis. Journal of Psychopharmacology, 33(2), 177–184. https://doi.org/10.1177/0269881118822167
589. Perahia D, Pritchett YL, Kajdasz DK, et al. A randomized, double-blind comparison of duloxetine and venlafaxine in the treatment of patients with major depressive disorder. J Psych Research, 2007.
590. Pharmacist's Letter / Prescriber's Letter May 2008 ~ Volume 24 ~ Number 240509
591. Gartlehner G, Gaynes BN, Hansen RA, et al. Comparative benefits and harms of second-generation antidepressants: background paper for the American College of Physicians. Ann Intern Med. 2008 Nov 18;149(10):734-50.
592. Iqbal SH, Prashker M. pharmacoeconomic evaluation of antidepressants: a critical appraisal of methods. Pharmacoeconomics 23(6):595-606, 2005.
593. Montgomery S, Doyle J, Stern L, et al. Economic Considerations in the Prescribing of Third-Generation Antidepressants. Pharmacoeconomics 2005;23(5):477-491.
594. Ereshefsky L, Jhee S, Grothe D. Antidepressant Drug-Drug Interaction Profile Update. Drugs in R&D 2005;6(6):323-336.
595. Norman TR and Olver JS. New Formulations of Existing Antidepressants: Advantages in the Management of Depression. CNS Drugs 2004;18(8):505-520.
596. Antidepressants: benefits overstated, harms understated? Inpharma Weekly 2004(April 24);1434:24.
597. Labbate LA, et al. Handbook of Psychiatric Drug Therapy, Sixth Edition (Lippincott Williams & Wilkins, Philadelphia, 2010, p. 54)
598. Goldberg JF. The Psychopharmacology of Depression: Strategies, Formulations, and Future Implications. Psychiatric Times 2019(7):9-14.
599. Suicide Statistics. The American Foundation for Suicide Prevention. https://afsp.org/about-suicide/suicide-statistics/ Accessed 12/11/19.
600. Thase ME. Effectiveness of Antidepressants: Comparative Remission Rates. Archives of General Psychiatry 2005;62(6):617-27
601. Stahl SM. Why Settle for Silver, When You Can Go for Gold? Response vs. Recovery as the Goal of Antidepressant Therapy. Available at: http://www.psychiatrist.com/pcc/brainstorm/br6004.htm Accessed on 10/18/2010.
602. Scheiderer DJ. Depression - PNIPs, SNPs, and Phenotypes. Psychiatric Times. Brief Communication 2014 (Sept.12). http://www.psychiatrictimes.com/uspc2014/pnips-snps-and-phenotypes?GUID=631E98CE-0053-4441-9560-14CD338CC37E&rememberme=1&ts=24092014#sthash.wgDlmqJD.dpuf Accessed on Sept. 24, 2014.
603. Sharpley CF, Bitsika V. Differences in neurobiological pathways of four "clinical content" subtypes of depression. Behav Brain Res. 2013;256(2013):368-376. doi:10.1016/j.bbr.2013.08.030
604. McGrath P, Khan A, Trivedi M, Stewart J, Morris DW, Wisniewski S, et al. "Response to a selective serotonin reuptake inhibitor (citalopram) in major depressive disorder with melancholic features: a STAR*D report." J Clin Psychiatry 2008;69:1847-55. doi:10.4088/jcp.v69n1201.
605. Radua J, Pertusa A, and Cardoner N. "Climatic relationships with specific clinical subtypes of depression". Psychiatry Research 2010(Feb 28);175(3):217–220. doi:10.1016/j.psychres.2008.10.025. PMID 20045197.
606. Cristancho MA, O'Reardon JP, and Thase ME. Atypical Depression in the 21st Century: Diagnostic and Treatment Issues. Psychiatric Times 2011;28(1):42-47.
607. Bunevicius R. Thyroid disorders in mental patients. Curr Opin Psychiatry 2009;22:391-395.
608. Zhuang S, Na M, Winkelman JW, et al. Association of Restless Legs Syndrome With Risk of Suicide and Self-harm. JAMA Netw Open. 2019;2(8):e199966. doi:10.1001/jamanetworkopen.2019.9966
609. Teasdale TW, Enberg AW. Suicide after a stroke: a population study. J Epidemiol Community Health 2001;55:863-866.
610. Samaan, Z et al. What is the role of vitamin D in depression. Psychiatric Times Web site. http://www.psychiatrictimes.com/depression/what-role-vitamin-d-depression Published April 21, 2014. Accessed April 8, 2015.
611. Puri BK. Medication- and substance-induced disorders. Textbook of Clinical Neuropsych and Beh Neurosci 2012;70(6):786-804.
612. A Head, M J Kendall, R Ferner, and C Eagles. Acute effects of beta blockade and exercise on mood and anxiety. Br J Sports Med. 1996 Sep; 30(3): 238–242. doi: 10.1136/bjsm.30.3.238
613. Molero Y, Larsson H, D'Onofrio BM, Sharp DJ, Fazel S. Associations between gabapentinoids and suicidal behaviour, unintentional overdoses, injuries, road traffic incidents, and violent crime: population based cohort study in Sweden. BMJ. 2019;365:l2147. doi:10.1136/bmj.l2147
614. Mollan KR, Smurzynski M, Eron JJ, et al. Association between efavirenz as initial therapy for HIV-1 infection and increased risk for suicidal ideation or attempted or completed suicide: an analysis of trial data. Ann Intern Med. 2014;161(1):1-10.
615. Kessing L V., Rytgaard HC, Gerds TA, Berk M, Ekstrøm CT, Andersen PK. New drug candidates for depression – a nationwide population-based study. Acta Psychiatr Scand. 2019;139(1):68-77. doi:10.1111/acps.13055
616. Bermond P. Therapy of side effects of oral contraceptive agents with vitamin B6. Acta Vitaminol Enzymol. 1982;4(1-2):45-54.
617. P.W. Adams, V. Wynn, D.P. Rose, et al. Effect of pyridoxine hydrochloride (vitamin B6) upon depression associated with oral contraception. The Lancet 1973(April 28); Volume 301, No. 7809, p897–904.
618. Leeton J. Depression Induced by Oral Contraception and the Role of Vit. B6 in its Management. Aust N Z J Psychiatry 1974;8(2):85-88.
619. Var C, Keller S, Tung R, et al. Supplementation with Vitamin B6 Reduces Side Effects in Cambodian Women Using Oral Contraception. Nutrients 2014;6:3353-3362; doi:10.3390/nu6093353.
620. Maxmen JS, Ward NG, Kilgus MD. Oral contraceptive and antihypertensive-induced depression. Essential Psychopathology and Its Treatment. 3rd Edition. W. W. Norton & Company; New York, NY. 2009.
621. Rappa LR, Larose-Pierre M, Branch E, Iglesias AJ, Norwood DA, Simon WA. Desperately seeking serendipity: The past, present, and future of antidepressant therapy. J Pharm Pract. 2001;14(6):560-569. doi:10.1177/089719001129040900
622. Musto DF. Historical Perspectives. Substance Abuse: A Comprehensive Textbook. 3rd Ed. 1997;1-9. Williams & Wilkinson, Baltimore, MD.
623. Cowen DL. Le Coquetier. Apothecary's Cabinet. 2000; 1:13.
624. King LJ. A Brief History of Psychiatry: Millennia Past and Present – Part IV. Ann Clin Psychiatry. 1999; 11(4):175-85.
625. HHH Shelton, Richard C. Treatment Options for Refractory Depression. J Clin Psychiatry. 1999; 60(4):57-61.
626. L Lader M. Introduction to Psychopharmacology. Kalamazoo, MI: Upjohn 1983.
627. Feighner JP. Mechanism of action of antidepressant medications. J Clin Psychiatry. 1999;60(SUPPL. 4):4-13.
628. Kline NS. USE OF RAUWOLFIA SERPENTINA BENTH. IN NEUROPSYCHIATRIC CONDITIONS. Ann N Y Acad Sci. 1954;59(1):107-132. doi:10.1176/ajp.122.5.509
629. Schildkraut JJ. The catecholamine hypothesis of affective disorders: a review of supporting evidence. Am J Psychiatry. 1965;122(5):509-522. doi:10.1176/ajp.122.5.509
630. Ames D. Reserpine exhumed. Br J Psychiatry. 1998;173(1958):440. doi:10.1192/bjp.173.5.440a
631. Lehmann HE, Ban TA. The history of the psychopharmacology of schizophrenia. Can J Psychiatry. 1997;42(2):152-163. doi:10.1177/070674379704200205
632. Vetulani J, Nalepa I. Antidepressants: past, present and future. Eur J Pharmacol. 2000;405:351-63.
633. Lemke TL, Williams DA, Roche, VF, Zito SW, eds. Foye's Principles of Medicinal Chemistry. 7th Edition. Publisher: Lippincott Williams & Wilkins. 2013. Baltimore, MD.
634. Schatzberg AF, Cole JO, and DeBattista C. Depression. Manual of Clinical Psychopharmacology, 7th ed. p.37-146. American Psychiatric Publishing, Inc. Arlington, VA. 2010.
635. Machado-Vieira R, Henter ID, Zarate CA Jr. New targets for rapid antidepressant action. Prog Neurobiol. 2017;152:21–37. doi:10.1016/j.pneurobio.2015.12.001
636. Kirsch I, Deacon BJ, Huedo-Medina TB, et al. Initial Severity and Antidepressant Benefits: A Meta-Analysis of Data Submitted to the Food and Drug Administration. PLoS Medicine 2008(Feb):5(2)e45:0620-0628. doi:10.1371/journal.pmed.0050045
637. Turner EH,Matthews AM, Linardatos E, et al. Selective Publication of Antidepressant Trials and Its Influence on Apparent Efficacy. N Engl J Med 2008;358:252-60.
638. Uguz F, Sahingoz M, Gungor B, et al. Weight gain and associated factors in patients using newer antidepressant drugs. General Hospital Psychiatry 2015;37(1);46-48.
639. Sheu Y, Lanteigne, A, Sturmer T, et al. SSRI use and risk of fractures among perimenopausal women without mental disorders. Inj Prev doi:10.1136/injuryprev-2014-041483. Published on-line first June 25, 2015.
640. Dragioti E, Solmi M, Favaro A, et al. Association of Antidepressant Use with Adverse Health Outcomes: A Systematic Umbrella Review. JAMA Psychiatry. 2019. doi:10.1001/jamapsychiatry.2019.2859
641. Bartels C, Wagner M, Wolfsgruber S, et al. Impact of SSRI therapy on risk of conversion from mild cognitive impairment to Alzheimer dementia in individuals with previous depression. Am J Psychiatry. 2018;175:232.
642. Collier TJ, Srivastava KR, Justman C, et al. Nortriptyline inhibits aggregation and neurotoxicity of alpha-synuclein by enhancing reconfiguration of the monomeric form. Neurobiol Dis. 2017;106:191-204. doi:https://doi.org/10.1016/j.nbd.2017.07.007
643. Paumier KL and Collier TJ. Disease-modifying Potential of Nortriptyline in Parkinson's Disease. Funded studies. Michael J. Fox Foundation.

167

https://www.michaelifox.org/grant/disease-modifying-potential-nortriptyline-parkinsons-disease Accessed on 9/30/19.

644. FDA News Release. FDA Launches a Multi-Pronged Strategy to Strengthen Safeguards for Children Treated With Antidepressant Medications. 10/15/04. Accessed on 2/26/15 at: http://www.fda.gov/newsevents/newsroom/pressannouncements/2004/ucm108363.htm.

645. Friedman RA. Antidepressants' black-box warning—10 years later. N Engl J Med. 2014;371(18):1666-8.

646. Keller MB, Ryan ND, Strober M et al. Efficacy of paroxetine in the treatment of adolescent major depression: a random-ized, controlled trial. J Am Acad Child Adolesc Psychiatry.2001; 40:762-72.

647. Mandoki MW, Tapia MR, Tapia MA et al. Venlafaxine in the treatment of children and adolescents with major depression. Psychopharmacol Bull.1997; 33:149-54.

648. Dopheide, JA. Recognizing and treating depression in children and adolescents: clinical review. AJHP 2006;63:233-43

649. Lu CY, Zhang F, Lakoma MD, et al. Changes in antidepressant use by young people and suicidal behavior after FDA warnings and media coverage: quasi-experimental study. BMJ. 2014;348:g3596.

650. FDA News Release. http://www.fda.gov/cder/drug/antidepressants_label_change_2007.pdf. Accessed 12/5/2008.

651. Statistics of Postpartum Depression. https://www.postpartumdepression.org/resources/statistics/ Accessed on 11/11/19.

652. US Food and Drug Administration MedWatch Safety information on antidepressants. http://www.fda.gov/Safety/MedWatch/SafetyInformation/ucm409855.htm Accessed on 2/23/15.

653. Keller, DM. Antidepressants at normal doses linked to first-time seizures. Medscape. Apr 06, 2015.

654. De Picker L, Van den eede F, Dumont G, Moorkens G, Sabbe BG. Antidepressants and the risk of hyponatremia: a class-by-class review of literature. Psychosomatics. 2014;55(6):536-47.

655. Allen SN, Fisher M, Phipps N. The correlation between depression and diabetes. US Pharm. 2014;39(10)(Diabetes suppl):12-15.

656. Hollon SD, Derubeis RJ, Fawcett J, et al. Effect of cognitive therapy with antidepressant medications vs antidepressants alone on the rate of recovery in major depressive disorder: a randomized clinical trial. JAMA Psychiatry. 2014;71(10):1157-64.

657. Lichtman JH, Froelicher ES, Blumenthal JA, et al. Depression as a risk factor for poor prognosis among patients with acute coronary syndrome: systematic review and recommendations: a scientific statement from the American Heart Association. Circulation. 2014;129(12):1350-69.

658. Preidt, Robert. Depression after heart attack may be more common for women. HealthDay Web site. http://consumer.healthday.com/mental-health-infomation-25/depression-news-176/depression-after-heart-attack-may-be-more-common-for-women-692894.html Updated October 22, 2014. Accessed April 8, 2015.

659. Zuidersma M, Conradi HJ, Van Melle JP, et al. Depression treatment after myocardial infarction and long-term risk of subsequent cardiovascular events and mortality: a randomized controlled trial. J Psychosom Res. 2013;74(1):25-30.

660. Casteel B. Antidepressants Linked with Improved Cardiovascular Outcomes. American College of Cardiology. Accessed 3/5/15 at: http://www.acc.org/about-acc/press-releases/2015/03/05/16/07/antidepressants-linked-with-improved-cardiovascular-outcomes.

661. Mamdani M, Gomes T, Greaves S, et al. Association Between Angiotensin-Converting Enzyme Inhibitors, Angiotensin Receptor Blockers, and Suicide. JAMA Netw open. 2019;2(10):e1913304. doi:10.1001/jamanetworkopen.2019.13304

662. Bushnell GA, Stürmer T, Gaynes BN, Pate V, Miller M. Simultaneous antidepressant and benzodiazepine new use and subsequent long-term benzodiazepine use in adults with depression, United States, 2001-2014. JAMA Psychiatry. 2017;74(7):747-755. doi:10.1001/jamapsychiatry.2017.1273

663. Koga M, Kodaka F, Miyata H, and Nakayama K. Symptoms of delusion: the effects of discontinuation of low-dose venlafaxine. Acta Psychiatr Scand. 2009 October; 120(4): 329–331.

664. Warner CH, Bobo W, Warner C, Reid S, Rachal J. Antidepressant discontinuation syndrome. Am Fam Physician 2006 Aug 1;74(3):449-56.

665. Haddad P, Lejoyeux M, Young A. Title Antidepressant discontinuation reactions: Are preventable and simple to treat. BMJ. 1998 April; 316(7138):1105-1106.

666. Muzina DJ. Discontinuing an antidepressant? Tapering tips to ease distressing symptoms. Current Psychiatry. 2010 March; 9(3):51-61.

667. Blier P and El Mansari M. Role of 5HT1A receptors in the mechanism of action of antidepressant treatments. Conference abstract from the 27th European College of Neuropsychopharmacology Congress. Berlin, Germany Oct. 18, 2014.

668. Phase IV: Safety and Efficacy of EMSAM in Adolescents With Major Depression. https://clinicaltrials.gov/ct2/show/NCT00531947 Accessed on 3/16/15.

669. Cipriani A, Funkawa TA, Salanti G, et al. Comparative efficacy and acceptability of 12 new-generation antidepressants: a multiple-treatments meta-analysis. Lancet 2009;373:746-758.

670. Young KC, Bai CH, Su HC, et al. Fluoxetine a novel anti-hepatitis C virus agent via ROS-, JNK-, and PPARβ/γ-dependent pathways. Antiviral Research (Available online August 21, 2014). DOI: 10.1016/j.antiviral.2014.08.002.

671. Newport DJ, Stowe ZN. Clinical management of perinatal depression: focus on paroxetine. Psychopharmacol Bull 2003;37(sup.1):148-66.

672. Khedezla™ Desvenlafaxine [package insert]. Wilmington, NC. Osmotica Pharmaceutical Corp.; 2013 July.

673. Pristiq shows low chance of sexual dysfunction in adults with MDD. MPR Web site. http://www.empr.com/pristiq-shows-low-chance-of-sexual-dysfunction-in-adults-with-mdd/article/379898/. Published October 29, 2014. Accessed April 8, 2015.

674. US Food and Drug Administration MedWatch Safety information on bupropion. http://www.fda.gov/Safety/MedWatch/SafetyInformation/ucm319241.htm Accessed on 2/23/15.

675. Ross C. Levomilnacipran (Fetzima™) for the Treatment of Major Depressive Disorder. Ment Health Clin. 2014;4(1):48.

676. Wesnes K, Gommoll C, and Chen C. Effects of levomilnacipran ER on measures of attention in a phase III trial of major depressive disorder. Conference abstract from the 27th European College of Neuropsychopharmacology Congress. Berlin, Germany Oct. 19, 2014.

677. Mohd S, Rizvi D, Shaikh S, et al. Fetzima (levomilnacipran), a Drug for Major Depressive Disorder as a Dual Inhibitor for Human Serotonin Transporters and Beta-Site Amyloid Precursor Protein Cleaving Enzyme-1. CNS & Neurological Disorders - Drug Targets 2014;13(8):1427-1431 DOI : 10.2174/1871527313666141023145703.

678. Ancona 2-2. Wyeth-Ayerst Drug Company. Information on file. September 11, 2000.

679. Stryjer R, Spivak B, Strous RD, et al. Trazodone for the treatment of sexual dysfunction induced by serotonin reuptake inhibitors: a preliminary open-label study. Clin Neuropharmacol. 2009 Mar;32(2):82-4. doi: 10.1097/WNF.0B013E31816D1CDC,

680. Fink HA, MacDonald R, Rutks IR, Wilt TJ. Trazodone for erectile dysfunction: a systematic review and meta-analysis. BJU Int. 2003 Sep;92(4):441-6.

681. Stryjer R, Spivak B, Strous RD, Shiloh R, Harary E, Polak L, Birgen M, Kotler M, Weizman A. Trazodone for the treatment of sexual dysfunction induced by serotonin reuptake inhibitors: a preliminary open-label study. Clin Neuropharmacol. 2009 Mar;32(2):82-4.

682. Jacobsen, P., Nomikos, G., Zhong, W., Cutler, A., Affinito, J., & Clayton, A. (n.d.). Clinical implications of directly switching antidepressants in well-treated depressed patients with treatment-emergent sexual dysfunction: A comparison between vortioxetine and escitalopram. CNS Spectrums, 1-14. doi:10.1017/S1092852919000750

683. Eslava-Kim L. Monthly Prescribing Reference. Brintellix sNDA Accepted for Labeling Update on Cognitive Effects. http://www.empr.com/drugs-in-the-pipeline/brintellix-snda-accepted-for-labeling-update-on-cognitive-effects/article/432007/?DCMP=EMC-MPR_DailyDose&cpn=emp_lathcp.mylan_2014.strib_pharm.strib_mobile&hmSubId=&hmEmail=phtCYW71bjQOffsCjTQl8t_fndfC6gdj0&NID=1922005446&dl=0&spMailingID=12113191&spUserID=NDc2NTIyMTYwNDES1&spJobID=600790467&spReportId=NjAwNzkwNDY3S0 Accessed on August 11, 2015.

684. Talmon M, Rossi S, Pastore A, Cattaneo CI, Brunelleschi S, Fresu LG. Vortioxetine exerts anti-inflammatory and immunomodulatory effects on human monocytes/macrophages. Br J Pharmacol. 2018;175(1):113-124. doi:10.1111/bph.14074

685. US Food and Drug Administration MedWatch Safety information on vilazodone tablets. http://www.fda.gov/Safety/MedWatch/SafetyInformation/ucm335517.htm Accessed on 2/23/15.

686. Hu LY, Liu CJ, Lu T, et al. Delayed onset urticaria in depressive patients with bupropion prescription: a nationwide population-based study. PLoS ONE. 2013;8(11):e80064.

687. US Food and Drug Administration MedWatch Safety information on bupropion. http://www.fda.gov/Safety/MedWatch/SafetyInformation/ucm229405.htm Accessed on 2/23/15.

688. Anttila SAK & Leinonen EVJ. A Review of the Pharmacological and Clinical Profile of Mirtazapine. CNS Drug Reviews 2001;7(3):249–264.

689. Abo-Zena RA, Bobek MB, Dweik RA. Hypertensive urgency induced by an interaction of mirtazapine and clonidine. Pharmacotherapy. 2000;20(4):476-478. doi:10.1592/phco.20.5.476.35061

690. Troncoso AL, Gill T. Hypertensive urgency with clonidine and mirtazepine [2]. Psychosomatics. 2004;45(5):449-450. doi:10.1176/appi.psy.45.5.449

691. E Huetteman. Clinical Psychiatry News. MDEdge Current Psychiatry. FDA overlooked red flags in esketamine testing. https://www.mdedge.com/psychiatry/article/202791/depression/fda-overlooked-red-flags-esketamine-testing Accessed on 6/13/19.

692. Daly EJ, Trivedi MH, Janik A, et al. Efficacy of Esketamine Nasal Spray Plus Oral Antidepressant Treatment for Relapse Prevention in Patients With Treatment-Resistant Depression: A Randomized Clinical Trial. JAMA Psychiatry. Published online June 05, 201976(9):893–903. doi:10.1001/jamapsychiatry.2019.1189

693. Altamura AC, Dell'Osso B, Buoli M, at el. Short-term intravenous citalopram augmentation in partial/nonresponders with major depression: a randomized placebo-controlled study. Int Clin Psychopharmacol. 2008 Jul;23(4):198-202.

694. Attard A, Ranjith G, Taylor D, et al. Alternative routes to oral antidepressant therapy: case vignette and literature review. J Psychopharmacol. 2010 Apr;24(4):449-54.

695. Koelle JS, Dimsdale JE. Antidepressants for the virtually eviscerated patient: options instead of oral dosing. Psychosom Med. 1998 Nov-Dec;60(6):723-5.

696. Mirassou MM. Rectal antidepressant medication in the treatment of depression. J Clin Psychiatry. 1998 Jan;59(1):29.

697. Storey P, Trumble M. Rectal doxepin and carbamazepine therapy in patients with cancer. N Engl J Med. 1992 Oct 29;327(18):1318-9.

698. Teter CJ, Phan KL, Cameron OG, et al. Relative rectal bioavailability of fluoxetine in normal volunteers. J Clin Psychopharmacol. 2005 Feb;25(1):74-8.

699. Kaminsky BM, Bostwick JR, and Guthrie SK. Alternate routes of administration of antidepressant and antipsychotic medications. Ann Pharmacother July 2015;49(7):808-817. doi: 10.1177/1060028015583893

700. Worsham J, Bishop JR, and Ellingrod VL. Antidepressant-Associated Sexual Dysfunction: A Review. The Journal of the College of Psychiatric and Neurologic Pharmacists 2007. https://cpnp.org/_docs/resource/jcpnp/sexual-dysfunction.pdf. Accessed 3/3/15.

701. Borg ER, Chavez B. Psychotropic-Induced Sexual Dysfunction. Ment Health Clin. 2014;4(3):78. http://cpnp.org/resource/mhc/2014/05/psychotropic-induced-sexual-dysfunction. Accessed May 19, 2014.

702. Baldwin DS and Foong T. Antidepressant drugs and sexual dysfunction. The British Journal of Psychiatry (2013) 202,396–397. doi: 10.1192/bjp.bp.112.110650

703. Ng A. Toolbox: Psychotropic Medications for Augmentation or Combination in Treatment-Resistant Depression. Ment Health Clin. 2014;4(5):85. http://cpnp.org/resource/mhc/2014/09/toolbox-psychotropic-medications-augmentation-or-combination-treatment Accessed September 15, 2014.

704. 6 Signs Your Patient is at Risk for Treatment-Resistant Depression. Psychiatric Times. http://www.psychiatrictimes.com/major-depressive-disorder/6-signs-your-patient-risk-treatment-resistant-depression?GUID=631E98CE-0053-4441-9560-14CD338CC37E&rememberme=1&ts=20082016. Accessed on 8/20/16.

705. Raison CL, Felger JC, Miller AH. Inflammation and treatment resistance in major depression: the perfect storm. Psychiatric Times Web site. http://www.psychiatrictimes.com/major-depressive-disorder/inflammation-and-treatment-resistance-major-depression-perfect-storm Published September 12, 2013. Accessed April 8, 2015.

706. Coryell W. The search for improved antidepressant strategies: is bigger better?. Am J Psychiatry. 2011;168(7):664-6.

707. PL Detail-Document, Combining and Augmenting Antidepressants. Pharmacist's Letter/Prescriber's Letter. September 2014.

708. Halpern R, Nadkarni A, Kalsekar I, et al. Medical costs and hospitalizations among patients with depression treated with adjunctive atypical antipsychotic therapy: an analysis of health insurance claims data. Ann Pharmacother. 2013;47(7-8):933-45.

709. Rapinesi C, Bersani FS, Kotzalidis GD, et al. Maintenance Deep Transcranial Magnetic Stimulation Sessions are Associated with Reduced Depressive Relapses in Patients with Unipolar or Bipolar Depression. Front Neurol. 2015;6:16.

710. Dunner DL. Transcranial Magnetic Stimulation for Depression: One-Year Durability of Response and Remission. Psychiatry Weekly 2014(Dec.15);9(12). http://www.psychweekly.com/aspx/article/articledetail.aspx?articleid=1687. Accessed on 3/2/15.

711. Sackeim HA. Modern electroconvulsive therapy: Vastly improved yet greatly underused. JAMA Psychiatry. 2017;74(8):779-780. doi:10.1001/jamapsychiatry.2017.1670

712. Sackeim HA. Modern Electroconvulsive Therapy: Vastly Improved yet Greatly Underused. JAMA Psychiatry. 2017;74(8):779-780. doi:10.1001/jamapsychiatry.2017.1670

713. Guinta GM, Graham RL. Special Populations: Treatment Resistant Mood Disorders. Ment Health Clin.2014;4(5):95.

714. Serretti A, Fabbri C. Factors That Predispose Patients to Treatment-Resistant Depression. Psychiatric Times 2014.

715. Waite R. Use of Second Generation Antipsychotics for Treatment-Resistant Major Depressive Disorder. Ment Health Clin. 2014;4(5)92.

716. Silverstein, W et al. The current status of transcranial direct current stimulation as a treatment for depression. Psychiatric Times Web site. http://www.psychiatrictimes.com/neuropsychiatry/current-status-transcranial-direct-current-stimulation-treatment-depression. Published February 27, 2014. Accessed April 8, 2015.

717. Crowell AL, Riva-Posse P, Holtzheimer PE, et al. Long-Term Outcomes of Subcallosal Cingulate Deep Brain Stimulation for Treatment-Resistant Depression. Am J Psychiatry. 2019;(19):appi.ajp.2019.1. doi:10.1176/appi.ajp.2019.18121427

718. Batya Swift Yasgur MA, LMSW. Monthly Prescribing Reference. Where Does CAM Fit in When Treating Mood, Anxiety Disorders? http://www.empr.com/features/where-does-cam-fit-in-when-treating-mood-anxiety-disorders/article/315857/ Accessed 10/17/13.

719. Phelps J. No Need for Blood: Nine Alternatives to the Antidepressant Debate. Psychiatric Times. January 23, 2014. http://www.psychiatrictimes.com/bipolar-disorder/no-need-blood-nine-alternatives-antidepressant-debate

720. Solomon D and Adams J. The use of complementary and alternative medicine in adults with depressive disorders. A critical integrative review. Journal of Affective Disorders 2015;179:101–113.

721. Andreescu C, Mulsant BH, and Emanuel JE. Complementary and alternative medicine in the treatment of bipolar disorder—A review of the evidence. Journal of Affective Disorders 2008;110:16–26.

722. Mischoulon D. Natural Medications in Psychiatry. https://psychopharmacologyinstitute.com/section/introduction-natural-medications-in-psychiatry-2066-4179 Accessed on 7/19/19.

723. Alan K. Davis, Sara So, Rafael Lancelotta, Joseph P. Barsuglia, Roland R. Griffiths. 5-methoxy-N,N-dimethyltryptamine (5-MeO-DMT) used in a naturalistic group setting is associated with unintended improvements in depression and anxiety. The American Journal of Drug and Alcohol Abuse, 2019; 1 DOI: 10.1080/00952990.2018.1545024

724. Brainard GC, Hanifin JR, Greeson JM, et al. Action spectrum for melatonin regulation in humans: Evidence for a novel circadian photoreceptor. J Neurosci. 2001;21(16):6405-6412. doi:10.1523/jneurosci.21-16-06405.2001

725. When the Light You See is not the Light You Want. Fact Sheet from CET. https://cet.org/wp-content/uploads/2017/12/When-the-Light-You-See-is-not-the-Light-You-Want.pdf Accessed on 10/26/19.

726. Lam RW, Levitt AJ, Levitan RD, et al. Efficacy of bright light treatment, fluoxetine, and the combination in patients with nonseasonal major depressive disorder a randomized clinical trial. JAMA Psychiatry. 2016;73(1):56-63. doi:10.1001/jamapsychiatry.2015.2235

727. Tuccori C, Benedetti F, Serfaty M, et al. Chronotherapy for the rapid treatment of depression: A meta-analysis. J Affect Disord. 2019. doi:10.1016/j.jad.2019.09.078

728. Chen C, Shan W. Pharmacological and non-pharmacological treatments for major depressive disorder in adults: A systematic review and network meta-analysis. Psychiatry Res. 2019;281(October):112595. doi:10.1016/j.psychres.2019.112595

729. Gordon BR, McDowell CP, Hallgren M, Meyer JD, Lyons M, Herring MP. Association of efficacy of resistance exercise training with depressive symptoms meta-analysis and meta-regression: Analysis of randomized clinical trials. JAMA Psychiatry. 2018;75(6):566-576. doi:10.1001/jamapsychiatry.2018.0572

730. Li LT, Wang SH, Ge HY, et al. The beneficial effects of the herbal medicine Free and Easy Wanderer Plus (FEWP) and fluoxetine on post-stroke depression. J Altern Complement Med. 2008 Sep;14(7):841-6. doi: 10.1089/acm.2008.0010.

731. Qin F, Wu XA, Tang Y, et al. Meta-analysis of randomized controlled trials to assess the effectiveness and safety of free and easy Wanderer plus, a polyherbal preparation for depressive disorders. Review Article. Journal of Psychiatric Research 2011;45(11):1518-1524.

732. Perez V, Alexander DD, Bailey WH. Air ions and mood outcomes: A review and meta-analysis. BMC Psychiatry. 2013;13(1):1. doi:10.1186/1471-244X-13-29

733. Brauser D. Fatty Fish May Boost Antidepressant Response. Medscape. October 22, 2014.

734. Mao JJ, Xie SX, Zee J, et al. Rhodiola rosea versus sertraline for major depressive disorder: A randomized placebo-controlled trial. Phytomedicine. 2015;22(3):394-399. doi:10.1016/j.phymed.2015.01.010

735. Qaseem A, Barry MJ, Kansagara D. Nonpharmacologic Versus Pharmacologic Treatment of Adult Patients With Major Depressive Disorder: A Clinical Practice Guideline From the American College of Physicians. Ann Intern Med. 2016;164(5):350. doi:10.7326/M15-2570

736. Najm WI, Reinsch S, Hoehler F, Tobis JS, Harvey PW. S-Adenosyl methionine (SAMe) versus celecoxib for the treatment of osteoarthritis symptoms: A double-blind cross-over trial. [ISRCTN36233495]. BMC Musculoskelet Disord. 2004;5(1). doi:10.1186/1471-2474-5-6

737. Hausenblas HA, Saha D, Dubyak PJ et al (2013) Saffron (Crocus sativus L.) and major depressive disorder: a meta-analysis of randomized clinical trials. J Integr Med 11:377–383.

738. Bangratz M, Abdellah SA, Berlin A, et al. A preliminary assessment of a combination of rhodiola and saffron in the management of mild–moderate depression. Neuropsychiatr Dis Treat. 2018;14:1821-1829. doi:10.2147/NDT.S169575

739. Hoban CL, Byard RW, and Musgrave IF. A comparison of patterns of spontaneous adverse drug reaction reporting with St. John's Wort and fluoxetine during the period 2000–2013. Clinical and Experimental Pharmacology and Physiology 2015;42:747–751. doi: 10.1111/1440-1681.12424.

740. Lopresti AL, Drummond PD (2017) Efficacy of curcumin, and a saffron/curcumin combination for the treatment of major depression: a randomised, double-blind, placebo-controlled study. J Affect Disord 207:188–196.

741. Ng QX, Koh SSH, Chan HW et al (2017) Clinical use of Curcumin in depression: a meta-analysis. J Am Med Dir Assoc 18:503–508.

742. Greenblatt BJM, To W, Dimino J. Evidence-Based Research on the Role of Zinc and Magnesium Deficiencies in Depression. Psychiatr Times. 2016;33(12):1-5.

743. Tarleton EK, Littenberg B, MacLean CD, Kennedy AG, Daley C. Role of magnesium in the treatment of depression. PLoS One. 2017;12(6 e0180067):1-15. doi:10.1371/journal.pone.0180067

744. 30+ New Antidepressants (2018): Drugs In Clinical Trials. https://mentalhealthdaily.com/2018/02/13/new-antidepressants-2018-drugs-in-clinical-trials/ Accessed on 8/3/19.

745. A Study of ALKS 5461 for the Treatment of Major Depressive Disorder (MDD) - FORWARD-5 Study. https://clinicaltrials.gov/ct2/show/study/NCT02218008?term=Alkermes&rank=5 Accessed on 6/29/15.

746. Yovell Y, Bar G, Mashiah M, et al. Ultra-Low-Dose Buprenorphine as a Time-Limited Treatment for Severe Suicidal Ideation: A Randomized Controlled Trial.[Erratum appears in Am J Psychiatry. 2016 Feb 1;173(2):198; PMID: 26844802]. Am J Psychiatry. 2016;173(5):491-498. doi:10.1176/appi.ajp.2015.15040535

747. Quiroz JA, Tamburri P, Deptula D, et al. Efficacy and safety of basimglurant as adjunctive therapy for major depression: A randomized clinical trial. JAMA Psychiatry. 2016;73(7):675-684. doi:10.1001/jamapsychiatry.2016.0838

748. Drewniany E, Han J, Hancock C, et al. Rapid-onset antidepressant action of ketamine: potential revolution in understanding and future pharmacologic treatment of depression. Journal of Clinical Pharmacy and Therapeutics, 2015, 40,125–130 doi: 10.1111/jcpt.12238.

749. Murrough JW, Iosifescu DV, Chang LC, et al. Antidepressant Efficacy of Ketamine in Treatment-Resistant Major Depression: A Two-Site Randomized Controlled Trial. American J Psychiatry 2013 (October);170(10):1134-1142.

750. DeWilde KE, Levitch CF, Murrough JW, et al. The promise of ketamine for treatment-resistant depression: current evidence and future directions. Ann. N.Y. Acad. Sci. 1345 (2015) 47–58. doi: 10.1111/nyas.12646.

751. Amidfar M, Khiabany M, Kohi A, et al. Effect of memantine combination therapy on symptoms in patients with moderate-to-severe depressive disorder: randomized, double-blind, placebo-controlled study. J Clin Pharm Ther. 2017;42(1):44-50. doi:10.1111/jcpt.12469

752. Dean OM, Kanchanatawan B, Ashton M, et al. Adjunctive minocycline treatment for major depressive disorder: A proof of concept trial. Aust New Zeal J Psychiatry. 2017;51(8):829-840. doi:10.1177/0004867417709357

753. Duman R, Kato T, Liu RJ, et al. "Sestrin 2 Modulator NV-5138 Shows Ketamine-Like Rapid Antidepressant Effects via Direct Activation of mTORC1 Signaling." Poster M130 at the ACNP 56th Annual Meeting of the American College of Neuropsychopharmacology. Neuropsychopharmacology (2017) 42,S111–S293.

754. Salagre E, Fernandes BS, Dodd S, Brownstein DJ, Berk M. Statins for the treatment of depression: A meta-analysis of randomized, double-blind, placebo-controlled trials. J Affect Disord. 2016;200:235-242. doi:10.1016/j.jad.2016.04.047

755. Köhler O, Gasse C, Petersen L, et al. The effect of concomitant treatment with SSRIs and statins: A population-based study. Am J Psychiatry. 2016;173(8):807-815. doi:10.1176/appi.ajp.2016.15040463

756. Jancin B/MDedge News. Statins may do double duty as antidepressants. Publish date: 9/10/19. The Hospitalist. https://www.the-hospitalist.org/hospitalist/article/207875/depression/statins-may-do-double-duty-antidepressants/page/0/2?channel=51329 Accessed 9/11/19.

757. Gardoni F, Di Luca M. New targets for pharmacological intervention in the glutamatergic synapse. Eur J Pharmacol. 2006;545(1):2-10. doi:10.1016/j.ejphar.2006.06.022

758. Hayasaka Y, Purgato M, Magni LR, et al. Dose equivalents of antidepressants: Evidence-based recommendations from randomized controlled trials. Journal of Affective Disorders 2015: 180;179–184.

759. de Abajo FJ, Garcia-Rodriguez LA. Risk of upper gastrointestinal tract bleeding associated with selective serotonin reuptake inhibitors and venlafaxine therapy. Arch Gen Psychiatry. 2008;65:795-803.

760. Hervas I, Vilaro MT, Romero L, Scorza MC, Mengod G, Artigas F. Desensitization of 5HT(1A) autoreceptors by a low chronic fluoxetine dose effect of the concurrent administration of WAY-100635. Neuropsychopharmacology 2001;24:11–20.

761. "Serotonin Receptors." Wikipedia. Wikimedia Foundation, 13 Jan. 2014. Web. 16 Jan. 2014. http://en.wikipedia.org/wiki/Serotonin_receptors.

762. "5HT Receptors." Tocris Bioscience. Tocris Bioscience, 2014. Web. 23 Jan. 2014. http://www.tocris.com/pharmacologicalBrowser.php?ItemId=5101.

763. Glennon, Richard A., Malgorzata Dukat, and Richard B. Westkaemper. "Serotonin Receptor Subtypes and Ligands." Serotonin Receptor Subtypes and Ligands. American College of Neuropsychopharmacology, 2000. Web. 24 Jan. 2014. http://www.acnp.org/g4/GN401000039/Ch039.html.

764. Artigas, Francesc. "Serotonin Receptors Involved in Antidepressant Effects." Pharmacology & Therapeutics 137.1 (2013): 119-31.

765. Hoyer, Daniel, David E. Clarke, John R. Fozard, Paul R. Hartig, and Greame R. Martin. "VII. International Union of Pharmacology Classification of Receptors for 5-Hydroxytryptamine (Serotonin)." Pharmacological Reviews 46.2 (1994): 163-85.

766. Frazer A, Hensler JG. Serotonin Receptors. In: Siegel GJ, Agranoff BW, Albers RW, et al., editors. Basic Neurochemistry: Molecular, Cellular and Medical Aspects. 6th edition. Philadelphia: Lippincott-Raven; 1999. Available from: http://www.ncbi.nlm.nih.gov/books/NBK28234

767. Golan, David E (editor). "Principles of Pharmacology: The Pathophysiologic Basis of Drug Therapy", 2nd edition. LWW: 2008.

768. Harvey, R; Champe, P (series editors). "Lippincott illustrated reviews: Pharmacology", 4th edition. LWW: 2009.

769. Viguier, Florent, et al. "Multiple roles of serotonin in pain control mechanisms–Implications of 5HT7 and other 5HT receptor types." European journal of pharmacology (2013).

770. Mendez-David I, David DJ, Darcet F, et al. Rapid anxiolytic effects of a 5-HT4 receptor agonist are mediated by a neurogenesis-independent mechanism. Neuropsychopharmacology. 2014;39(6):1366-1378. doi:10.1038/npp.2013.332

771. Dunkley EJ, Isbister GK, Sibbritt D, Dawson AH, Whyte IM (September 2003). "The Hunter Serotonin Toxicity Criteria: simple and accurate diagnostic decision rules for serotonin toxicity". QJM 96 (9): 635–42. doi:10.1093/qjmed/hcg109. PMID 12925718

772. Sternbach H. The serotonin syndrome. Am J Psychiatry. 1991;148:705–713.

773. Werneke U, et al. Conundrums in neurology: Diagnosing serotonin syndrome – a meta-analysis of cases. BMC Neurology 2016;16:97.

774. Turner AH, Kim JJ, and McCarron RM. Differentiating serotonin syndrome and neuroleptic malignant syndrome. Current Psychiatry. 2019 February;18(2):30-36.

775. Ables AZ, Nagubilli R. Prevention, recognition, and management of serotonin syndrome. Am Fam Physician.2010 May 1;81(9):1139-42.

776. Rushton WF, Charlton NP. Dexmedetomidine in the treatment of serotonin syndrome. Ann Pharmacother. 2014;48(12):1651-4.

777. Ultram® (tramadol) [package insert]. Raritan, NJ; Ortho-McNeil Pharmaceutical, Inc.; 2007 Feb.

778. Keegan MT, Brown DR, Rabinstein AA. Serotonin syndrome from the interaction of cyclobenzaprine with other serotonergic drugs. Anesth Analg 2006;103:1466-8.

779. Silberstein S, Loder E, Diamond S, et al. Probable migraine in the United States: Results of the American Migraine Prevalence and Prevention (AMPP) study. Cephalalgia. 2007;27:220-234.

780. Gillman PK. Triptans, Serotonin Agonists, and Serotonin Syndrome (Serotonin Toxicity): A Review. Headache. 2010 Feb;50(2):264-72. Epub 2009 Nov 17.

781. Leung M, Ong M. Lack of an interaction between sumatriptan and selective serotonin reuptake inhibitors. Headache 1995;35:488-9.

782. Ables AZ and Nagubilli R. Prevention, recognition, and management of serotonin syndrome. American Family Physician 2010 May 1;81(9):1139-42.

783. Keegan MT, Brown DR, Rabinstein AA. Serotonin syndrome from the interaction of cyclobenzaprine with other serotoninergic drugs. Anesth Analg 2006;103:1466-8.

784. PROVAYBLUE® (methylene blue) injection [package insert]. CENEXI, Fontenay sous Bois, France. May 2018.

785. Schutte-Rodin S, Broch L, Buysse D, et al. Clinical guideline for the evaluation and management of chronic in-somnia in adults. J Clin Sleep Med 2008;4(5):487-504.

786. SJ Wilson, DJ Nutt, C Alford, et al. British Association for Psychopharmacology consensus statement on evidence-based treatment of insomnia, parasomnias and circadian rhythm disorders. Journal of Psychopharmacology 2010;24(11):1577–1600. sagepub.co.uk/journals DOI: 10.1177/0269881110379307.

787. Fisher HL, Lereya ST, Thompson A, Lewis G, Zammit S, Wolke D. Childhood parasomnias and psychotic experiences at age 12 years in a United Kingdom birth cohort. Sleep. 2014;37(3):475-82.

788. American Academy of Sleep Medicine Avoid sleeping pills for children with insomnia. http://www.choosingwisely.org/patient-resources/avoid-sleeping-pills-for-children-with-insomnia/ Accessed on 9/30/19.

789. Academy A, Medicine S. American Academy of Sleep Medicine Five Things Physicians and Patients Should Question. Am Acad Sleep Med. 2014:10-11. Choosing Wisely update June 1, 2017.

790. Sateia MJ, Buysse DJ, Krystal AD, Neubauer DN, Heald JL. Clinical Practice Guideline for the Pharmacologic Treatment of Chronic Insomnia in Adults: An American academy of sleep medicine clinical practice guideline. J Clin Sleep Med. 2017;13(2):307-349. doi:10.5664/jcsm.6470

791. Qaseem A, Kansagara D, Forciea MA, et al. Management of chronic insomnia disorder in adults: A clinical practice guideline from the American college of physicians. Ann Intern Med. 2016;165(2):125-133. doi:10.7326/M15-2175

792. Wilson SJ, Nutt DJ, Alford C, et al. British association for psychopharmacology consensus statement on evidence-based treatment of insomnia, parasomnias and circadian rhythm disorders. J Psychopharmacol. 2010;24(11):1577-1600.

793. Buscemi N, Vandermeer B, Friesen C, et al. The efficacy and safety of drug treatments for chronic insomnia in adults: a meta-analysis of RCTs. Journal of General Internal Medicine 2007;22(9):1335–50.

794. Parrino L, Terzano MG. Polysomnographic effects of hypnotic drugs. A review. Psychopharmacology 1996;126(1):1–16.

795. Young CA. Common prescription insomnia drugs have new boxed warning for serious injuries, death. Pharmacy Today 2019;25(7):19.

796. Huedo-Medina TB, Kirsch I, Middlemass J, Klonizakis M, Siriwardena AN. Effectiveness of non-benzodiazepine hypnotics in treatment of adult insomnia: meta-analysis of data submitted to the Food and Drug Administration. BMJ. 2012;345:e8343.

797. Rappa LR, Larose-Pierre M, Payne DR, Eraikhuemen NE, Lanes DM, and Kearson ML. "Detoxification from high dose zolpidem using diazepam" – Ann Pharmacother April 2004;38: 590-594. DOI 10.1345/aph.1D339.

798. Heesch CB. The Long-term Use of Sedative Hypnotics in Chronic Insomnia. Ment Health Clin. 2014; 4(2):54.

http://cpnp.org/resource/mhc/2014/03/long-term-use-sedarive-hypnotics-chronic-insomnia. Accessed March 03, 2014.

799. Jeffery S. FDA Recommends Lower Bedtime Dose for Zolpidem. Medscape website. http://www.medscape.com/viewarticle/777431. Accessed April 12, 2015

800. Harnod T, Li YF, Lin CL, et al. Higher-dose uses of zolpidem will increase the subsequent risk of developing benign brain tumors. J Neuropsychiatry Clin Neurosci. 2015 Spring;27(2):e107-11. doi: 10.1176/appi.neuropsych.14010006.

801. Tomor H, Yu-Fen L, Cheng-Li L, Shin-Ni C, Fung-Chang S, Chia-Hung, K. Higher-Dose Uses of Zolpidem Will Increase the Subsequent Risk of Developing Benign Brain Tumors. The Journal of Neuropsychiatry. http://neuro. psychiatryonline.org/doi/10.1176/appi.neuropsych.14010006. Accessed April 12, 2015.

802. Bomalaski MN, Claflin ES, Townsend W, Peterson MD. Zolpidem for the Treatment of Neurologic Disorders: A Systematic Review. JAMA Neurol. 2017;74(9):1130-1139. doi:10.1001/jamaneurol.2017.1133

803. Patel KV, Aspesi AV, Evoy KE. Suvorexant - A Dual Orexin Receptor Antagonist for the Treatment of Sleep Onset and Sleep Maintenance Insomnia. doi: 10.1177/1060028015570467 Ann Pharmacother April 2015;49(4):477-483.

804. Dubey AK, Handu SS, and Mediratta PK. Suvorexant: The first orexin receptor antagonist to treat insomnia. J Pharmacol Pharmacother 2015 Apr-Jun; 6(2):118–121.doi: 10.4103/0976-500X.155496. PMCID: PMC4419247.

805. Katwala J, Kumar AK, Sejpal JJ, Terrence M, Mishra M. Therapeutic rationale for low dose doxepin in insomnia patients. Asian Pacific J Trop Dis. 2013;3(4):331-336. doi:10.1016/S2222-1808(13)60080-8

806. Richardson GS, Roehrs TA, Rosenthal L, Koshorek G, Roth T. Tolerance to daytime sedative effects of H1 antihistamines. J Clin Psychopharmacol. 2002;22(5):511-5. DOI: 10.1097/00004714-200210000-00012.

807. Nazarian PK, Park SH. Antidepressant Management of Insomnia Disorder in the Absence of a Mood Disorder. Ment Health Clin [Internet]. 2014;4(2):41-6. Available from: http://dx.doi.org/10.9740/mhc.n188364

808. Alexander B, Lund BC, Bernardy NC, et al. Early Discontinuation and Suboptimal Dosing of Prazosin: A Potential Missed Opportunity for Veterans with Posttraumatic Stress Disorder. J Clin Psychiatry 2015;76(5):e639–e644. 10.4088/JCP.14m09057.

809. Morin AK. Off-Label Use of Atypical Antipsychotic Agents for Treatment of Insomnia. Ment Health Clin. 2014;4(2):46. http://cpnp.org/resource/mhc/2014/03/label-use-atypical-antipsychotic-agents-treatment-insomnia. Accessed April 12, 2015.

810. Anderson SL, Vande Griend JP. Quetiapine for insomnia: A review of the literature. Am J Health Syst Pharm 2014;71(5):394-402.

811. Arendt J. Safety in melatonin in long-term use. J Biol rhythms. 1997 Dec;12(6):673-81.

812. Role in therapy of melatonin for the treatment of insomnia in children and adults. Trends in sedative-hypnotic therapy. Mental Health Clinician 2014 (March);4(2):52-58. doi: http://dx.doi.org/10.9740/mhc.n190085.

813. Adib-Hajbaghery M, Mousavi SN (2017) The effects of chamomile extract on sleep quality among elderly people: a clinical trial. Complement Ther Med 35:109–114.

814. Möller HJ, Volz HP, Dienel A et al (2017) Efficacy of Silexan in subthreshold anxiety: meta-analysis of randomised, placebo-controlled trials. Eur Arch Psychiatry Clin Neurosci. 2019 10.1007/ s00406-017-0852-4

815. Nematolahi P, Mehrabani M, Karami-Mohajeri S et al (2018) Effects of Rosmarinus officinalis L. on memory performance, anxiety, depression, and sleep quality in university students: a randomized clinical trial. Complement Ther Clin Pract 30:24–28.

816. Fox M. Brain Zap Could Help You Control Your Dreams. NBC News website. http://www.nbcnews.com/health-news/brain-zap-could-help-you-control-your-dreams-n101736. Accessed 4/1215.

817. Vanover KE, Davis RE. Role of 5HT2A receptor antagonists in the treatment of insomnia. Nat Sci Sleep. 2010;2:139-150.

818 Eisai Inc. A multicenter, randomized, double-blind, placebo-controlled, active comparator, parallel-group study of the efficacy and safety of lemborexant in subjects 55 years and older with insomnia disorder. (E2006-G000-304). (Clinicaltrials.gov Identifier NCT02783729). 2018. Unpublished data on file.

Eisai Inc. A long-term multicenter, randomized, double-blind, controlled, parallel-group study of the safety and efficacy of lemborexant in subjects with insomnia disorder (E2006-G000-303). (Clinicaltrials.gov Identifier NCT02952820). 2018. Unpublished data on file.

Margaret Moline, Patricia Murphy, Jane Yardley, Dinesh Kumar, Kate Pinner, Carlos Perdomo, Russell Rosenberg, Gary Zammit, 0368 Efficacy and Tolerability of Lemborexant in Female and Male Subjects with Insomnia, Sleep, Volume 42, Issue Supplement_1, April 2019, Page A150, https://doi.org/10.1093/sleep/zsz067.367

819. Bhattarai J, Sumerall S. Current and future treatment options for narcolepsy: A review. Sleep Sci. 2017;10(1):19-27. doi:10.5935/1984-0063.20170004

820. Orlovska S, Vestergaard CH, Bech BH, Nordentoft M, Vestergaard M, Benros ME. Association of streptococcal throat infection with mental disorders: Testing key aspects of the PANDAS hypothesis in a nationwide study. JAMA Psychiatry. 2017;74(7):740-746. doi:10.1001/jamapsychiatry.2017.0995

821. Clomipramine [package insert]. Hazelwood, MO: Mallinckrodt Inc.; 2007

822. Mataix-Cols D, De La Cruz LF, Monzani B, et al. D-cycloserine augmentation of exposure-based cognitive behavior therapy for anxiety, obsessive-compulsive, and posttraumatic stress disorders a systematic review and meta-analysis of individual participant data. JAMA Psychiatry. 2017;74(5):501-510. doi:10.1001/jamapsychiatry.2016.3955

823. Paydary K, Akamaloo A, Ahmadipour A, Pishgar F, Emamzadehfard S, Akhondzadeh S. N-acetylcysteine augmentation therapy for moderate-to-severe obsessive-compulsive disorder: Randomized, double-blind, placebo-controlled trial. J Clin Pharm Ther. 2016;41(2):214-219. doi:10.1111/jcpt.12370

824. Grant JE, Chamberlain SR, Redden SA, Leppink EW, Odlaug BL, Kim SW. N -Acetylcysteine in the Treatment of Excoriation Disorder. JAMA Psychiatry. 2016;73(5):490. doi:10.1001/jamapsychiatry.2016.0060

825. Odlaug, BL and Grant JE. N-Acetyl Cysteine in the Treatment of Grooming Disorders. Letters to the Editor. J Clin Psychopharmacol 2007;27(2):227.

826. Koran LM. Refractory OCD? Consider opioids, amphetamines, caffeine. Clinical Psychiatry News. MDedge Conference Coverage from the APA 2019 annual meeting in San Francisco, CA. May 28, 2019.

827. Hirschtritt ME, Bloch MH, Mathews CA. Obsessive-compulsive disorder advances in diagnosis and treatment. JAMA - J Am Med Assoc. 2017;317(13):1358-1367. doi:10.1001/jama.2017.2200

828. PL Detail-Document,Off-Label Use of Atypical Antipsychotics in Adults. Pharmacist's Letter/Prescriber's Letter. July 2015.

829. National Collaborating Centre for Mental Health. Borderline Personality Disorder: The NICE GUIDELINE on Treatment and Management. National Clinical Practice Guideline No. 78. British Psychological Society & Royal College of Psychiatrists, 2009. London, England.

830. Xenitidis K and Campbell C, eds. Pharmacotherapy for borderline personality disorder: NICE guideline. The British Journal of Psychiatry 2010;196:158–160.

831. Kendall T, Burbeck R, and Bateman A. Correspondence - Pharmacotherapy for borderline personality disorder: NICE guideline. The British Journal of Psychiatry 2010;196:158–160. doi: 10.1192/bjp.196.2.158.

832. Zanarini MC, Frankenburg FR, Hennen J, et al. Mental health service utilization by borderline personality disorder patients and Axis II comparison subjects followed prospectively for 6 years. Journal of Clinical Psychiatry 2004;65:28–36.

833. Black DW, Zanarini MC, Romine A, et al. Comparison of Low and Moderate Dosages of Extended-Release Quetiapine in Borderline Personality Disorder. A Randomized, Double-Blind, Placebo-Controlled Trial. Am J Psychiatry. 2014 Jun 27. doi: 10.1176/appi.ajp.2014.13101348. [Epub ahead of print]

834. Oldham JM, Gabbard GO, Goin MK, et al. Practice Guideline for the Treatment of Patients with Borderline Personality. American Psychiatric Association 2001. 1-82.

835. National Health and Medical Research Council. Clinical practice guideline for the management of borderline personality disorder. Melbourne (Australia): National Health and Medical Research Council; 2012. 166 p. [278 references].

836. Ali S, Findlay C. A review of NICE guidelines on the management of borderline personality disorder. Br J Med Pract. 2016;9(1).

837. Monti JM. Serotonin control of sleep-wake behavior. Sleep Med Rev. 2011;15(4):269-281.

838. Hendrickson RC, Raskind MA. Noradrenergic dysregulation in the pathophysiology of PTSD. Exp Neurol. 2016;284(Pt B):181-195.

839. Krystal AD, Richelson E, Roth T. Review of the histamine system and the clinical effects of H1 antagonists: basis for a new model for understanding the effects of insomnia medications. Sleep Med Rev. 2013;17(4):263-272.

840. VA/DoD Clinical Practice Guideline for Management of Post-Traumatic Stress. Version 2.0 – 2010. http://www.healthquality.va.gov/PTSD-full-2010c.pdf Accessed on 6/26/15.

841. Argolo FC, Cavalcanti-Ribeiro P, Netto LR, Quarantini LC. Prevention of posttraumatic stress disorder with propranolol: A meta-analytic review. J Psychosom Res. 2015;79(2):89-93. doi:10.1016/j.jpsychores.2015.04.006

842. Kindt M, Soeter M, Sevenster D. Disrupting reconsolidation of fear memory in humans by a noradrenergic β-blocker. J Vis Exp. 2014;(94):1-8. doi:10.3791/52151

843. Brunet A, Saumier D. Reduction of PTSD Symptoms With Pre- Reactivation Propranolol Therapy : A Randomized Controlled Trial Reduction of PTSD Symptoms With Pre-Reactivation Propranolol Therapy : A Randomized Controlled Trial. 2018;(January):17050481. doi:10.1176/appi.ajp.2017.17050481

844. Guina J, Rossetter SR, DeRhodes BJ, et al. Benzodiazepines for PTSD: A Systematic Review and Meta-Analysis. Journal of Psychiatric Practice 2015 (Jul);21(4):281-303.

845. Keeshin, B. R., and J. R. Strawn. Psychological and pharmacologic treatment of youth with posttraumatic stress disorder: An evidence-based

review. Child Adolescent Psychiatric Clinics of North American 2014;23: 399–411.

846. Koola MM, Varghese SP, Fawcett JA. High-dose prazosin for the treatment of post-traumatic stress disorder. Ther Adv Psychopharmacol. 2014;4(1):43–47. doi:10.1177/2045125313500982

847. Raskind MA, Peskind ER, Chow B, et al. Trial of Prazosin for Post-Traumatic Stress Disorder in Military Veterans. N Engl J Med. 2018;378(6):507-517. doi:10.1056/NEJMoa1507598

848. Singh B, Hughes AJ, Mehta G, et al. Prim Care Companion CNS Disord 2016;18(4) doi:10.4088/PCC.16r01943

849. Slomski A. Ketamine Effective in Treating PTSD. JAMA 2014;312(4):327. doi:10.1001/jama.2014.9149.

850. Feder A, Parides MK, Murrough JW. Efficacy of intravenous ketamine for treatment of chronic posttraumatic stress disorder: a randomized clinical trial. JAMA Psychiatry. 2014 April 16. [Epub ahead of print].

851. Chedekel L. Yale: 'Magic' Antidepressant May Hold Promise For PTSD. June 03, 2012. The Hartford Courant. Accessed on 6/27/15. http://articles.courant.com/2012-06-03/health/hc-yale-drug-research-20120601_1_ptsd-debilitating-anxiety-disorder-ketamine.

852. Han DH. Benefits of blueberries for PTSD explored in study. http://www.empr.com/news/benefits-of-blueberries-for-post-traumatic-stress-disorder-explored-in-study/article/405810/. Accessed on 3/30/15.

853. Tonmya® for PTSD. https://www.tonixpharma.com/pipeline/tonmya-for-ptsd. Accessed on 8/18/19.

854. Rautaharju PM, Surawicz B, Gettes LS. AHA/ACCF/HRS recommendations for the standardization and interpretation of the electrocardiogram, part IV: the ST segment, T and U waves, and the QT interval: a scientific statement from the American Heart Association Electrocardiography and Arrhythmias Committee, Council on Clinical Cardiology; the American College of Cardiology Foundation; and the Heart Rhythm Society. Circulation.2009;119:e241–e250.

855. Hincapie-Castillo JM, Staley B, Henriksen C, et al. Development of a predictive model for drug-associated QT prolongation in the inpatient setting using electronic health record data. Am J Health-Syst Pharm.2019;76:1059-1070

856. Document E 14: Clinical Evaluation of QT/QTc Interval Prolongation and Proarrhythmic Potential of Non-Antiarrhythmic Drugs. Rockville, MD: US Department of Health and Human Services, Food and Drug Administration; October 2005.

857. Crouch MA, Limon L, Cassano AT. Clinical relevance and management of drug-related QT interval prolongation. Pharmacotherapy 2003;23(7):881-908.

858. Post-graduate Healthcare Education. Power-Pak CE. Medication-induced QT interval prolongation. http://www.powerpak.com/course/print/108469. Accessed on 8/23/2012.

859. Wenzel-Seifert K, Wittmann M, Haen E. QTc prolongation by psychotropic drugs and the risk of Torsade de Pointes. Dtsch Arztebl Int. 2011;108(41):687-93.

860. Beach SR, Celano CM, Noseworthy PA, Januzzi JL, Huffman JC. QTc prolongation, torsades de pointes, and psychotropic medications. Psychosomatics. 2013;54(1):1-13.

861. Zemrak WR, Kenna GA. Association of antipsychotic and antidepressant drugs with Q-T interval prolongation. Am J Health Syst Pharm. 2008;65(11):1029-38.

862. Harrigan EP, Miceli JJ, Anziano R, et al. A randomized evaluation of the effects of six antipsychotic agents on QTc, in the absence and presence of metabolic inhibition. J Clin Psychopharmacol. 2004;24(1):62-9.

863. PL Detail-Document #280111, Drug-induced Long QT Interval. Pharmacist's Letter/Prescriber's Letter. January 2012.

864. FDA Guidance Document: E14 Clinical Evaluation of QT-QTc Interval Prolongation and Proarrhythmic Potential for Non-Antiarrhythmic Drugs - Questions and Answers (R3) - Guidance for Industry. June 2017. https://www.fda.gov/media/71379/download Accessed on 10/21/19.

865. Funk MC, Beach SR, Bostwick JR, et al: American Psychiatric Association resource document QTc prolongation and psychotropic medications. Washington, DC, American Psychiatric Association, 2018. http://www.psychiatry.org/File%20Library/Psychiatrists/Directories/Library-and-Archive/resource_documents/Resource-Document-2018-QTc-Prolongation-and-Psychotropic-Med.pdf. Accessed July 29, 2019.

866. Sala M, Vincentini A, Brambilla P, et al. QT interval prolongation related to psychoactive drug treatment: a comparison of monotherapy versus polytherapy. Ann Gen Psychiatry 2005;4:1. http://www.annals-general-psychiatry.com/content/4/1/1

867. Van der Sijs H, Kowlesar R, Klootwijk APJ, et al. Clinically relevant QTc prolongation due to overridden drug-drug interaction alerts: a retrospective cohort study. Br J Clin Pharmacol 2009;67(3):347-354.

868. van Noord C, Straus SMJM, Sturkenboom MCJM, et al. Psychotropic Drugs Associated With Corrected QT Interval Prolongation. J Clin Psychopharmacol 2009;29:9-15.

869. Castro VM, Clements CC, Murphy SN, et al. QT interval and antidepressant use: a cross sectional study of electronic health records. BMJ 2013;346;f288:1-11. doi: 10.1136/bmj.f288.

870. Choi S, Bostwick JR, Murphy LR. QT Prolongation and Antidepressants There is a better solution to. 2018;(March):21-22.

871. Jasiak NM, Bostwick JR. Risk of QT/QTc prolongation among newer non-SSRI antidepressants. Ann Phamacother. 2014;48(12):1620-8.

872. Straus SM, Bleumink GS, Dieleman JP, et al. Antipsychotics and the risk of sudden cardiac death. Arch Intern Med 2004 Jun 28;164(12):1293-7.

873. Gardner D, Murphy A, O'Donnell H, et al. International consensus study of antipsychotic dosing. Am J Psychiatry. 2010; 167:686-93.

874. Tauscher J and Kapur S. Choosing the right dose of antipsychotics in schizophrenia: lessons from neuroimaging studies. CNS Drugs 2001;15(9):671-8.

875. Agid O, Kapur S, Remington G. Emerging drugs for schizophrenia. Expert Opinion on Emerging Drugs. 13(3):479-95, September 2008.

876. Bishara D, Taylor D. Upcoming agents for the treatment of schizophrenia: mechanism of action, efficacy and tolerability. Drugs 2008 (May);68(16):2269-92,.

877. Stahl SM. Describing an atypical antipsychotic: receptor binding and its role in pathophysiology. Primary Care Companion J Clin Psychiatry 2003;5[suppl3]:9-13.

878. Kishi T, Oya K, Iwata N. Long-acting injectable antipsychotics for the prevention of relapse in patients with recent-onset psychotic disorders: A systematic review and meta-analysis of randomized controlled trials. Psychiatry Res. 2016;246(August 2016):750-755. doi:10.1016/j.psychres.2016.10.053

879. Kristen A. Woodberry, Anthony J. Giuliano, Larry J. Seidman Premorbid IQ in Schizophrenia: A Meta-Analytic Review Published Online:1 May 2008. The Am J Psychiatry 2008 May;165(5):579-587 https://doi.org/10.1176/appi.ajp.2008.07081242

880. Sullivan PF. The genetics of schizophrenia. PLoS Med. 2005;2(7):0614-0618. doi:10.1371/journal.pmed.0020212

881. Rabinowicz EF, Silipo C, Goldman R, Javitt DC. Auditory sensory dysfunction in schizophrenia: imprecision or distractibility? Arch Gen Psychiatry. 2000 Dec;57(12):1149-55. https://www.nature.com/articles/nrn4002

882. Hamilton HK, Williams TJ, Ventura J, Jasperse LJ, Owens EM, Miller GA, Subotnik KL, Nuechterlein KH, Yee CM. Clinical and Cognitive Significance of Auditory Sensory Processing Deficits in Schizophrenia. Am J Psychiatry. 2018 Mar 1;175(3):275-283. doi: 10.1176/appi.ajp.2017.16111203. Epub 2017 Dec 5.

883. Daniel C. Javitt and Robert A. Sweet. Auditory dysfunction in schizophrenia: integrating clinical and basic features. Nat Rev Neurosci. 2015 September ; 16(9) 535–550. doi:10.1038/nrn4002.

884. Bedi G, Carrillo F, Cecchi GA, et al. Automated analysis of free speech predicts psychosis onset in high-risk youths. NPJ Schizophrenia (2015) 1, Article number: 15030; doi:10.1038/npjschz.2015.30; published online 26 August 2015.

885. Brauser D. Retinal Imaging May Identify Schizophrenia. Medscape at: http://www.medscape.com/viewarticle/818774. Accessed 4/10/15.

886. Minichino A, Senior M, Brondino N, et al. Measuring Disturbance of the Endocannabinoid System in Psychosis: A Systematic Review and Meta-analysis. JAMA Psychiatry. Published online June 05, 201976(9):914–923. doi:10.1001/jamapsychiatry.2019.0970

887. Di Forti M, Marconi A, Carra E, et al. Proportion of patients in south London with first-episode psychosis attributable to use of high potency cannabis: A case-control study. The Lancet Psychiatry. 2015;2(3):233-238. doi:10.1016/S2215-0366(14)00117-5

888. Di Forti M, Quattrone D, Freeman TP, et al. The contribution of cannabis use to variation in the incidence of psychotic disorder across Europe (EU-GEI): a multicentre case-control study. The Lancet Psychiatry. 2019;6(5):427-436. doi:10.1016/S2215-0366(19)30048-3

889. Morrison AP, Turkington D, Pyle M, et al. Cognitive therapy for people with schizophrenia spectrum disorders not taking antipsychotic drugs: a single-blind randomised controlled trial. Lancet. 2014;383(9926):1395-1403.

890. Kety SS, Wender PH, Jacobsen B, et al. Mental illness in the biological and adoptive relatives of schizophrenic adoptees. Replication of the Copenhagen Study in the rest of Denmark. Arch Gen Psychiatry. 1994 Jun. 51(6):442-55.

891. Frankenburg FR. Schizophrenia. Mar 16, 2018. https://emedicine.medscape.com/article/288259-print Accessed on 3/5/19.

892. Cardno AG, Owen MJ. Genetic relationships between schizophrenia, bipolar disorder, and schizoaffective disorder. Schizophr Bull. 2014;40(3):504-515. doi:10.1093/schbul/sbu016

893. NeuroscienceNews.com. Researchers identify master gene regulator that could contribute to Schizophrenia. http://neurosciencenews.com/schizophrenia-gene-regulator-2067/ Accessed on May 30, 2015.

894. Schizophrenia Working Group on the Psychiatric Genomics Consortium. Biological insights from 108 schizophrenia-associated genetic loci. Nature 2014;511(7510):421-427.

895. New Clues to Schizophrenia Pathogensis. Medscape. Jul 9, 2015. Report from the 12th World Congress of Biological Psychiatry. Abstract S-37:004. Presented 6/17/15. www.medscape.com/viewarticle/847695_print. Accessed on 7/10/15.

896. University of Pennsylvania. "Parasite-schizophrenia connection: One-fifth of schizophrenia cases may involve the parasite T. gondii." ScienceDaily. ScienceDaily, 29 October 2014. <www.sciencedaily.com/releases/2014/10/141029133448.htm>.

897. Brooks M. Aspirin May Have Beneficial Effects in Schizophrenia: Study. http://www.psychcongress.com/article/aspirin-may-have-beneficial-effects-schizophrenia-study-19349. Accessed on Oct. 28, 2014.

898. Çakici N, van Beveren NJM, Judge-Hundal G, Koola MM, Sommer IEC. An update on the efficacy of anti-inflammatory agents for patients with schizophrenia: a meta-analysis. Psychol Med. 2019;49(14):2307-2319. doi:10.1017/s0033291719001995

899. Dickerson F, Jones-brando L, Ford G, et al. Schizophrenia is Associated With an Aberrant Immune Response to Epstein – Barr Virus. Schizophr Bull. 2018:1-8. doi:10.1093/schbul/sby164

900. Javitt DC. Glutamate and Schizophrenia: From Theory to Treatment Implications. Psychiatric Times website. http://www.psychiatrictimes.com/cme/glutamate-and-schizophrenia-theory-treatment-implications. Accessed on 04/12/2015.

901. Miller B. Toward Biological Subtypes in Schizophrenia: Potential Role of NMDA-Receptor Antibodies. Psychiatric Times. http://www.psychiatrictimes.com/schizophrenia/toward-biological-subtypes-schizophrenia. Accessed on 6/10/15.

902. Valipour G, Saneei P, and Esmaillzadeh A. Serum Vitamin D Levels in Relation to Schizophrenia: A Systematic Review and Meta-Analysis of Observational Studies. J Clin Endocrinol Metab 2014;99:3863–3872.

903. Nasrallah HA. Haloperidol clearly is neurotoxic. Should it be banned? Curr Psychiatry 2013(July);12(7):7-8 plus on-line supplement table

904. Nichols TA. Anti-NMDA receptor encephalitis: An emerging differential diagnosis in the psychiatric community. Ment Heal Clin. 2016;6(6):297-303. doi:10.9740/mhc.2016.11.297

905. M.W. J. Implications for atypical antipsychotics in the treatment of schizophrenia: Neurocognition effects and a neuroprotective hypothesis. Pharmacotherapy. 2004;24(12 I):1759-1783. doi:10.1592/phco.24.17.1759.52346

906. He J, Kong J, Tan QR, Li XM. Neuroprotective effect of atypical antipsychotics in cognitive and non-cognitive behavioral impairment in animal models. Cell Adhes Migr. 2009;3(1):129-137. doi:10.4161/cam.3.1.7401

907. Nasrallah HA. Editor A decade after the CATIE study , the focus has shifted from effectiveness to neuroprotection Remarkable findings emerge. Curr Psychiat. 2015;14(12):19-21.

908. Kusumi I, Boku S, Takahashi Y. Psychopharmacology of atypical antipsychotic drugs: From the receptor binding profile to neuroprotection and neurogenesis. Psychiatry Clin Neurosci. 2015;69(5):243-258. doi:10.1111/pcn.12242

909. Nasrallah HA. Impaired Neuroplasticity in Schizophrenia and the Neuro-regenerative Effects of Atypical Antipsychotics. https://www.medscape.org/viewarticle/569521. Accessed on 9/27/18.

910. Kamal SM, Dine SE (2015) Neuroplasticity and Antipsychotics in Treatment of Schizophrenia. J Neurol Disord 3:232. doi: 10.4172/2329-6895.1000232

911. He J, Kong J, Tan QR, Li XM. Neuroprotective effect of atypical antipsychotics in cognitive and non-cognitive behavioral impairment in animal models. Cell Adhes Migr. 2009;3(1):129-137. doi:10.4161/cam.3.1.7401

912. Joa I, Gisselgård J, Brønnick K, et al. Primary Prevention of Psychosis Through Interventions in the Symptomatic Prodromal Phase, a Pragmatic Norwegian Ultra High Risk Study. BMC Psychiatry. 2015;15(89).

913. Grunze H. Differentiating schizoaffective and bipolar disorder: a dimensional approach. ECNP Berlin 2014. http://www.ecnp.eu/presentationpdfs/7/S_05_04.pdf. Accessed on Oct. 20, 2014.

914. Stahl S. Stahl's Essential Psychopharmacology Online, 4th Ed. Accessed on 5/28/15. http://stahlonline.cambridge.org/essential_4th_chapter.jsf?page=chapter5_summary.htm&name=Chapter%205&title=Summary.

915. Drug Safety Information for Healthcare Professionals: Updated Information on Leukotriene Inhibitors. FDA (Food & Drug Administration) at: http://www.fda.gov/Drugs/DrugSafety/PostmarketDrugSafetyInformationforPatientsandProviders/DrugSafetyInformationforHeathcareProfessionals/ucm165489.htm Accessed on 3/11/15.

916. Buckley PF. Receptor-binding profiles of antipsychotics: clinical strategies when switching between agents. J Clin Psychiatry 2007;68 [suppl 6]:5-9.

917. Richtand NM, Welge JA, Logue AD, et al. Dopamine and Serotonin Receptor Binding and Antipsychotic Efficacy. Neuropsychopharmacology (2007) 32:1715–1726.

918. Poster presented at the 2012 NEI Global Psychopharmacology Congress. Receptor Binding Profiles of Atypical Antipsychotics: Mechanisms of Therapeutic Actions and Adverse Side Effects. http://seragpsych.com/wordpress/wp-content/uploads/2013/06/50188_nei_009_bindings.pdf. Accessed on 5/28/15.

919. Kroeze WK, Hufeisen SJ, Popadak BA, et al. H1-Histamine Receptor Affinity Predicts Short-Term Weight Gain for Typical and Atypical Antipsychotic Drugs. Neuropsychopharmacology 3002;28:519-526; doi:10.1038/sj.npp.1300027.

920. Wu C-S, Wang S-C, Gau SS, et al. Association of stroke with receptor-binding profiles of antipsychotics - A case-crossover study. Biol Psychiatry 2013;73:414-421.

921. Hwang YJ, Dixon SN, Reiss JP, et al. Atypical antipsychotic drugs and the risk for acute kidney injury and other adverse outcomes in older adults: a population-based cohort study. Ann Intern Med. 2014;161(4):242-8.

922. Fraser LA, Liu K, Naylor KL, et al. Falls and fractures with atypical antipsychotic medication use: a population-based cohort study. JAMA Intern Med. 2015;175(3):450-2.

923. Woods SW. Chlorpromazine equivalent doses for the newer atypical antipsychotics. J Clin Psychiatry. 2003;64(6):663-7.

924. Manzella F, Maloney SE, Taylor GT. Smoking in schizophrenic patients: A critique of the self-medication hypothesis. World J Psychiatr 2015 March 22; 5(1): 35-46

925. Hsieh A. A Phase IIb, Randomized, Double-blind, Placebo-controlled, 12-week Study of Encenicline, an α7 Nicotinic Acetylcholine Receptor Partial Agonist, for Cognitive Impairment in Patients with Schizophrenia. Poster presentation at the CPNP (College of Psychiatric and Neurologic Pharmacists) 4/2015.

926. Prickaertsb J, van Goethemb NP, Chesworth R, et al. EVP-6124, a novel and selective α7 nicotinic acetylcholine receptor partial agonist, improves memory performance by potentiating the acetylcholine response of α7 nicotinic acetylcholine receptors. Neuropharmacology 2012 (Feb);62(2):1099–1110.

927. Leucht S, Leucht C, Huhn M, et al. Sixty Years of Placebo-Controlled Antipsychotic Drug Trials in Acute Schizophrenia: Systematic Review, Bayesian Meta-Analysis, and Meta-Regression of Efficacy Predictors. Am J Psychiatry. 2017;174(10):927-942. doi:10.1176/appi.ajp.2017.16121358

928. Haddad PM, Correll CU. The acute efficacy of antipsychotics in schizophrenia : a review of recent meta-analyses. 2018;(December 2017):303-318. doi:10.1177/2045125318781475.

929. Shalev A, Hermesh H, Rothberg J, Munitz H. Poor neuroleptic response in acutely exacerbated schizophrenic patients. Acta Psychiatr Scand 1993;87:86–91

930. Harding CM. Changes in Schizophrenia Across Time: Pardoxes, Patterns and Predictors. In: Cohen CI, ed Schizophrenia into later life: Treatment, research and policy. Arlington, VA: American Psychiatric Publishing, Inc.; 2003:19-41.

931. Leucht S, Cipriani A, Spineli L, Mavridis D, Orey D, Richter F, Samara M, Barbui C, Engel RR, Geddes JR, Kissling W, Stapf MP, Lässig B, Salanti G, Davis JM (September 2013). "Comparative efficacy and tolerability of 15 antipsychotic drugs in schizophrenia: a multiple-treatments meta-analysis". Lancet. 382 (9896): 951–62. doi:10.1016/S0140-6736(13)60733-3. PMID 23810019.

932. Leucht S, Corves C, Arbter D, Engel RR, Li C, and Davis JM. Second-generation versus first-generation antipsychotic drugs for schizophrenia: a meta-analysis. Lancet. 2009; 373: 31-41

933. Zhu Y, Krause M, Huhn M, et al. Antipsychotic drugs for the acute treatment of patients with a first episode of schizophrenia: a systematic review with pairwise and network meta-analyses. Lancet Psychiatry2017; 4: 694–705.

934. Leucht S, Rossum IW, Heres S, et al. The Optimization of Treatment and Management of Schizophrenia in Europe (OPTiMiSE) Trial: Rationale for Its Methodology and a Review of the Effectiveness of Switching Antipsychotics. 2015;41(3):549-558. doi:10.1093/schbul/sbv019

935. Heres S, Meliu Cirjaliu D, Dehelean L, et al. The SWITCH study: rationale and design of the trial. Eur Arch Psychiatry Clin Neurosci 2015. DOI 10.1007/s00406-015-0624-y. Published on-line: 31 Jul 2015.

936. Samara MT, Leucht C, Leeflang MM, et al. Early Improvement as a Predictor of Later Response to Antipsychotics in Schizophrenia: A Diagnostic Test Review. Am J Psychiatry 2015 July;172(7):617-629. http://dx.doi.org/10.1176/appi.ajp.2015.14101329.

937. Remington G, Addington D, Honer W, Ismail Z, Raedler T, Teehan M. Guidelines for the Pharmacotherapy of Schizophrenia in Adults. Can J Psychiatry. 2017;62(9):604-616. Doi: 10.1177/0706743717720448.

938. DaSilva J, Houle S, Zipursky R. High levels of dopamine D2 receptor occupancy with low dose haloperidol treatment: a PET study. Am J Psychiatry 1996;153:948-50.

939. Tauscher J and Kapur S. Choosing the right dose of antipsychotics in schizophrenia: lessons from neuroimaging studies. CNS Drugs. 2001;15(9):671-8.

940. Farde L, Nyberg S, Oxenstierna G, et al. Positron emission tomography studies on D2 and 5HT2 receptor binding in risperidone-treated schizophrenic patients. J Clin Psychopharmacol 1995;15:19SY23S.

941. Kapur S, Zipursky R, Jones C, et al. Relationship between dopamine D(2) occupancy, clinical response, and side effects: a double-blind PET study of first-episode schizophrenia. Am J Psychiatry 2000;157:514-520.

942. Uchida H, Kapur S, Mulsant BH, et al. Sensitivity of older patients to antipsychotic motor side effects: a PET study examining potential mechanisms. Am J Geriatr Psychiatry 2009;17:255-263.

943. Uchida H, Kapur S, Pollock BG, et al. Optimal dosing of antipsychotic drugs in older patients with schizophrenia: PET investigations. Int J Neuropsychopharm 2008;11(suppl 1):136

944. Uchida H, Takeuchi H, Graff-Guerrero A, et al. Dopamine D2 receptor occupancy and clinical effects: a systematic review and pooled analysis. J Clin Psychopharmacology 2011 Aug;31(4):497-502.

945. Madras BK. History of the discovery of the antipsychotic dopamine D2 receptor: a basis for the dopamine hypothesis of schizophrenia. J Hist Neurosci. 2013;22(1):62-78. doi: 10.1080/0964704X.2012.678199.
946. Pierre JM, Wirshing DA, and Wirshing WC. High-dose antipsychotics: Desperation or data-driven? Current Psychiatry 2004;3(8):30-37.
947. Gisev N, Bell JS, Chen TF. Factors associated with antipsychotic polypharmacy and high-dose antipsychotics among individuals receiving compulsory treatment in the community. J Clin Psychopharmacol. 2014;34(3):307-12.
948. Hasan A, Falkai P, Wobrock T, et al. World Federation of Societies of Biological Psychiatry (WFSBP) Guidelines for Biological Treatment of Schizophrenia, Part 1: Update 2012 on the acute treatment of schizophrenia and the management of treatment resistance. World J Biol Psychiatry. 2012;13(5):318-378. doi:10.3109/15622975.2012.696143
949. Deutch S. Psychosis and Antipsychotic Medication Can be Neurotoxic. Psychiatry Weekly 2013; 16(8). http://www.psychweekly.com/aspx/article/articledetail.aspx?articleid=1597 Accessed on 12/26/2014.
950. D Velligan, N Maples, and J Pokorny. 2019 Congress of the Schizophrenia International Research Society – Orlando, FloridaPoster S118. The assessment of adherence to oral antipsychotic medications: what has changed in the past decade? Schizophrenia Bulletin, Volume 45, Issue Supplement 2, April 2019, Page NP, https://doi.org/10.1093/schbul/sbz019.
951. Zipursky RB, Menezes NM, and Streiner DL. Risk of symptom recurrence with medication discontinuation in first-episode psychosis: A systematic review. Schizophrenia Research 2014;152(2):408–414.
952. Robinson D, Woerner MG, Alvir JM, et al. Predictors of relapse following response from a first episode of schizophre-nia or schizoaffective disorder. Arch Gen Psychiatry. 1999;56(3):241-247.
953. Llorca PM, Abbar M, Courtet P, Guillaume S, Lancrenon S, Samalin L. Guidelines for the use and management of long-acting injectable antipsychotics in serious mental illness. BMC Psychiatry 2013;13:340.
954. Subotnik KL, Casaus LR, Ventura J, et al. Long-Acting Injectable Risperidone for Relapse Prevention and Control of Breakthrough Symptoms After a Recent First Episode of Schizophrenia: A Randomized Clinical Trial. JAMA Psychiatry. doi:10.1001/jamapsychiatry.2015.0270. Published online June 24, 2015.
955. Stetka BS and Correll CU. Psychiatry Practice Changers 2014. Medscape. Dec 08, 2014.
956. Kishimoto T, Nitta M, Borenstein M, Kane JM, Correll CU. Long-acting injectable versus oral antipsychotics in schizophrenia: a systematic review and meta-analysis of mirror-image studies. J Clin Psychiatry. 2013;74:957-965.
957. Many First-Episode Psychosis Txs Not Following Guidelines. MPR website. http://www.empr.com/many-first-episode-psychosis-treatments-not-following-guidelines/article/386746/. Accessed on 04/12/2015.
958. Correll CU, Frederickson AM, Kane JM, et al. Does antipsychotic polypharmacy increase the risk for metabolic syndrome? Schizophrenia Research 2007:89:91–100.
959. Procyshyn RM, Honer WG, Wu TK, et al. Persistent antipsychotic polypharmacy and excessive dosing in the community psychiatric treatment setting: a review of medication profiles in 435 Canadian outpatients. J Clin Psychiatry 2010;71(5):566-573.
959. Skalli L, Skalli L, Lalonde P, et al. Benefits and Risks of Antipsychotic Polypharmacy: An Evidence-Based Review of the Literature. Drug Safety. 31(1):7-20, January 2008.
960. Girgis R, Javitch J, Lieberman J, et al. Antipsychotic drug mechanisms: links between therapeutic efficacy, metabolic side effects and the insulin signaling Pathway. Molecular Psychiatry. 13(10):918-929, October 2008.
961. Nasrallah, H. Atypical antipsychotic-induced metabolic side effects: insights from receptor-binding profiles. Molecular Psychiatry 13(1):27-35, January 2008.
962. Ito H, Koyoma A, Higuchi T. Polypharmacy and excessive dosing: psychiatrists' perceptions of antipsychotic drug prescription. British Journal of Psychiatry. 187(3):243-247, September 2005.
963. Tiihonen J, Taipale H, Mehtälä J, et al. Association of antipsychotic polypharmacy vs monotherapy with psychiatric rehospitalization among adults with schizophrenia. JAMA Psychiatry doi:10.1001/jamapsychiatry.2018.4320. 2019 30785608 (Published online February 20, 2019).
964. Correll CU, Rubio JM, Inczedy-Farkas G, Birnbaum ML, Kane JM, Leucht S. Efficacy of 42 pharmacologic cotreatment strategies added to antipsychotic monotherapy in schizophrenia: Systematic overview and quality appraisal of the meta-analytic evidence. JAMA Psychiatry. 2017;74(7):675-684. doi:10.1001/jamapsychiatry.2017.0624
965. Kreyenbuhl J, Buchanan RW, Dickerson FB, Dixon LB. The Schizophrenia Patient Outcomes Research Team (PORT): updated treatment recommendations 2009. Schizophr Bull 2010;36(1):94-103.
966. National Collaborating Centre for Mental Health. Psychosis and schizophrenia in adults: treatment and management. NICE Guidel. 2014;(February):Feb 54 Clinical Guidelines n° 178. doi:10.1002/14651858.CD010823.pub2.
967. Schmidt SJ, Schultzelutter F, Schimmelmann BG, et al. EPA guidance on the early intervention in clinical high risk states of psychoses. 2015;30:388-404. doi:10.1016/j.eurpsy.2015.01.013
968. American Psychiatric Association. Practice guideline for the treatment of patients with schizophrenia, 2004, Second Edition. http://psychiatryonline.org/pb/assets/raw/sitewide/practice_guidelines/guidelines/schizophrenia.pdf Accessed on 7/9/15.
969. Keepers GA, Fochtmann LJ, Anzia JM et al. The American Psychiatric Association Practice Guideline For The Treatment of Patients With Schizophrenia. Draft 5/13/19. https://www.psychiatry.org/File%20Library/Psychiatrists/Practice/Clinical%20Practice%20Guidelines/APA-Draft-Schizophrenia-Treatment-Guideline.pdf. Accessed on 7/16/19.
970. Stilwell EN, Yates SE, Brahm NC. Violence among persons diagnosed with schizophrenia: How pharmacists can help. Res Soc Adm Pharm. 2011;7(4):421-429. doi:10.1016/j.sapharm.2010.11.002
971. Pies RW. How antipsychotic medication may save lives. Psychiatric Times. June 1, 2016.
972. Mohr P, Knytl P, Voráčková V, Bravermanová A, Melicher T. Long-acting injectable antipsychotics for prevention and management of violent behaviour in psychotic patients. Int J Clin Pract. 2017;71(9):1-7. doi:10.1111/ijcp.12997
973. Hor K, Taylor M. Review: Suicide and schizophrenia: a systematic review of rates and risk factors. J Psychopharmacol. 2010;24(4_suppl):81-90. doi:10.1177/1359786810385490
974. Lindenmayer JP, Liu-Seifert H, Kulkarni PM, et al. Medication non-adherence and treatment outcome in patients with schizophrenia or schizoaffective disorder with suboptimal prior response. J Clin Psychiatry. 2009;70:990-996
975. Fazel S, Zetterqvist J, Larsson H, et al. Antipsychotics, mood stabilizers, and risk of violent crime. Lancet 2014;384(May 8):1206–1214.
976. Neurolepsis. Mosby's Medical Dictionary, 8th edition. © 2009, Elsevier. http://medical-dictionary.thefreedictionary.com/neurolepsis Accessed on 5/31/15.
977. Diphenhydramine HCL Injection USP. [package insert]. Fresenius Kabi USA, LLC, 5/2018.
978. Lorazepam injection [package insert]. Hospira, Inc., Lake Forest, IL. 5/2019.
979. Diphenhydramine (systemic): Drug information UpToDate. Waltham, MA: UpToDate Inc. https://www.uptodate.com/contents/diphenhydramine-systemic-drug-information Accessed on 8/1/2019.
980. Aminoff MJ "Pharmacologic Management of Parkinsonism & Other Movement Disorders" (Chapter 28). In: Katzung BG: Basic & Clinical Pharmacology, 13e. 2015. Katzung BG, Masters SB, Trevor AJ (Editors). McGraw-Hill / Lange.
981. Tachere RO, Modirrousta M. Beyond anxiety and agitation: A clinical approach to akathisia. Aust Fam Physician. 2017;46(5):296-298.
982. Carbon, M., Kane, J. M., Leucht, S. and Correll, C. U. (2018), Tardive dyskinesia risk with first- and second-generation antipsychotics in comparative randomized controlled trials: a meta-analysis. World Psychiatry, 17: 330-340. doi:10.1002/wps.20579
983. Miller BJ. Tardive Dyskinesia: A Review of the Literature. Psychiatr Times, a Suppl. 2017;July:1-6. http://images.ubmmedica.com/psychiatrictimes/pdfs/2017PT_TDSupplement.pdf.
984. Robert L. Tardive Dyskinesia Facts and Figures. Psychiatric Times May 30, 2019. https://www.psychiatrictimes.com/tardive-dyskinesia/tardive-dyskinesia-facts-and-figures Accessed 6/25/19.
985. Bhidayasiri R, Fahn S, Weiner WJ, et al. Evidence-based guideline: treatment of tardive syndromes: report of the Guideline Development Subcommittee of the American Academy of Neurology. Neurology. 2013;81(5):463-9.
986. Inder, W. J., & Castle, D. (2011). Antipsychotic-Induced Hyperprolactinaemia. Australian & New Zealand Journal of Psychiatry, 45(10), 830–837. doi:10.3109/00048674.2011.589044
987. Strawn JR, Keck PE, and Caroff SN. Neuroleptic malignant syndrome: Answers to 6 tough questions. http://www.nmmis.org/content.asp?type=publications&src=pages/nms_answers.asp&title=Neuroleptic+malignant+syndrome:+Answers+to+6+tough+questions. Accessed on 5/15/15.
988. Benzer TI, Mancini MC, Tarabar A, et al. Neuroleptic Malignant Syndrome. Medscape Reference. Updated Feb. 12, 2015. http://emedicine.medscape.com/article/816018-overview Accessed on 5/15/15.
989. Zarrouf FA, Bhanot V. Neuroleptic malignant syndrome: don't let your guard down yet. Current Psychiatry 2007;6(8):89-95.
990. Pileggi DJ, Cook AM. Neuroleptic Malignant Syndrome: Focus on Treatment and Rechallenge. Ann Pharmacother. 2016;50(11):973-981. doi:10.1177/1060028016657553
991. FDA Adverse Event Reporting System (FAERS) Public Dashboard. https://www.fda.gov/Drugs/GuidanceCompliance RegulatoryInformation/Surveillance/AdverseDrugEffects/ucm070093.htm Accessed on 4/18/19.
992. Elbe D, Condé C. Visual Compatibility of Various Injectable Neuroleptic Agents with Benztropine and Lorazepam in Polypropylene Syringes. The Canadian Journal of Hospital Pharmacy. 2001;54:104-107.
993. Sikich L, Frazier JA, McClellan J, Findling RL, Vitiello B, Ritz L, Ambler D, Puglia M, Maloney AE, Michael E, De Jong S, Slifka K, Noyes N, Hlastala S, Pierson L, McNamara NK, Delporto-Bedoya D, Anderson R, Hamer RM, Lieberman JA: Double-blind comparison of first- and second-generation antipsychotics in early-onset schizophrenia and schizo-affective disorder: findings from the Treatment of Early Onset Schizophrenia Spectrum Disorders (TEOSS) study. Am J Psychiatry 2008; 165:1420–1431.

174

994. Apiquian R, Fresán A, Herrera K, et al. Minimum effective doses of haloperidol for the treatment of first psychotic episode: a comparative study with risperidone and olanzapine. Int J Neuropsychopharmacol. 2003;6(4):S1461145703003742. doi:10.1017/S1461145703003742

995. Anderson BP. Low-dose Strategy Can Benefit Schizophrenics. The Medical Post. Aug. 6, 1996. http://www.mentalhealth.com/mag1/p5m-sc03.html Accessed on 5/24/16.

996. Trissel L. Handbook on Injectable Drugs. 15th edition. Maryland: American Society of Health-System Pharmacists; 2009.

997. Sesame Now the 9th Most Common Food Allergy in the U.S. Study presented at the 2019 Annual Meeting of the American Academy of Allergy, Asthma & Immunology (AAAAI). https://www.aaaai.org/about-aaaai/newsroom/news-releases/sesame Accessed 12/10/19.

998. Svendsen O, Aaes-Jørgensen T. Studies on the Fate of Vegetable Oil after Intramuscular Injection into Experimental Animals. Acta Pharmacol Toxicol (Copenh). 1979;45(5):352-378. doi:10.1111/j.1600-0773.1979.tb02404.x

999. Results from First-of-Kind Abilify Maintena Study Announced. MPR website. http://www.empr.com/results-from-first-of-kind-abilify-maintena-study-announced/article/380997/. Accessed on 04/12/2015.

1000. This $1,650 pill will tell your doctors whether you've taken it. Is it the future of medicine? https://www.washingtonpost.com/business/economy/this-1650-pill-will-tell-your-doctors-whether-youve-taken-it-is-it-the-future-of-medicine/2019/04/28/393281b2-4c10-11e9-b79a-961983b7e0cd_story.html?utm_term=.5172568b6af9 Accessed on 5/6/19.

1001. Alkermes Presents Phase III Data From Successful Pivotal Study of Aripiprazole Lauroxil for Treatment of Schizophrenia at ASCP Annual Meeting. http://investor.alkermes.com/phoenix.zhtml?c=92211&p=irol-newsArticle&ID=1940691 Accessed on June 9, 2015.

1002. Meltzer HY, Risinger RS, Nasrallah HA, et al. A Randomized, Double-Blind, Placebo-Controlled Trial of Aripiprazole Lauroxil in Acute Exacerbation of Schizophrenia. Online ahead of print: June 9, 2015 (doi:10.4088/JCP.14m09741).

1003. FDA Medwatch. Saphris (asenapine) sublingual tablets. http://www.fda.gov/safety/medwatch/safetyinformation/ucm271083.htm Accessed on April 21, 2013.

1004. Matthew D. FDA declines to approve Forest/Gedeon Richter's antipsychotic cariprazine, seeks more clinical data. First World Pharma 2013.

1005. Coronas V, Bantubungi K, Fombonne J, et al. Dopamine D3 receptor stimulation promotes the proliferation of cells derived from the post-natal subventricular zone. J Neurochem. 2004;91:1292-1301.

1006. Citrome L. Cariprazine: chemistry, pharmacodynamics, pharmacokinetics, and metabolism, clinical efficacy, safety, and tolerability. Expert Opin Drug Metab Toxicol. 2013 Feb;9(2):193-206. doi: 10.1517/17425255.2013.759211.

1007. Németh G, Laszlovszky I, Czobor P, et al. Cariprazine versus risperidone monotherapy for treatment of predominant negative symptoms in patients with schizophrenia: a randomised, double-blind, controlled trial. Lancet. 2017;389(10074):1103-1113.

1008. Brooks M. Clozapine 'Vastly' Underutilized for Resistant Schizophrenia. Medscape. http://www.medscape.com/viewarticle/820547_print Accessed on Feb 12, 2014.

1009. Stanton RJ II, Paxos C, Geldenhuys WJ, Boss JL, Muntez M, Darvesh AS. Clozapine underutilized in treatment-resistant schizophrenia. Ment Health Clin [Internet]. 2015;5(2):63-7.

1010. Meltzer HY. Treatment of the neuroleptic-nonresponsive schizophrenic patient. Schizophr Bull1992;18:515–42.

1011. Tiihonen J, Mittendorfer-Rutz E, Majak M, et al. Real-world effectiveness of antipsychotic treatments in a nationwide cohort of 29 823 patients with schizophrenia. JAMA Psychiatry. 2017;74(7):686-693. doi:10.1001/jamapsychiatry.2017.1322

1012. Masuda T, Misawa F, Takase M, Kane JM, Correll CU. Association With Hospitalization and All-Cause Discontinuation Among Patients With Schizophrenia on Clozapine vs Other Oral Second-Generation Antipsychotics. JAMA Psychiatry. 2019;11004:1-11. doi:10.1001/jamapsychiatry.2019.1702

1013 Tiihonen J, Lönnqvist J, Wahlbeck K, et al. 11-year follow-up of mortality in patients with schizophrenia: a population-based cohort study (FIN11 study). Lancet 2009; 374:620–627.

1014. Devinsky O, Honigfeld G, Patin J. Clozapine-related seizures. Neurology. 41:369-371.

1015. Trompicamide. https://www.drugbank.ca/drugs/DB00809 Accessed on 9/24/19.

1016. Cuvposa® (glycopyrrolate) oral solution [package insert]. Merz Pharmaceuticals, LLC, Raleigh, NC, 2/2018.

1017. FDA Drug Safety Communication: FDA modifies monitoring for neutropenia associated with schizophrenia medicine clozapine; approves new shared REMS program for all clozapine medicines at: http://www.fda.gov/Drugs/DrugSafety/ucm461853.htm. Accessed on 9/15/15.

1018. Personal communication with representative, Denisha, from the Clozapine REMS program at (844)267-8678 on 9/16/15.

1019. Beutler E and West C. Hematologic differences between African-Americans and whites: the roles of iron deficiency and α-thalassemia on hemoglobin levels and mean corpuscular volume. Blood. 2005 Jul15;106(2):740–745. doi:10.1182/blood-2005-02-0713. PMCID: PMC1895180.

1020. McKee JR, Wall T, Owensby J. Impact of Complete Blood Count Sampling Time Change on White Blood Cell and Absolute Neutrophil Count Values in Clozapine Recipients. Clinical Schizophrenia & Related Psychoses 2011 Apr;5(1):26-32. doi: 10.3371/CSRP.5.1.4.

1021. Nielsen J, Correll CU, Manu P, and Kane JM. Termination of Clozapine Treatment Due to Medical Reasons: When Is It Warranted and How Can It Be Avoided? J Clin Psychiatry 2013;74(6):603-613. 10.4088/JCP.12r08064.

1022. Rajagopal S. Clozapine, agranulocytosis, and benign ethnic neutropenia. Editorial Postgrad Med J 2005;81:545-546 doi:10.1136/pgmj.2004.031161.

1023. Lim E-M, Cembrowski G, Cembrowski M, et al. Race-specific WBC and neutrophil count refererence intervals. Int Jnl Lab Hem 2010;32:590–597. doi:10.1111/j.1751-553X.2010.01223.x.

1024. Lim EM, Cembrowski G, Cembrowski M, Clarke G. Race-specific WBC and neutrophil count reference intervals. Int J Lab Hematol. 2010;32(6 PART 2):590-597. doi:10.1111/j.1751-553X.2010.01223.x

1025. Sennels HP, Jørgensen HL, Hansen ALS, et al. Diurnal variation of hematology parameters in healthy young males: The Bispebjerg study of diurnal variations. Scandinavian Journal of Clinical & Laboratory Investigation, 2011; 71: 532–541. doi:10.3109/00365513.2011.602422.

1026. Sporn A, Gogtay N, Ortiz-Aguayo R, et al. Clozapine-induced neutropenia in children: management with lithium carbonate. J Child Adolesc Psychopharmacol. 2003 Fall;13(3):401-4.

1027. Esposito D, Rouillon F, Limosin F. Continuing clozapine treatment despite neutropenia. Eur J Clin Pharmacol. 2005 Jan;60(11):759-64. Epub 2004 Nov 30.

1028. Pinninti NR, Houdart MP, Strouse EM. Case report of long-term lithium for treatment and prevention of clozapine-induced neutropenia in an African American male. J Clin Psychopharmacol. 2010;30(2):219-21.

1029. Kutscher EC, Robbins GP, Kennedy WK, Zebb K, Stanley M, Carnahan RM. Clozapine-induced leukopenia successfully treated with lithium. Am J Health Syst Pharm. 2007;64(19):2027-31.

1030. Nykiel S, Henderson D, Bhide G, Freudenreich O. Lithium use clozapine prescribing in benign ethnic neutropenia. Clin Schizophr Relat Psychoses. 2010 Jul;4(2):138-40. doi: 10.3371/CSRP.4.2.5.

1031. Perry PJ, Miller DD. The clinical utility of plasma concentrations. In: Marder SR, Davis JM, Janiack PG(eds). Clinical use of neuroleptic plasma levels. Arlington, VA: American Psychiatric Association. 1993;85-100.

1032 Schulte P. What is an adequate trial with clozapine? Therapeutic drug monitoring and time to response in treatment-refractory schizophrenia. Clin Pharmacokinet2003; 42: 607–618

1033. Hasegawa M, Guitierrez-Esteinou R, Way L, et al. Relationship between clinical efficacy and clozapine concentrations in plasma in schizophrenia: effect of smoking. J Clin Psychopharmacol. 1993; 13:83-90.

1034. Kronig MH, Munne RA, Szymanski S, et al. Plasma clozapine levels and clinical response for treatment refractory schizophrenic patients. Am J Psychiatry. 1995; 152:179-82.

1035. Perry PJ, Miller DD, Arndt SV, et al. Clozapine and norclozapine concentrations and clinical response of treatment-refractory schizophrenic patients. Am J Psychiatry. 1991; 148:231-5.

1036. Potkin SG, Bera R, Gulasekaram B, et al. Plasma clozapine concentrations predict clinical response in treatment-resistant schizophrenia. J Clin Psychiatry. 1994; 55(Suppl B):133-6.

1037. Miller DD, Fleming F, Holman TL, et al. Plasma clozapine concentrations as a predictor of clinical response: a follow-up study. J Clin Psychiatry. 1994; 55(Suppl B):117-21.

1038. PR Newswire. Vanda Pharmaceuticals Announces U.S. Patent Allowance for a Long-Acting Injectable Formulation of Fanapt(TM) (iloperidone) in the U.S. http://www.prnewswire.com/news-releases/vanda-pharmaceuticals-announces-us-patent-allowance-for-a-long-acting-injectable-formulation-of-fanapttm-iloperidone-in-the-us-85395607.html Accessed on March 30, 2015.

1039. New Data on Latuda for Schizophrenia Announced. MPR website. http://www.empr.com/new-data-on-latuda-for-schizophrenia-announced/article/378362/. Accessed on 04/12/2015.

1040. Han DH. Latuda for MDD With Mixed Features: New Results Announced. MPR News. http://www.empr.com/news/latuda-versus-placebo-for-mdd-with-mixed-features/article/415708/ Accessed on May 21, 2015.

1041. Haslemo T, et al. Valproic Acid Significantly Lowers Serum Concentrations of Olanzapine - An Interaction Effect Comparable With Smoking. Therapeutic Drug Monitoring Oct. 2012;34(5):512-517.

1042. Martel ML, Klein LR, Rivard RL, Cole JB. A large retrospective cohort of patients receiving intravenous olanzapine in the emergency department. Acad Emerg Med. 2016;23(1):29-35. doi:10.1111/acem.12842

1043. Khorassani F, Saad M. Intravenous Olanzapine for Management of Agitation: Review of the Literature. Ann Pharmacother. 2019. doi:10.1177/1060028019831634

1044. FDA Drug Safety Communication: FDA review of study sheds light on two deaths associated with the injectable schizophrenia drug Zyprexa Relprevv (olanzapine pamoate). http://www.fda.gov/Drugs/DrugSafety/ucm439147.htm. Accessed on 04/12/2015.

1045. Lauriello J, Lambert T, Andersen S, Lin D, Taylor CC, McDonnell D. An 8-week, double-blind, randomized, placebo-controlled study of olanzapine long-acting injection in acutely ill patients with schizophrenia. J Clin Psychiatry 2008;69:790–9.

1046. Modabbernia A, Heidari P, Soleimani R, et al. Melatonin for prevention of metabolic side-effects of olanzapine in patients with first-episode schizophrenia: randomized double-blind placebo-controlled study. J Psychiatr Res. 2014 Jun;53:133-40. doi: 10.1016/j.jpsychires.2014.02.013. Epub 2014 Feb 24.

1047. Hahn MK, Wolever TM, Arenovich T, et al. Acute effects of single-dose olanzapine on metabolic, endocrine, and inflammatory markers in healthy controls. J Clin Psychopharmacol. 2013;33(6):740-6.

1048. Berwaerts J, Liu Y, Gopal S, et al. Efficacy and Safety of the 3-Month Formulation of Paliperidone Palmitate vs Placebo for Relapse Prevention of Schizophrenia: A Randomized Clinical Trial. JAMA Psychiatry. Published online March 29, 2015. doi:10.1001/jamapsychiatry.2015.0241.

1049. Subotnik KL, Casaus LR, Ventura J, et al. Long-acting injectable risperidone for relapse prevention and control of break-through symptoms after a recent first episode of schizophrenia: a randomized clinical trial. JAMA Psychiatry. 2015;72(8):822-829.

1050. U.S. Food and Drug Administration. http://www.fda.gov/Drugs/DrugSafety/ucm426391.htm. Accessed on 12/16/14.

1051. 20+ New Schizophrenia Medications In Development (2015). https://mentalhealthdaily.com/2015/09/09/20-new-schizophrenia-medications-in-development-2015/ Accessed on 8/2/19.

1052. Fellner C. New Schizophrenia Treatments Address Unmet Clinical Needs. P T. 2017;42(2):130-134. http://www.ncbi.nlm.nih.gov/pubmed/28163559%0Ahttp://www.pubmedcentral.nih.gov/articlerender.fcgi?artid=PMC5265239.

1053. Abruzzo A, Cerchiara T, Luppi B, Bigucci F. Transdermal Delivery of Antipsychotics: Rationale and Current Status. CNS Drugs. 2019;(0123456789). doi:10.1007/s40263-019-00659-7

1054. ADX-1149. https://www.addextherapeutics.com/en/news-and-events/press-releases/addex-selective-mglu2-pam-adx71149-included-review-highlighting-promising-investigative-drugs-epilepsy/ Accessed on 8/2/19.

1055. C Correll. Phase III study of ALKS 3831 for schizophrenia yields positive results https://www.healio.com/psychiatry/schizophrenia/news/online/%7b969abf36-4736-463e-bac6-0debbb237ab1%7d/phase-3-study-of-alks-3831-for-schizophrenia-yields-positive-results Accessed on 8/2/19.

1056. Umbricht D, Alberati D, Martin-Facklam M, et al. Effect of bitopertin, a glycine reuptake inhibitor, on negative symptoms of schizophrenia: A randomized, double-blind, proof-of-concept study. JAMA Psychiatry. 2014;71(6):637-646. doi:10.1001/jamapsychiatry.2014.163

1057. Kishi T, Matsuda Y, Nakamura H, and Iwata N. Blonanserin for schizophrenia: Systematic review and meta-analysis of double-blind, randomized, controlled trials. J Psychiatric Res 2013(Feb);47(2):149–154. DOI: http://dx.doi.org/10.1016/j.jpsychires.2012.10.011

1058. Brauser D. Warfarin for Long-term Psychosis Remission? Medscape website. http://www.medscape.com/viewarticle/825210. Accessed April 12, 2015.

1059. Concert Pharmaceuticals Reports Positive Results from Phase I Studies Evaluating CTP-692 in Healthy Volunteers. https://ir.concertpharma.com/news-releases/news-release-details/concert-pharmaceuticals-reports-positive-results-phase-1-studies. Accessed on June 26, 2019. {Happy 100th birthday Grandma Rappa}

1060. Wilborn RJ, Hall CP, Fuller MA. Recycling N-acetylcysteine: A review of evidence for adjunctive therapy in schizophrenia. Ment Heal Clin. 2019;9(3):116-123. doi:10.9740/mhc.2019.05.116

1061. Lin C-H, Lin C-H, Chang Y-C, et al. Sodium Benzoate, a D-amino Acid Oxidase Inhibitor, Added to Clozapine for the Treatment of Schizophrenia: A Randomized, Double-Blind, Placebo-Controlled Trial. Biol Psychiatry. 2017:1-11. doi:10.1016/j.biopsych.2017.12.006

1062. A Study of Paliperidone Palmitate 6-Month Formulation. https://www.centerwatch.com/clinical-trials/listings/160465/schizophrenia-study-paliperidone-palmitate-6-month  Accessed 11/22/19.

1063 Curtis, D. (n.d.). A possible role for sarcosine in the management of schizophrenia. The British Journal of Psychiatry, 1-2. doi:10.1192/bjp.2019.194.

1064. Earnst D. Novel Treatment for Schizophrenia Gets FDA's Breakthrough Therapy Designation. https://www.empr.com/home/news/drugs-in-the-pipeline/novel-treatment-for-schizophrenia-gets-fdas-breakthrough-therapy-designation. Accessed on June 27, 2019.

1065. Campbell P. SEP- 363856 for Treatment of Schizophrenia. May 26, 2019. https://www.mdmag.com/medical-news/sep363856-for-treatment-of-schizophrenia Accessed on 8/2/19.

1066. Wang AM, Pradhan S, Coughlin JM, et al. Assessing Brain Metabolism With 7-T Proton Magnetic Resonance Spectroscopy in Patients With First-Episode Psychosis. JAMA Psychiatry. 2019;76(3):314–323. doi:https://doi.org/10.1001/jamapsychiatry.2018.3637

1067. Weiser M, Levi L, Zamora D, et al. Effect of Adjunctive Estradiol on Schizophrenia Among Women of Childbearing Age: A Randomized Clinical Trial. JAMA Psychiatry. Published online July 31, 2019. doi:10.1001/jamapsychiatry.2019.1842

1068. Ballon JS. Management of Treatment-Refractory Schizophrenia. Psychiatric Times website. http://www.psychiatrictimes.com/special-reports/management-treatment-refractory-schizophrenia. Accessed on 04/12/2015.

1069. American Diabetes Association, American Psychiatric Association, American Association of Clinical Endocrinologists, and North American Association for the study of Obesity. Consensus Development Conference on Antipsychotic Drugs and Obesity and Diabetes. Diabetes Care 2004;27(2):596-601).

1070. Cohn T. Metabolic Monitoring for Patients on Antipsychotic Medications. Psychiatric Times 2013:30(12). http://www.psychiatrictimes.com/cme/metabolic-monitoring-patients-antipsychotic-medications Accessed 11/26/18.
Bostwick JR and Murphy LR. Metabolic Monitoring of Antipsychotic Medications: What Psychiatrists Need to Know. Psychiatric Times 2017:34(5). https://www.psychiatrictimes.com/psychopharmacology/metabolic-monitoring-antipsychotic-medications-what-psychiatrists-need-know Accessed 12/1/19.

1071. Ihara H, Arai H. Ethical dilemma associated with the off-label use of antipsychotic drugs for the treatment of behavioral and psychological symptoms of dementia. Psychogeriatrics. 8(1):32-37, March 2008.

1072. Holt R, Peveler R. Association between antipsychotic drugs and diabetes. Diabetes, Obesity & Metabolism. 8(2):125-135, March 2006.

1073. Neil W, Curran S, Wattis J, et al. Antipsychotic prescribing in older people. Age & Aging. 32(5):475-483, September 2003.

1074. Lieberman JA, Stroup TS, Mcevoy JP, et al. Effectiveness of antipsychotic drugs in patients with chronic schizophrenia. N Engl J Med. 2005;353(12):1209-23.

1075. Dahl SG. Plasma Level Monitoring of Antipsychotic Drugs Clinical Utility. Clin Pharmacokinet. 1986;11(1):36-61. doi:10.2165/00003088

1076. Schulz and Schmoldt. "Therapeutic and Toxic Blood Concentrations of More than 800 Drugs and Other Xenobiotics." Latest TOC RSS, Avoxa - Mediengruppe Deutscher Apotheker GmbH, 1 July 2003, www.ingentaconnect.com/content/govi/pharmaz/2003/00000058/00000007/art00001.

1077. McCutcheon R, Beck K, D'Ambrosio E, et al. Antipsychotic plasma levels in the assessment of poor treatment response in schizophrenia. Acta Psychiatr Scand. 2018;137(1):39-46. doi:10.1111/acps.12825

1078. Midha K, Korchinski E, Verbeeck R, et al. Kinetics of oral trifluoperazine disposition in man. Br J Clin Pharmacol. 1983;15(3):380-382. doi:10.1111/j.1365-2125.1983.tb01515.x -198611010-00003 30:388-404. doi:10.1016/j.eurpsy.2015.01.013

1079. Mazzola, C. D. et al. "Loxapine Intoxication: Case Report and Literature Review". Journal of Analytical Toxicology, vol 24, no. 7, 2000, pp. 638-641. Oxford University Press (OUP), doi:10.1093/jat/24.7.638. Accessed 25 Mar 2019.

1080. Ziprasidone, aripiprazole, & quetiapine, Serum or Plasma. https://www.labcorp.com/test-menu/38741/ziprasidone-serum-or-plasma Accessed on 7/22/19.

1081. Meyer J. Antipsychotic Plasma Levels and Adherence. Psychopharmacology Institute. https://goo.gl/N5ytnD Accessed on 1/4/19.

1082. Hiemke C, Bergemann N, Clement HN, Conca A, Deckert J, Domschke K, et al. Consensus guidelines for therapeutic drug monitoring in neuropsychopharmacology: update 2017. Pharmacopsychiatry. 2018;51:9-62. DOI:10.1055/s-0043-116492. PubMed PMID:28910830.

1083. Noel C. A review of a recently published guidelines' "strong recommendation" for therapeutic drug monitoring of olanzapine, haloperidol, perphenazine, and fluphenazine. Ment Health Clin [Internet]. 2019;9(4):287-93. DOI: 10.9740/mhc.2019.07.287.

1084. Washington NB, Brahm NC, and Kissack J. Which psychotropics carry the greatest risk of QTc prolongation? Current Psychiatry Oct. 2012;11(10):36-39.

1085. Rubin DM and Feudtner C. Risk for Incident Diabetes Mellitus Following Initiation of Second-Generation Antipsychotics Among Medicaid-Enrolled Youths. JAMA Pediatr. 2015;169(4):e150285. doi:10.1001/jamapediatrics.2015.0285.

1086. David SR, Taylor CC, Kinon BJ, et al. The effects of olanzapine, risperidone, and haloperidol on plasma prolactin levels in patients with schizophrenia. Clinical Therapeutics 2000;22(9):1085-1096.

1087. Rummel-Kluge C, Komossa K, Schwarz S, et al. Second-Generation Antipsychotic Drugs and Extrapyramidal Side Effects: A Systematic Review and Meta-analysis of Head-to-Head Comparisons. Schizophr Bull 2012 Jan;38(1):167–177. doi: 10.1093/schbul/sbq042.

1088. Newman-Tancredi A, Kleven MS. Comparative pharmacology of antipsychotics possessing combined dopamine D2 and serotonin 5HT1A receptor properties. Psychopharmacology (Berl). 2011 Aug;216(4):451-73. doi: 10.1007/s00213-011-2247-y. Epub 2011 Mar 11.

1089. Citrome L. Activating and sedating adverse effects of second-generation antipsychotics in the treatment of schizophrenia and major depressive disorder: Absolute risk increase and number needed to harm. J Clin Psychopharmacol. 2017;37(2):138-147. doi:10.1097/JCP.0000000000000665

1090. Pillinger T, McCutcheon RA, Vano L, et al. Comparative effects of 18 antipsychotics on metabolic function in schizophrenia, predictors of metabolic dysregulation, and association with psychopathology: a systematic review and network meta-analysis. Lancet Psychiatry. 2020;7(1):64-77. doi:10.1016/S2215-0366(19)30416-X

1091. Gray R, Spilling R, Burgess D, et al. Antipsychotic long-acting injections in clinical practice: medication management and patient choice. Br J Psychiatry Suppl. 2009;52:S51-56.

1092. Cocoman A, Murray J. Intramuscular injections; a review of best practices for mental health nurses. J Psychiatr Ment Health Nurs 2008;15(5):424-434.
1093. Wynaden D, Landsborough I, McGowans S, et al. Best practice guidelines for the administration of intramuscular injections in the mental health setting. Int J Ment Health Nurs. 2006;15(3):195-200.
1094. Eerdekens M, Van Hove I, Remmerie B, et al. Pharmacokinetics and Tolerability of Long-Acting Risperidone in Schizophrenia. Schizophr Res 2004;70:91-100.
1095. Goldenberg MM. Overview of Drugs Used For Epilepsy and Seizures: Etiology, Diagnosis, and Treatment. P&T July 2010;35(7):392-415.
1096. Ochoa JG. Antiepileptic Drugs. http://emedicine.medscape.com/article/1187334. Accessed on 8/26/15.
1097. Gidal BE. Psychiatric Aspects of Epilepsy: Implications for Pharmacotherapy. Live presentation on 4/3/11 at the 2011 Annual CPNP (College of Psychiatric and Neurologic Pharmacists Meeting in Phoenix, AZ.
1098. Eudy AE and Bainbridge JL. Clinical pearls for chronic use of antiepileptic drugs. Mental Health Clinician 2012 (Nov);2(5):124-126.
1099. Thigpen J, Miller SE, and Pond BB. Behavioral Side Effects of Antiepileptic Drugs. US Pharmacist. 2013;38(11):HS15-HS20.
1100. St. Louis EK. Monitoring Antiepileptic Drugs: A Level-Headed Approach. Curr Neuropharmacol 2009 Jun;7(2):115-119. doi: 10.2174/157015909788848938. PMCID: PMC2730002.
1101. American Academy of Neurology. Practice Guideline Update: Efficacy and Tolerability of the New Antiepileptic Drugs II: Treatment-resistant Epilepsy. 2018:1. www.aappublications.org/news/2016/04/06/FDAUpdate040616.
1102 Kanner AM, Ashman E, Gloss D, et al. Practice guideline update summary: Efficacy and tolerability of the new antiepileptic drugs I: Treatment of new-onset epilepsy: Report of the Guideline Development, Dissemination, and Implementation Subcommittee of the American Acade. Neurology. 2018;91(2):74-81. doi:10.1212/WNL.0000000000005755. Epilepsy Curr. 2018;18(4):260-268. doi:10.5698/1535-7597.18.4.260
1103. Knezevic CE, Marzinke MA. Clinical Use and Monitoring of Antiepileptic Drugs. J Appl Lab Med. 2018;3(1):115-127. doi:10.1373/jalm.2017.023689
1104. Patsalos PN, Berry DJ, Bourgeois BFD, et al. Antiepileptic drugs - Best practice guidelines for therapeutic drug monitoring: A position paper by the subcommission on therapeutic drug monitoring, ILAE Commission on Therapeutic Strategies. Epilepsia. 2008;49(7):1239-1276. doi:10.1111/j.1528-1167.2008.01561.x
1105. Krumholz A, Wiebe S, Gronseth G, et al. Practice parameter: Evaluating an apparent unprovoked first seizure in adults (an evidence-based review): Report of the Quality Standards Subcommittee of the American Academy of Neurology and the American Epilepsy Society. Neurology. 2007;69(21):1996-2007. doi:10.1212/01.wnl.0000285084.93652.43
1106. Glauser T, Ben-Menachem E, Bourgeois B, et al. Updated ILAE evidence review of antiepileptic drug efficacy and effectiveness as initial monotherapy for epileptic seizures and syndromes. Epilepsia. 2013;54(3):551-563. doi:10.1111/epi.12074
1107. Practice Guideline : Sudden Unexpected Death in Epilepsy Incidence Rates and Risk Factors Generalized tonic-clonic seizures. Neurology 2017(4).
1108. Hamed SA. Psychiatric symptomatologies and disorders related to epilepsy and antiepileptic medications. Expert Opin Drug Saf. 2011;10(6):913-934. doi:10.1517/14740338.2011.588597
1109. Glauser T, Shinnar S, Gloss D, et al. Evidence-based guideline: Treatment of convulsive status epilepticus in children and adults: Report of the guideline committee of the American epilepsy society. Epilepsy Curr. 2016;16(1):48-61. doi:10.5698/1535-7597-16.1.48
1110. Cassard L, Hegde M, Gidal BE, et al. Levetiracetam versus sodium channel blockers as first prescribed antiepileptic drug: Data from the Human Epilepsy Project. Abstract #1.318 presented at the 2019 Annual American Epilepsy Society (AES). https://www.aesnet.org/meetings_events/annual_meeting_abstracts/view/2421313 Accessed 12/20/19.
1111. POTIGA (ezogabine) [package insert]. GlaxoSmithKline, Research Triangle Park, NC, May 2015.
1112. GlaxoSmithKline: Trobalt®/Potiga® Discontinuation - Important Reminder. Accessible at: www.ilae.org/files/dmfile/GSK_RetigabineTrobalt-Reminder.pdf Accessed on 9/24/19.
1113. NICE, National Institute for Health and Care Excellence. Epilepsies: Diagnosis and Management Clinical Guideline [CG137].; 2019. www.nice.org.uk/guidance/cg137.
1114. FDA Safety Information. Dilantin-125 (phenytoin) Oral Suspension. FDA website. http://www.fda.gov/Safety/MedWatch/safetyinformation/ucm286345.htm Accessed April 10, 2015.
1115. Knezevic CE, Marzinke MA. Clinical Use and Monitoring of Antiepileptic Drugs. J Appl Lab Med. 2018;3(1):115-127. doi:10.1373/jalm.2017.023689
1116. St. Louis E. Monitoring Antiepileptic Drugs: A Level-Headed Approach. Curr Neuropharmacol. 2009;7(2):115-119. doi:10.2174/157015909788848938
1117. Marvanova M. Pharmacokinetic characteristics of antiepileptic drugs (AEDs). Ment Heal Clin. 2016;6(1):8-20. doi:10.9740/mhc.2015.01.008
1118. Lee DJ and Lozano AM. Deep Brain Stimulation for Memory Deficits. October 24, 2017. Psychiatric Times. http://www.psychiatrictimes.com/special-reports/deep-brain-stimulation-memory-deficits Accessed on 12/8/2017.
1119. "Zogenix drug cuts seizure rate in patients with severe epilepsy". statnews.com. 29 September 2017. Archived from the original on 30 April 2018. Retrieved 9 May 2018.
1120. Antipsychotics drugs class labeling change treatment during pregnancy and potential risk to newborns. Food and Drug Administration, Feb. 2011. http://www.fda.gov/safety/medwatch/safetyinformation/safetyalertsforhumanmedicalproducts/ucm244175.htm.
1121. Arnon J, Shechtman S, Ornoy A. The use of psychotropic drugs in pregnancy and lactation. Isr J Psychiatry Relat Sci. 2000;37(3):205-22.
1122. Pedersen CA. Postpartum mood and anxiety disorders: a guide for the nonpsychiatric clinician with an aside on thyroid associations with postpartum mood. Thyroid. 1999 Jul;9(7):691-7.
1123. Trixler M, Tényi T. Antipsychotic use in pregnancy. What are the best treatment options? Drug Saf. 1997 Jun;16(6):403-10.
1124. Kuller JA, Katz VL, McMahon MJ, Wells SR, Bashford RA. Pharmacologic treatment of psychiatric disease in pregnancy and lactation: fetal and neonatal effects. Obstet Gynecol. 1996 May;87(5 Pt 1):789-94.
1125. Menon SJ. Psychotropic medication during pregnancy and lactation. Arch Gynecol Obstet 2008 Jan;277(1):1-13.
1126. Gentile S. The safety of newer antidepressants in pregnancy and breastfeeding. Drug Saf. 2005;28(2):137-52.
1127. Levey L, Ragan K, Hower-Hartley A, et al. Psychiatric disorders in pregnancy. Neurol Clin 2004 Nov;22(4):863-93.
1128. Iqbal MM, Aneja A, Fremont WP. Effects of chlordiazepoxide (Librium) during pregnancy and lactation. Conn Med. 2001;39(4):381-92.
1129. Iqbal MM, Sobhan T, Aftab SR, et al. Diazepam use during pregnancy: a review of the literature. Del Med J 2002 Mar;74(3):127-35.
1130. Spigset O and Hagg S. Excretion of Psychotropic Drugs into Breast Milk. Pharmacokinetic Overview and Therapeutic Implications. CNS Drugs 1998 (Feb);9(2):111-134.
1131. Freeland KN and Shealy KM. Toolbox: Psychotropic use in pregnancy and lactation-Psychotropics and treatment of the child-bearing woman. Mental Health Clinician August 2013;3(2):45-57. doi: http://dx.doi.org/10.9740/mhc.n164620
1132. Centers for Disease Control and Prevention. Unintended Pregnancy Prevention. http://www.cdc.gov/reproductivehealth/unintendedpregnancy/index.htm Accessed on 10/15/19.
1133. Centers for Disease Control and Prevention. Data and Statistics on Use of Medication in Pregnancy. http://www.cdc.gov/pregnancy/meds/treatingfortwo/data.html Accessed on 6/27/15.
1134. Singh A, Hughes GJ, and Mazzola N. New Changes in Pregnancy and Lactation Labeling. US Pharm. 2014;39(10):40-43.
1135. Fokina, Valentina M. et al. Bupropion therapy during pregnancy: the drug and its major metabolites in umbilical cord plasma and amniotic fluid. American Journal of Obstetrics & Gynecology, Volume 215, Issue 4, 497.e1 - 497.e7
1136. Huybrechts KF, Bateman BT, Palmsten K, et al. Antidepressant Use Late in Pregnancy and Risk of Persistent Pulmonary Hypertension of the Newborn. JAMA. 2015;313(21):2142-2151. doi:10.1001/jama.2015.5605
1137. Chambers CD, Hernandez-Diaz S, Van Marter LS, et al. Selective serotonin-reuptake inhibitors and risk of persistent pulmonary hypertension of the newborn. N Engl J Med 2006;354:579-587.
1138. Grigoriadis S, Vonderporten EH, Mamisashvili L, et al. Prenatal exposure to antidepressants and persistent pulmonary hypertension of the newborn: systematic review and meta-analysis. BMJ. 2014;348:f6932.
1139. Nörby U, Forsberg L, Wide K, Sjörs G, Winbladh B, Källén K. Neonatal morbidity after maternal use of antidepressant drugs during pregnancy. Pediatrics. 2016;138(5). doi:10.1542/peds.2016-0181
1140. Huybrechts KF, Palmsten K, Avorn J, et al. Antidepressant use in pregnancy and the risk of cardiac defects. NEJM 2014;370(25):2397-407.
1141. El Marroun H. Maternal SSRI Use During Pregnancy: New Findings on Fetal Development. Psychiatry Weekly 2012, May 21, Volume 7, Issue 10 Accessed at http://www.psychweekly.com/aspx/article/articledetail.aspx?articleid=1450 on 6/4/2012.
1142. El Marroun, H, Jaddoe VWV, Hudziak JJ, et al. Maternal Use of Selective Serotonin Reuptake Inhibitors, Fetal Growth, and Risk of Adverse Birth Outcomes. Arch Gen Psychiatry. July 2012;69(7):706-714 doi:10.1001/archgenpsychiatry.2011.2333
1143. Yonkers KA, Gilstad-Hayden K, Forray A, Lipkind HS. Association of Panic Disorder, Generalized Anxiety Disorder, and Benzodiazepine Treatment During Pregnancy With Risk of Adverse Birth Outcomes. JAMA psychiatry. 2017;74(11):1145-1152. doi:10.1001/jamapsychiatry.2017.2733
1144. Levinson-Castiel R, Merlob P, Linder N, et al. Neonatal abstinence syndrome after in utero exposure to selective serotonin reuptake inhibitors in term infants. Arch Pediatr Adolesc Med 2006;160:173-176.
1145. Knickmeyer RC, Meltzer-brody S, Woolson S, et al. Rate of Chiari I malformation in children of mothers with depression with and without prenatal SSRI exposure. Neuropsychopharmacology. 2014;39(11):2611-21.

1146. Andersen JT, Andersen NL, Horwitz H, Poulsen HE, Jimenez-Solem E. Exposure to selective serotonin reuptake inhibitors in early pregnancy and the risk of miscarriage. Obstet Gynecol. 2014;124(4):655-61.
1147. Reefhuis J, Devine O, Friedman JM, et al. Specific SSRIs and birth defects: bayesian analysis to interpret new data in the context of previous reports. BMJ 2015;350:h3190. doi: 10.1136/bmj.h3190
1148. Hviid A, Melbye M, Pasternak B. Use of selective serotonin reuptake inhibitors during pregnancy and risk of autism. N Engl J Med. 2013;369(25):2406-15.
1149. Rai D, Lee BK, Dalman C, Golding J, Lewis G, Magnusson C. Parental depression, maternal antidepressant use during pregnancy, and risk of autism spectrum disorders: population based case-control study. BMJ. 2013;346:f2059.
1150. Harrington RA, Lee LC, Crum RM, et al. Prenatal SSRI use and offspring with autism spectrum disorder or developmental delay. Pediatrics. 2014;133(5):e1241-8.
1151. Andrade C. Antidepressant exposure during pregnancy and risk of autism in the offspring, 1: Meta-review of meta-analyses. J Clin Psychiatry. 2017;78(8):e1047-e1051. doi:10.4088/JCP.17f11903
1152. Brown AS, Gyllenberg D, Malm H, et al. Association of selective serotonin reuptake inhibitor exposure during pregnancy with speech, scholastic, and motor disorders in offspring. JAMA Psychiatry. 2016;73(11):1163-1170. doi:10.1001/jamapsychiatry.2016.2594
1153. Malm, H., Artama, M., Gissler, M., & Ritvanen, A. Selective serotonin reuptake inhibitors and risk for major congenital anomalies . Obstetrics & Gynecology 2011;118(1):111-120.
1154. Eberhard-Gran M, Eskild A, and Opjordsmoen S. Use of Psychotropic Medications in Treating Mood Disorders during Lactation. CNS Drugs 2006(Mar);20(3):187-198.
1155. Gorman JR, Kao K, Chambers CD. Breastfeeding among women exposed to antidepressants during pregnancy. J Hum Lact. 2012;28(2):181-8.
1156. Sheehy O, Zhao J, Bérard A. Association Between Incident Exposure to Benzodiazepines in Early Pregnancy and Risk of Spontaneous Abortion. JAMA Psychiatry. Published online May 15, 201976(9):948–957. doi:10.1001/jamapsychiatry.2019.0963
1157. Roakis T and Williams KE. During Pregnancy: Make decisions based on available evidence, individualized risk/benefit analysis. Current Psychiatry 2013;12(7):12-20 (+ Suppl A&B).
1158. Wisner KL, Jeong H, Chambers C. Use of antipsychotics during pregnancy: Pregnant women get sick-sick women get pregnant. JAMA Psychiatry. 2016;73(9):901-903. doi:10.1001/jamapsychiatry.2016.1538
1159. Vigod SN, Gomes T, and Wilton AS. Antipsychotic drug use in pregnancy: high dimensional, propensity matched, population based cohort study. BMJ 2015;350:h2298 doi: 10.1136/bmj.h2298. http://dx.doi.org/10.1136/bmj.h2298.
1160. Kulkarni J, Worsley R, Gilbert H, et al. A prospective cohort study of antipsychotic medications in pregnancy: the first 147 pregnancies and 100 one year old babies. PLoS One. 2014 May 2;9:e94788. doi: 10.1371/journal.pone.0094788. eCollection 2014.
1161. Cohen LS, Viguera AC, McInemey KA, et al. Establishment of the National Pregnancy Registry for Atypical Antipsychotics. Published on-line ahead of print. J Clin Psychiatry 2015. 10.4088/JCP.14br09418.
1162. Windhager E, Kim S-W, Saria A, et al. Perinatal Use of Aripiprazole: Plasma Levels, Placental Transfer, and Child Outcome in 3 New Cases. Journal of Clinical Psychopharmacology 2014 (Oct);34(5):637–641. doi: 10.1097/JCP.0000000000000171.
1163. Deligiannidis KM, Byatt N, Freeman MP. Pharmacotherapy for mood disorders in pregnancy: a review of pharmacokinetic changes and clinical recommendations for therapeutic drug monitoring. J Clin Psychopharmacol. 2014;34(2):244-55.
1164. Patorno E, Huybrechts KF, Bateman BT, et al. Lithium use in pregnancy and the risk of cardiac malformations. N Engl J Med. 2017;376(23):2245-2254. doi:10.1056/NEJMoa1612222
1165. Munk-Olsen T, Liu X, Viktorin A, et al. Maternal and infant outcomes associated with lithium use in pregnancy: an international collaborative meta-analysis of six cohort studies. The Lancet Psychiatry. 2018;5(8):644-652. doi:10.1016/S2215-0366(18)30180-9
1166. Moretti, M.E., Koren, G., Verjee, Z. & Ito, S. Monitoring lithium in breast milk: An individualized approach for breast-feeding mothers. Therapeutic Drug Monitoring 2003;25(3):364–366.
1167. Rebecca L. Newmark, Debra L. Bogen, Katherine L. Wisner, Mariana Isaac, Jody D. Ciolino & Crystal T. Clark (2019) Risk-Benefit assessment of infant exposure to lithium through breast milk: a systematic review of the literature, International Review of Psychiatry, 31:3, 295-304, DOI: 10.1080/09540261.2019.1586657
1168. Christensen J, Grønborg TK, Sørensen MJ, et al. Prenatal valproate exposure and risk of autism spectrum disorders and childhood autism. JAMA. 2013;309(16):1696-703.
1169. Shallcross R, Bromley RL, Cheyne CP, et al. In utero exposure to levetiracetam vs valproate: development and language at 3 years of age. Neurology. 2014;82(3):213-21.
1170. Bloti P. Risks of 23 speci fi c malformations associated with prenatal exposure to 10 antiepileptic drugs. 2019;(November 2017). doi:10.1212/WNL.0000000000007696
1171. Schwenkhagen AM, Stodieck SR. Which contraception for women with epilepsy? Seizure. 2008 Mar;17(2):145-50. Epub 2008 Jan 4.
1172. Maust DT, Gerlach LB, Gibson A, Kales HC, Blow FC, Olfson M. Trends in Central Nervous System–Active Polypharmacy Among Older Adults Seen in Outpatient Care in the United States. JAMA Intern Med. 2017;177(4):583–585. doi:10.1001/jamainternmed.2016.9225
1173. Haddad YK, Luo F, Karani M V., Marcum ZA, Lee R. Psychoactive medication use among community-dwelling Americans. J Am Pharm Assoc. 2019;59(5):686-690. doi:10.1016/j.japh.2019.05.001
1174. Gurwitz JH. Bonner A and Berwick DM. Reducing Excessive Use of Antipsychotic Agents in Nursing Homes. JAMA July 11, 2017;318(2):118-119.
1175. Weintraub D, Chiang C, Kim HM, et al. Association of antipsychotic use with mortality risk in patients with Parkinson disease. JAMA Neurol. 2016;73(5):535-541. doi:10.1001/jamaneurol.2016.0031
1176. Beers MH et al. Explicit criteria for determining inappropriate medication in nursing home residents. Arch Int Med 1991;151:1825-32.
1177. Fick DM, Semla TP, Steinman M, et al. American Geriatrics Society 2019 Updated AGS Beers Criteria® for Potentially Inappropriate Medication Use in Older Adults. J Am Geriatr Soc. 2019;67(4):674-694. doi:10.1111/jgs.15767
1178. Parameswaran N, Chalmers L, Peterson GM, et al. Hospitalization in older patients due to adverse drug reactions–the need for a prediction tool. Clin Interv Aging. 2016;11:497-505. doi:10.2147/CIA. S99097
1179. Sobieraj DM, Baker WL, Martinez BK, et al. Adverse Effects of Pharmacologic Treatments of Major Depression in Older Adults. Advers Eff Pharmacol Treat Major Depress Older Adults. 2019;1-11. doi:10.1111/jgs.15966
1180. Lenze EJ. Psychotropic Drugs and Falls in Older Adults: What Do We Do Now? Psychiatric Times 2018(3):19-20.
1181. Gallagher P and O'Mahony D. STOPP (Screening Tool of Older Persons' potentially inappropriate Prescriptions): application to acutely ill elderly patients and comparison with Beers' criteria. Age Ageing (2008) 37 (6): 673-679. doi: 10.1093/ageing/afn197.
1182. D O'Mahony and O'Sullivan D. STOPP/START criteria for potentially inappropriate prescribing in older people: version 2. Age Ageing (2015) 44 (2): 213-218. doi: 10.1093/ageing/afu145.
1183. Gurwitz Field JH, Judge TS, J, et al. The incidence of adverse drug events in two large academic long-term care facilities. Am J Med March 2005;118(3);251–258. DOI: http://dx.doi.org/10.1016/j.amjmed.2004.09.018.
1184. Billioti de Gage S, Begaud B, Bazin F, et al. Benzodiazepine use and risk of dementia: prospective population based study. BMJ 2012;345:e6231 doi:1136/bmj.e6231 (Published 27 September 2012)
1185. Donnelly K, Bracchi R, Hewitt J, Routledge PA, Carter B. Benzodiazepines, Z-drugs and the risk of hip fracture: A systematic review and meta-analysis. PLoS One. 2017;12(4). doi:10.1371/journal.pone.0174730
1186. Pavon JM, Zhao Y, McConnell E, et al. Identifying risk of readmission in hospitalized elderly adults through inpatient medication exposure. J Am Geriatr Soc. 2014 Jun;62(6):1116-21. doi: 10.1111/jgs.12829. Epub 2014 May 6.
1187. Yokoi Y, Misal M, Oh E, et al. Benzodiazepine discontinuation and patient outcome in a chronic geriatric medical/psychiatric unit: a retrospective chart review. Geriatr Gerontol Int. 2014 Apr;14(2):388-94. doi: 10.1111/ggi.12113. Epub 2013 Nov 8.
1188. Gray SL, Anderson ML, Dublin S, et al. Cumulative Use of Strong Anticholinergics and Incident Dementia: A Prospective Cohort Study. JAMA Intern Med 2015;175(3):401-407. doi:10.1001/jamainternmed.2014.7663.
1189. Coupland CAC, Hill T, Dening T, Morriss R, Moore M, Hippisley-Cox J. Anticholinergic Drug Exposure and the Risk of Dementia: A Nested Case-Control Study. JAMA Intern Med. 2019;179(8):1084-1093. doi:10.1001/jamainternmed.2019.0677
1190. Boudreau DM, Yu O, Gray SL, et al. Concomitant use of cholinesterase inhibitors and anticholinergics: prevalence and outcomes. J Am Geriatr Soc. 2011 Nov;59(11):2069-76. doi: 10.1111/j.1532-5415.2011.03654.x. Epub 2011 Oct 22.
1191. Campbell N, Boustani M, Lane K, et al. Use of anticholinergics and the risk of cognitive impairment in an African-American population. Neurology. 2010;75:152-159.
1192. Fox C, Richardson K, Maidment I, et al. Anticholinergic medication use and cognitive impairment in the older population: the Medical Research Council Cognitive Function and Ageing Study. Journal of the American Geriatric Society. 2011; 59(8): 1477-1483.
1193. Ruxton K, Woodman RJ, Mangoni AA. Drugs with anticholinergic effects and cognitive impairment, falls and all-cause mortality in older adults: A systematic review and meta-analysis. Br J Clin Pharmacol. 2015 Aug;80(2):209-20. doi: 10.1111/bcp.12617. Epub 2015 May 20.
1194. Salahudeenet MS, Duffull SB, Nishtala PS. Anticholinergic burden quantified by anticholinergic risk scales and adverse outcomes in older people: a systematic review. BMC Geriatrics 2015;15(31):1-14. DOI 10.1186/s12877-015-0029-9.
1195. West T, Pruchnicki MC, Porter K, et al. Evaluation of anticholinergic burden of medications in older adults. J Am Pharm Assoc 2013;53:496–504. doi: 10.1331/JAPhA.2013.12138.

178

1196. Sakel M, Boukouvalas A, Buono R, et al. Does anticholinergics drug burden relate to global neuro-disability outcome measures and length of hospital stay? Brain Injury, Ahead of Print : Pages 1-5. Posted online on August 5, 2015. doi: 10.3109/02699052.2015.1060358. Read More: http://informahealthcare.com/doi/abs/10.3109/02699052.2015.1060358
1197. Hoeft D. An Overview of Clinically Significant Drug Interactions between Medications Used to Treat Psychiatric and Medical Conditions. Ment Health Clin. 2014;4(3):71. http://cpnp.org/resource/mhc/2014/05/overview-clinically-significant-drug-interactions-between-medications-used Accessed May 12, 2014.
1198. Orzechowski RF, Currie DS, and Valancius CA. Comparative anticholinergic activities of 10 histamine H1 receptor antagonists in two functional models. European Journal of Pharmacology 2005 (Jan);506(3):257–264.
1199. Tune L, Carr S, Hoag E, et al. Anticholinergic effects of drugs commonly prescribed for the elderly. Am J Psych 1992; 149:1393-1394.
1200. Trevisan LA. Update on Geriatric Depression and Anxiety. Published on Psychiatric Times. http://www.psychiatrictimes.com/apa-2015-MDD/update-geriatric-depression-and-anxiety?GUID=631E98CE-0053-4441-9560-14CD338CC37E&rememberme=1&ts=16062015 Accessed on 6/16/15.
1201. Abdelmalik PA, Draghic N, Ling GSF. Management of moderate and severe traumatic brain injury. Transfusion. 2019;59(S2):1529-1538. doi:10.1111/trf.151712.
1202. Woodard TJ, Hill AM, and Bell-Lynum KS. Managing Neuropsychiatric Symptoms in Traumatic Brain Injury. U.S. Pharmacist 2015;40(11):HS-3-HS-9.
1203. Silver JM. Traumatic Brain Injury - Neuropsychiatry of TBI: an update. Psychiatric Times 2019;4:15-25. • Rao V and Vaishnavi S. Pharmacological Management of the Psychiatric Aspects of Traumatic Brain Injury. Psychiatric Times 2019;4:16-19. • Brenner LA, Grassmeyer RP, and Kelly JP. Preventing Suicide When Caring for Patients With a History of TBI. Psychiatric Times 2019;4:20-22. • Narapareddy BR, Richy LN, and Peters ME. TBI in Older Adults: A Growing Epidemic. Psychiatric Times 2019;4:23-24. • Jones M and Jorge RE. Depression Following TBI Can It Be Prevented? Psychiatric Times 2019;4:24-25.
1204. Carney N, Totten AM, O'Reilly C, et al. Guidelines for the Management of Severe Traumatic Brain Injury, Fourth Edition. Neurosurgery. 2016;80(1):6-15. doi:10.1227/NEU.0000000000001432
1205. The CRASH-3 trial collaborators. Effects of tranexamic acid on death , disability , vascular occlusive events and other morbidities in patients with acute traumatic brain injury ( CRASH-3 ): a randomised , Lancet. 2019;6736(19). doi:10.1016/S0140-6736(19)32233-0
1206. Bhatti Junaid, Nascimento Barto, Akhtar Umbreen, Rhind Shawn G., Tien Homer, Nathens Avery, et al. Systematic Review of Human and Animal Studies Examining the Efficacy and Safety of N-Acetylcysteine (NAC) and N-Acetylcysteine Amide (NACA) in Traumatic Brain Injury: Impact on Neurofunctional Outcome and Biomarkers of Oxidative Stress and Inflammation. Frontiers in Neurology. 2018. 8:744.
1207. Hammond FM, et al. Effectiveness of amantadine hydrochloride in the reduction of chronic traumatic brain injury irritability and aggression. J Head Trauma Rehabil 2013 Nov 20; [e-pub ahead of print]. http://dx.doi.10.HTR.0000438116.56228.de
1208. Hammond FM et al. Effectiveness of amantadine hydrochloride in the reduction of chronic traumatic brain injury irritability and aggression. J Head Trauma Rehabil 2013 Nov 20; [e-pub ahead of print]. (http://dx.doi.org/10.1097/01.HTR.0000438116.56228.de)
1209. VA/DoD Clinical Practice Guideline for Management of Concussion/Mild Traumatic Brain Injury (mTBI). Version 1.0 – 2009. http://www.healthquality.va.gov/guidelines/Rehab/mtbi/concussion_mtbi_full_1_0.pdf Accessed on 2/27/15.
1210. Lequerica A, Jasey N, Portelli Tremont JN, et al. Pilot Study on the Effect of Ramelteon on Sleep Disturbance After Traumatic Brain Injury: Preliminary Evidence From a Clinical Trial. Archives of Physical Medicine and Rehabilitation 2015. Published Online: May 27, 2015 DOI: http://dx.doi.org/10.1016/j.apmr.2015.05.011.
1211. Neurobehavioral Guidelines Working Group, Warden DL, Gordon B, et al. Guidelines for the pharmacologic treatment of neurobehavioral sequelae of traumatic brain injury. J Neurotrauma 2006 Oct;23(10):1468-501.
1212. Traumatic Brain Injury - TBI – Neurovive. http://www.neurovive.com/research-overview/traumatic-brain-injury-tbi/ Accessed on 8/3/19
1213. Howard R, McShane R, Lindesay J, et al. Donepezil & memantine for moderate-to-severe Alzheimer's disease. NEJM 2012;366:893-903.
1214. Knight R, Khondoker M, Magill N, et al. A systematic review and meta-analysis of the effectiveness of acetylcholinesterase inhibitors and memantine in treating the cognitive symptoms of dementia. Dement Geriatr Cogn Disord. 2018;45(3-4):131-151. doi:10.1159/000486546
1215. Maust DT, Kim HM, Seyfried LS, et al. Antipsychotics, Other Psychotropics, and the Risk of Death in Patients with Dementia Number Needed to Harm. JAMA Psychiatry 2015;72(5):438-445. doi:10.1001/jamapsychiatry.2014.3018.
1216. Lopez OL, Becker JT, Chang YF, et al. The long-term effects of conventional and atypical antipsychotics in patients with probable Alzheimer's disease. Am J Psychiatry 2013;170(9):1051-1058.
1217. Ruthirakuhan, M. T., Herrmann, N., Abraham, E. H., Chan, S., & Lanctôt, K. L. Pharmacological interventions for apathy in Alzheimer's disease. Cochrane Database Syst Rev. 2018 May 4;5:CD012197. doi: 10.1002/14651858.CD012197.pub2.
1218. Knight R, Khondoker M, Magill N, Stewart R, Landau S. A systematic review and meta-analysis of the effectiveness of acetylcholinesterase inhibitors and memantine in treating the cognitive symptoms of dementia. Dement Geriatr Cogn Disord. 2018;45(3-4):131-151. doi:10.1159/000486546
1219. Sharma K. Cholinesterase inhibitors as Alzheimer's therapeutics (Review). Mol Med Rep. 2019;20(2):1479-1487. doi:10.3892/mmr.2019.10374
1220. Press D and Alexander M. Treatment of dementia. UpToDate. Waltham, MA: UpToDate Inc. https://www.uptodate.com/contents/treatment-of-dementia. Updated 6/19/19. Accessed 10/22/19.
1221. Kessing LV, Gerds TA, Knudsen N, et al. Association of lithium in drinking water with the incidence of dementia. JAMA Psychiatry. 2017;74(10):1005-1010. doi:10.1001/jamapsychiatry.2017.2362
1222. Sheline YI, West T, Yarasheski K, et al. An antidepressant decreases CSF Ab production in healthy individuals and in transgenic AD mice. Science Translational Medicine, online May 14, 2014.
1223. Gauthier S, Feldman HH, Schneider LS, et al. Efficacy and safety of tau-aggregation inhibitor therapy in patients with mild or moderate Alzheimer's disease: a randomised, controlled, double-blind, parallel-arm, phase 3 trial. Lancet. 2016;388(10062):2873-2884. doi:10.1016/S0140-6736(16)31275-2
1224. Wilcock GK, Gauthier S, Frisoni GB, et al. Potential of Low Dose Leuco-Methylthioninium Bis(Hydromethanesulphonate) (LMTM) Monotherapy for Treatment of Mild Alzheimer's Disease: Cohort Analysis as Modified Primary Outcome in a Phase III Clinical Trial. J Alzheimer's Dis. 2018;61(1):435-457. doi:10.3233/JAD-170560
1225. Craft S, et al "Open Label Extension Results from a Phase II/III Trial of Intranasal Insulin" AAIC 2019; Abstract 35542. Alzheimer's Association 2019 International Conference. https://eventpilotadmin.com/web/page.php?page=IntHtml&project=AAIC19&id=35542 Accessed 9/24/19.
1226. Zaugg J and Peng J. (CNN) China approves seaweed-based Alzheimer's drug. It's the first new one in 17 years. https://amp-cnn-com.cdn.ampproject.org/c/s/amp.cnn.com/cnn/2019/11/03/health/china-alzheimers-drug-intl-hnk-scli/index.html Accessed on 11/7/19
1227. European Parkinson's Disease Association. https://www.epda.eu.com/ Accessed on 10/10/19
1228. Parkinson's Foundation. https://www.parkinson.org/ Accessed on 10/10/19
1229. Clinical manifestations of Parkinson's Disease. UpToDate. Waltham, MA: UpToDate Inc. https://www.uptodate.com/contents/clinical-manifestations-of-parkinson-disease Accessed 10/9/19.
1230. James Parkinson. Project Gutenberg's An Essay on the Shaking Palsy. http://www.gutenberg.org/files/23777/23777-h/23777-h.htm Accessed on 10/10/19.
1231. Tysnes, OB. & Storstein, A. Epidemiology of Parkinson's disease. J Neural Transm 2017;124:901. https://doi.org/10.1007/s00702-017-1686-y
1232. Ascherio A and Schwarzschild MA. The epidemiology of Parkinson's disease: risk factors and prevention. Lancet Neurol 2016;15(12):1257-1272. https://doi.org/10.1016/S1474-4422(16)30230-7
1233. Lee A and Gilbert RM. Epidemiology of Parkinson Disease. Neurol Clin 2016;34(4):955–965 https://doi.org/10.1016/j.ncl.2016.06.012
1234. Postuma RB, Berg D, Stern M, Poewe W, Marek K, Litvan I. CME MDS Clinical Diagnostic Criteria for Parkinson's Disease Centrality of Motor Syndrome — Parkinsonism and PD Criteria Benchmark — The Expert Examination. Mov Disord. 2015;30(12):1591-1599. doi:10.1002/mds.26424
1235. Gomperts SN. "Lewy Body Dementias: Dementia With Lewy Bodies and Parkinson Disease Dementia". CONTINUUM: Lifelong Learning in Neurology 2016(April);22(2, Dementia):435–463. doi:10.1212/CON.0000000000000309. PMID 27042903
1236. Lawson RA, Yarnall AJ, Johnston F, et al. Cognitive impairment in Parkinson's disease: impact on quality of life of caregivers. Int J Geriatr Psychiatry. 2017;32(12):1362–1370. doi:10.1002/gps.4623
1237. Parkinsonism Treatments. https://www.empr.com/home/clinical-charts/parkinsonism-treatments/ Accessed 8/20/19
1238. Northera® (droxidopa) Lundbeck, Deerfield, IL [package insert]. 7/2019.
1239. Warren Olanow, C, Torti, M, Kieburtz, K et al. Continuous versus intermittent oral administration of levodopa in Parkinson's disease patients with motor fluctuations: A pharmacokinetics, safety, and efficacy study. Mov Disord, 2019;34:425-429. doi:10.1002/mds.27610
1240. "Synthesis of deuterium-labelled analogues of NLRP3 inflammasome inhibitor MCC950", Manohar Sallaai; Mark S.Butler; Nicholas L.Massey; Janet C. Reid; Matthew A. Cooper; Avril A. B. Robertson, Bioorganic & Medicinal Chemistry Letters, 2018, DOI: 10.1016/j.bmcl.2017.12.054
1241. Opicapone. https://www.neurocrine.com/pipeline/opicapone/ Accessed on 10/8/19.
1242. Murata M, Odawara T, Hasegawa K, et al. Adjunct zonisamide to levodopa for DLB parkinsonism. Neurology. 2018;0:10.1212 /WNL.0000000000005010. doi:10.1212/WNL.0000000000005010
1243. Gibbons, RD, Mann, JJ. The relationship between antidepressant initiation & suicide risk. Psychiatric Times. Published 12/31/14.

179

http://www.psychiatrictimes.com/special-reports/relationship-between-antidepressant-initiation-and-suicide-risk Accessed 4/8/15.

1244. Coupland C, Hill T, Morriss R, Arthur A, Moore M, Hippisley-cox J. Antidepressant use and risk of suicide and attempted suicide or self harm in people aged 20 to 64: cohort study using a primary care database. BMJ. 2015;350:h517.

1245. Nock MK, Green JG, Hwang I, et al. Prevalence, correlates, and treatment of lifetime suicidal behavior among adolescents: results from the National Comorbidity Survey Replication Adolescent Supplement. JAMA Psychiatry. 2013;70(3):300-10.

1246. Wasserman D, Rihmer Z, Rujescu D, et al. [The European Psychiatric Association (EPA) guidance on suicide treatment and prevention]. Neuropsychopharmacol Hung. 2012; 14(2):113-36.

1247. American Association of Suicidology - Facts and Statistics at: http://www.suicidology.org/resources/facts-statistics. Accessed on 6/15/15.

1248. Nierenberg AA, Gray SM, Grandin LD. Mood disorders and suicide. J Clin Psychiatry. 2001;62(suppl 25):27–30.

1249. Gören JL, Parks JJ, and Ghinassi FA, et al. When is antipsychotic polypharmacy supported by research evidence? Implications for QI. The Joint Commission Journal on Quality and Patient Safety 2008;34(10):571-82.

1250. Maglione M, Ruelaz Maher A, Hu J, et al. Off-label use of atypical antipsychotics: an update. Comparative Effectiveness Review No. 43. (Prepared by the Southern California/RAND Evidence-based Practice under Contract No. HHSA290-2007-10062-1.) AHRQ Publication No.11-ECH087-EF. Rockville, MD: Agency for Healthcare Research and Quality. September 2011. http://www.effectivehealthcare.ahrq.gov/reports/final.cfm

1251. Gugger JJ and Cassagnol M. Low-Dose Quetiapine Is Not a Benign Sedative-Hypnotic Agent. The American Journal on Addictions 2008;17:454–455.

1252. Correll CU, Rummel-Kluge C, Corves C, et al. Antipsychotic Combinations vs Monotherapy in Schizophrenia: A Meta-analysis of Randomized Controlled Trials. Schizophrenia Bulletin 2009;35(2):443–457, doi:10.1093/schbul/sbn018.

1253. Burghart SM. Antipsychotic polypharmacy and Joint Commission quality measures: Implications to the psychiatric pharmacist. Ment Health Clin. 2013;3(1):100.

1254. Barbui C, Signoretti A, Mulè S, Boso M, Cipriani A. Does the addition of a second antipsychotic drug improve clozapine treatment? Schizophr Bull. 2009;35(2):458-68.

1255. Faries D. et al. Antipsychotic monotherapy and polypharmacy in the naturalistic treatment of schizophrenia with atypical antipsychotics. BMC Psychiatry 2005;5:26.

1256. Blier P, Ward HE, Tremblay P, et al. Combination of Antidepressant Medications From Treatment Initiation for Major Depressive Disorder: A Double-Blind Randomized Study. Am J Psychiatry 2010;167:281-8.

1257. Rush AJ, Trivedi MH, Stewart JW, et al. Combining medications to enhance depression outcomes (CO-MED): acute and long-term outcomes of a single-blind randomized study. Am J Psychiatry 2011 Jul;168(7):689-701. doi: 10.1176/appi.ajp.2011.10111645.

1258. Nelson JC, Mazure CM, Jatlow PI, et al. Combining norepinephrine and serotonin reuptake inhibition mechanisms for treatment of depression: a double-blind, randomized study. Biol Psychiatry 2004;55(3):296-300.

1259. Citrome L. Combination Treatments: Your Individual Mileage May Vary. Posted at www.medscape.com/viewarticle/746887 on 8/9/2011.

1260. Stahl SM. Novel therapeutics for depression: L-methylfolate as a trimonoamine modulator and antidepressant-augmenting agent. CNS Spectr 2007;12:739–744.

1261. Kingsbury SJ, Lotito ML. Psychiatric polypharmacy: the good, the bad, and the ugly. Psychiatr Times. 2007;24(4):1–3.

1262. Sarwer DB, Faulconbridge LF, Steffen KJ, et al. Bariatric Procedures: Managing Patients After Surgery. Curr Psychiatry 2011;10(1):18-30.

1263. Seaman JS, Bowers SP, Dixon P, et al. Dissolution of common psychiatric medications in a Roux-en-Y gastric bypass model. Psychosomatics 2005;46:250-253.

1264. Julius RJ, Novitsky MA Jr, Dubin WR. Medication adherence: a review of the literature and implications for clinical practice. J Psychiatr Pract. 2009;15:34-44.

1265. Newcomer JW, Hennekens CH. Severe mental illness and risk of cardiovascular disease. JAMA. 2007;298:1794-1796. Abstract

1266. Druss BG, Bradford WD, Rosenheck RA, Radford MJ, Krumholz HM. Quality of medical care and excess mortality in older patients with mental disorders. Arch Gen Psychiatry 2001;58:565-572.

1267. 5 Things to Know About Eating Disorders. http://www.psychiatrictimes.com/eating-disorders/5-things-know-about-eating-disorders?GUID=631E98CE-0053-4441-9560-14CD338CC37E&rememberme=1&ts=27022015#sthash.i1sXyj1I.dpuf. Accessed on 2/27/15.

1268. Ward DJ, Rodriguez P, Wright DR, Austin SB, Long MW. Estimation of Eating Disorders Prevalence by Age and Associations With Mortality in a Simulated Nationally Representative US Cohort. JAMA Netw Open. 2019;2(10):e1912925. doi:10.1001/jamanetworkopen.2019.12925

1269. Brownley KA, Berkman ND, Peat CM, et al. Binge-eating disorder in adults a systematic review and meta-analysis. Ann Intern Med. 2016;165(6):409-420. doi:10.7326/M15-2455

1270. Citrome L, et al "Effect of dasotraline on body weight in patients with binge-eating disorders" Psych Congress 2019; Poster 143. Citrome L, et al "Dasotraline for treatment of adults with binge-eating disorder: effect on binge-related obsessions and compulsions" Psych Congress 2019; Poster 240.

1271. Walter K. FDA Considering Sunovion Drug Application to Treat Binge Eating Disorder. https://www.mdmag.com/medical-news/fda-sunovion-drug-application-binge-eating-disorder. Accessed on 8/2/19

1272. U.S. Preventive Services Task Force. Screening for thyroid disease: recommendation statement. Ann Intern Med 2004(Jan);140(2):125-7.

1273. Lefevre ML et al. Screening for thyroid dysfunction: U.S. Preventive Services Task Force recommendation statement. Ann Intern Med 2015 Mar 24; [e-pub]. (http://dx.doi.org/10.7326/M15-0483).

1274. Cappola AR & Cooper DS. Screening and treating subclinical thyroid disease: getting past the impasse. Ann Intern Med 2015(3/24) [e-pub].

1275. Garber, JR; Cobin, RH; Gharib, H; et al. (December 2012). Clinical Practice Guidelines for Hypothyroidism in Adults. Thyroid 2012(12);22:1200–1235. doi:10.1089/thy.2012.0205. PMID 22954017.

1276. Longo, DL; Fauci, AS; Kasper, DL; Hauser, SL; Jameson, JL; Loscalzo, J (2011) "341: disorders of the thyroid gland" in Harrison's principles of internal medicine. (18th ed.). New York City: McGraw-Hill ISBN: 007174889X.

1277. Bahn Chair RS; Burch HB; Cooper DS, et al. "Hyperthyroidism and other causes of thyrotoxicosis: management guidelines of the American Thyroid Association and American Association of Clinical Endocrinologists.". Thyroid : official journal of the American Thyroid Association 2011(June);21(6):593–646. PMID 21510801.

1278. Melanie Cupp, Pharm.D., BCPS PL Detail-Document, Comparison of Atypical Antipsychotics. Pharmacist's/Prescriber's Letter. July 2015.

1279. Larson AM. Drugs and the liver. Metabolism and mechanisms of injury. . UpToDate. Waltham, MA: UpToDate Inc. 2019.

1280. Caudle K, Klein T, Hoffman J, et al. Incorporation of Pharmacogenomics into Routine Clinical Practice: the Clinical Pharmacogenetics Implementation Consortium (CPIC) Guideline Development Process. Curr Drug Metab. 2014;15(2):209-217. doi:10.2174/1389200215666140130124910

1281. Wijesinghe R. A review of pharmacokinetic and pharmacodynamic interactions with antipsychotics. Ment Heal Clin. 2016;6(1):21-27. doi:10.9740/mhc.2016.01.021

1282. Ingelman-Sundberg M. Genetic polymorphisms of cytochrome P450 2D6 (CYP2D6): clinical consequences, evolutionary aspects and functional diversity. The Pharmacogenomics Journal 2005;5,6–13. doi:10.1038/sj.tpj.6500285.

1283. Ma MK, Woo MH, Mcleo HL. Genetic Basis of Drug Metabolism. Am J Health Syst Pharm. 2002;59(21). http://www.medscape.com/viewarticle/444804 Accessed on 8/1/15.

1284. Pharmacology Weekly. What are common medications that may be impacted by known genetic polymorphisms of CYP1A2 enzyme? http://www.pharmacologyweekly.com/articles/medications-affected-genetic-polymorphisms-CYP1A2 What are the common genetic polymorphisms to cytochrome P450 (CYP) 2C19 that could impact drug metabolism.pdf http://www.pharmacologyweekly.com/articles/cytochrome-p450-CYP-2C19-genetic-polymorphism-SNP What common genetic polymorphisms of the CYP1A2 enzyme have the potential to influence drug efficacy and/or safety.pdf http://www.pharmacologyweekly.com/articles/genetic-polymorphisms-cytochrome-P450-CYP1A2-enzyme What medications used in clinical practice are likely to be influenced by the presence of genetic polymorphisms to CYP2D6.pdf What genetic polymorphisms of the CYP3A4 enzyme have the potential to influence drug efficacy and /or safety.pdf http://www.pharmacologyweekly.com/articles/CYP2D6-genetic-polymorphisms-medication-substrates Accessed 8/1/15.

1285. Preissner SC, Hoffmann MF, Preissner R, Dunkel M, Gewiess A, et al. (2013) Polymorphic Cytochrome P450 Enzymes (CYPs) and Their Role in Personalized Therapy. PLoS ONE 8(12): e82562. doi:10.1371/journal.pone.0082562.

1286. PL Detail-Document, Cytochrome P450 Drug Interactions. Pharmacist's Letter/Prescriber's Letter. October 2013.

1287. Flockhart DA, MD, PhD. Drug Interactions: Cytochrome P450s Drug Interaction Table. Indiana University Department of Medicine. www.drug-interactions.com or http://medicine.iupui.edu/clinpharm/ddis Accessed on 7/31/15.

1288. Fuller MA, Sajatovic M. Drug Information Handbook for Psychiatry, 5th ed. Hudson, OH.: Lexi Comp, 2004.

1289. Barkin RL and Barkin S. Pharmacologic Management of Acute and Chronic Pain: Focus on Drug Interactions and Patient-Specific Pharmacotherapeutic Selection. South Med J 94(8):756-812, 2001.

1290. Harvey AT, Preskorn SH, Cytochrome P450 enzymes: interpretation of their interactions with selective serotonin reuptake inhibitors. Part I. J Clin Psychopharmacol. 1996;16:273-285.

1291. Zhou SF, Xue CC, Yu XQ, et al. Clinically Important Drug Interactions Potentially Involving Mechanism-based Inhibition of Cytochrome P4503A4 and the Role of Therapeutic Drug Monitoring. Ther Drug Monit 2007;29:687–710.

1292. Michalets EL. Update: Clinically Significant Cytochrome P-450 Drug Interactions. Pharmacotherapy 1998;18(1):84–112.

1293. Lin JH, Lu AY. Inhibition and induction of cytochrome P450 and the clinical implications. Clin Pharmacokinet 1998 Nov;35(5):361-390.

1294. Sachse C, Brockmoller J, Bauer S, et al. Cytochrome P450 2D6 Variants in a Caucasian Population: Allele Frequencies and Phenotypic Consequences. Am. J. Hum. Genet. 1997;60:284-295.
1295. Nelson, DR (2009) The Cytochrome P450 Homepage. Human Genomics 4, 59-65. http://drnelson.uthsc.edu/CytochromeP450.html Accessed on July 31, 2015.
1296. Cytochrome P450 Polymorphisms and Drug Metabolism. Pharmacogenomics Course. Spring 2008. Arthur I. Cederbaum, PhD. Professor, Dept of Pharmacology, Mount Sinai School of Medicine. bcny.org/Pdfs/Pharmacogenomics/p450.pdf. Accessed on 8/1/15.
1297. Flockhart DA, Tanus-Santos JE. Implications of cytochrome P450 interactions when prescribing medication for hypertension. Arch Intern Med 2002;405-12.
1298. Seredina TA, Goreva OB, Talaban VO, et al. Association of cytochrome P450 genetic polymorphisms with neoadjuvant chemotherapy efficacy in breast cancer patients. BMC Medical Genetics 2012, 13:45 doi:10.1186/1471-2350-13-45.
1299. Thea R. Moore, Angela M. Hill and Siva K. Panguluri. Pharmacogenomics in Psychiatry: Implications for Practice. Recent Patents on Biotechnology 2014,8,152-159.
1300. Fabbri C, Serretti A. Overcoming Treatment Resistance. Can Pharmacogenetics Help? Psychiatr Times. 2019;(June):14-16.
1301. Verbelen M, Weale ME, Lewis CM. Cost-effectiveness of pharmacogenetic-guided treatment: Are we there yet? Pharmacogenomics J. 2017;17(5):395-402. doi:10.1038/tpj.2017.21
1302. Holden C. Behavioral genetics. Getting the short end of the allele. Science. 2003 Jul 18;301(5631):291-3.
1303. Sharpley CF, Palanisamy SKA, Glyde NS, et al. An update on the interaction between the serotonin transporter promoter variant (5HTTLPR), stress and depression, plus an exploration of non-confirming findings. Behavioural Brain Research 2014;273:89–105.
1304. Caspi A, Sugden K, Moffitt TE, et al. Influence of life stress on depression: moderation by a polymorphism in the 5HTT gene. Science 2003 (July 18);301:386-389.
1305. Holden C. Getting the short end of the allele. (Behavioral Genetics). Science (July 18, 2003);301(5631):291.
1306. Nucleic Acid Based Tests. https://www.fda.gov/medical-devices/vitro-diagnostics/nucleic-acid-based-tests. Accessed on 8/2/19.
1307. Raghava KM, Lakshmi PK. Overview of P-glycoprotein inhibitors: A rational outlook. Brazilian J Pharm Sci. 2012;48(3):353-367. doi:10.1590/S1984-82502012000300002
1308. Carpenter M, Berry H, Pelletier AL. Clinically Relevant Drug-Drug Interactions in Primary Care. Am Fam Physician. 2019;99(9):558-564. http://www.ncbi.nlm.nih.gov/pubmed/31038898.
1309. Nikolic B, Jankovic S, Stojanov O, Popovic J. Prevalence and predictors of potential drug-drug interactions. Cent Eur J Med. 2014;9(2):348-356. doi:10.2478/s11536-013-0272-4
1310. Rainone A, De Lucia D, Morelli CD, Valente D, Catapano O, Caraglia M. Clinically Relevant of Cytochrome P450 Family Enzymes for Drug-Drug Interaction in Anticancer Therapy. World Cancer Res J. 2015;2(2):1-7.
1311. Carpenter M, Berry H, Pelletier AL. Clinically Relevant Drug-Drug Interactions in Primary Care. Am Fam Physician. 2019;99(9):558-564. http://www.ncbi.nlm.nih.gov/pubmed/31038898.
1312. Lister JF. Pharmacogenomics: A focus on antidepressants and atypical antipsychotics. Ment Health Clin [Internet]. 2016;6(1):48-53. DOI:10.9740/
1313. de Leon J, Armstrong SC, Cozza KL. Clinical guidelines for psychiatrists for the use of pharmacogenetic testing for CYP4502D6 and CYP450 2C19. Psychosomatics. 2006;47(1):75-85. DOI: 10.1176/appi.psy.47.1.75. PubMed PMID: 16384813
1314. Palleria C, Di Paolo A, Giofrè C, et al. Pharmacokinetic drug-drug interaction and their implication in clinical management. J Res Med Sci. 2013;18(7):601-610. https://www.ncbi.nlm.nih.gov/pubmed/24516494.
1315. FDA. Drug Development and Drug Interactions: Table of Substrates, Inhibitors and Inducers. https://www.fda.gov/drugs/drug-interactions-labeling/drug-development-and-drug-interactions-table-substrates-inhibitors-and-inducers Accessed on 11/29/19.
1316. Markowitz JS. Drug Metabolism: Beyond CYP450. Non-CYP metabolism relevant to clinical psychopharmacology. Presentation for CPNP at www.cpnp.org Accessed 10/1/19.
1317. FDA. Drug Development and Drug Interactions: Table of Substrates, Inhibitors and Inducers. https://www.fda.gov/drugs/drug-interactions-labeling/drug-development-and-drug-interactions-table-substrates-inhibitors-and-inducers Accessed on 11/29/19.

*Everyone we meet is fighting a battle we know nothing about.*
*Make your own life better by making someone else's life better.*

Made in the USA
Coppell, TX
28 April 2021